Recent Results in Cancer Research 106

Recent Results in Cancer Research

Volume 96: Adjuvant Chemotherapy of Breast Cancer
Edited by H.-J. Senn
1984. 98 figures, 91 tables. X, 243. ISBN 3-540-13738-6

Volume 97: Small Cell Lung Cancer
Edited by S. Seeber
1985. 44 figures, 47 tables. VII, 166. ISBN 3-540-13798-X

Volume 98: Perioperative Chemotherapy
Edited by U. Metzger, F. Largiadèr, H.-J. Senn
1985. 48 figures, 45 tables. XII, 157. ISBN 3-540-15124-9

Volume 99: Peptide Hormones in Lung Cancer
Edited by K. Havemann, G. Sorenson, C. Gropp
1985. 100 figures, 63 tables. XII, 248. ISBN 3-540-15504-X

Volume 100: Therapeutic Strategies in Primary and
Metastatic Liver Cancer
Edited by Ch. Herfarth, P. Schlag, P. Hohenberger
1986. 163 figures, 104 tables. XIV, 327. ISBN 3-540-16011-6

Volume 101: Locoregional High-Frequency Hyperthermia
and Temperature Measurement
Edited by G. Bruggmoser, W. Hinkelbein, R. Engelhardt,
M. Wannenmacher
1986. 96 figures, 8 tables. IX, 143. ISBN 3-540-15501-5

Volume 102: Epidemiology of Malignant Melanoma
Edited by R. P. Gallagher
1986. 15 figures, 70 tables. IX, 169. ISBN 3-540-16020-5

Volume 103: Preoperative (Neoadjuvant) Chemotherapy
Edited by J. Ragaz, P. R. Band, J. H. Goldie
1986. 58 figures, 49 tables. IX, 162. ISBN 3-540-16129-5

Volume 104: Hyperthermia and the Therapy of Malignant Tumors
Edited by C. Streffer
1987. 52 figures, 63 tables. IX, 207. ISBN 3-540-17250-5

Volume 105: Breast Cancer
Edited by S. Brünner and B. Langfeldt
1987. 59 figures, 43 tables. IX, 132. ISBN 3-540-17301-3

E. Grundmann L. Beck (Eds.)

Minimal Neoplasia

Diagnosis and Therapy

With 82 Figures and 61 Tables

Springer-Verlag
Berlin Heidelberg New York
London Paris Tokyo

Professor Dr. Ekkehard Grundmann
Gerhard-Domagk-Institut für Pathologie
Westfälische Wilhelms-Universität Münster
Domagkstraße 17, 4400 Münster, FRG

Professor Dr. Lutwin Beck
Frauenklinik, Medizinische Einrichtungen
Universität Düsseldorf
Moorenstraße 5, 4000 Düsseldorf, FRG

ISBN-13:978-3-642-83247-5 e-ISBN-13:978-3-642-83245-1
DOI: 10.1007/978-3-642-83245-1

Library of Congress Cataloging-in-Publication Data. Minimal neoplasia. (Recent results in cancer research; 106) Includes bibliographies and index. 1. Carcinogenesis. 2. Tumors-Growth. 3. Cancer-Pathophysiology. I. Grundmann, E. (Ekkehard) II. Beck, Lutwin. III. Series. [DNLM: 1. Neoplasms-diagnosis. 2. Neoplasms-therapy. 3. Precancerous Conditions-diagnosis. 4. Precancerous Conditions-therapy. W1 RE106P v. 106 / QZ 200 M665] RC261.R35 vol. 106 616.99'4 s 87-32198 [RC268.5] [616.99'4]

Softcover reprint of the hardcover 1st edition 1988

2125/3140-543210

Preface

The genesis of malignant tumors is currently viewed as a multistep phenomenon with regard to both molecular biology and morphology. In histology and cytology, premalignant lesions are of diagnostic relevance for the early recognition of malignancy.

The present volume focuses on another definite phase in the process of malignant growth, i.e. when a lesion has passed both the potentially premalignant and the in situ stages and can just be recognized as an early invasive tumor. As in the terminology of premalignant lesions, gynecology has been the pioneer in this field with the concept of "microcarcinoma", proposed in 1947 by G. Mestwerdt. These very early stages of invasion have also been appraised as "incipient neoplasia" or "minimal neoplasia". Our preference for the last term is based on the idea that all the histologic criteria of malignant growth are present, albeit with minimal expression. These phases, visualized with increasing accuracy by modern diagnostic techniques, represent an important challenge for truly early cancer detection.

Consequently, the volume has two main parts: The first meets the challenge by providing a general survey of the biology and pathology of early malignant invasion, while the second deals with the minimal forms of neoplasia in tumors in various organs. A display of histologic manifestations is followed, as far as possible, by the current spectrum of therapeutic consequences. Cryptic gliomas are also included as a very special form of minimal neoplasia. With several papers on the cytogenetics, histology and cytology of preleukemia and incipient lymphoma, the volume closes with a complex for which definition and therapeutic consequences are still somewhat controversial.

Our overview of the present state of knowledge on minimal neoplasia is by no means comprehensive. We have attempted to assemble some established concepts of biology, pathology, and clinical medicine in order to provide a useful basis for diagnosis and therapy. This book may also be seen as a contribution to the rapid development of early cancer detection and the ensuing therapeutic consequences.

November 1987

E. Grundmann
L. Beck

Contents

*List of Contributors**

* The address of the principal author is given on the first page of each contribution.

[1] Page on which contribution begins.

General Aspects

Minimal Neoplasia as a Challenge for Early Cancer Detection

L. G. Koss

Department of Pathology, Montefiore Medical Center, Henry and Lucy Moses Hospital Division, 111 East 210th Street, Bronx, NY 10467, USA

Introduction

The topic of this volume belongs to the most difficult in human pathology and represents a challenge of definition, scientific understanding, and clinical significance. What is minimal neoplasia, how is it defined, and what does it mean? I gave a great deal of thought to the definition and finally decided that the simplest way of describing the target of these deliberations would be to define it as "small cancers that have progressed beyond their site of primary origin into the surrounding tissue." The definition is relatively simple for tumors derived from flat epithelia, which are separated from their underlying stroma by a basement membrane. The name of microinvasive carcinoma has been attached to such lesions (Burghardt and Holzer 1982; Henson and Albores-Saavedra 1986). Current evidence suggests that malignant processes begin by a transformation of the epithelium into a carcinoma in situ, or morphologically related entities, sometimes named dysplasia or intraepithelial neoplasia, whence cancer cells will cross the basement membrane and invade the stroma. It is known today that the basement membrane is a complex structure that regulates epithelial regeneration (Vracko and Benditt 1972) and is composed of two morphologic components: the basement lamina, derived from the epithelial cells, and the reticular lamina, which is the product of connective tissue cells (Porter and Whelan 1984). It is also known that the biochemical makeup of the basement membrane is very complex: it is composed of the glycoprotein laminin, collagen types IV and V, and a large number of other proteins not all of which have been identified or characterized as yet (Madri et al. 1984).

In spite of extensive work at the molecular level there is still very little known about biologic mechanisms of transition of a lesion still confined to the epithelium of origin to invasive carcinoma. Several options may be proposed (Fig. 1):

1. The transformed epithelial cells acquire proteolytic enzymes or other characteristics, which give them the ability to penetrate through the basement membrane (Liotta et al. 1984).
2. The proteins of the basement membrane may become weakened or acquire a different physicochemical configuration so that they can no longer contain the epithelial cells from spreading into the stroma.
3. The stromal infiltrate composed of leukocytes and macrophages, that conceivably may act to prevent the extension of an intraepithelial malignant process into the sur-

Recent Results in Cancer Research, Vol. 106

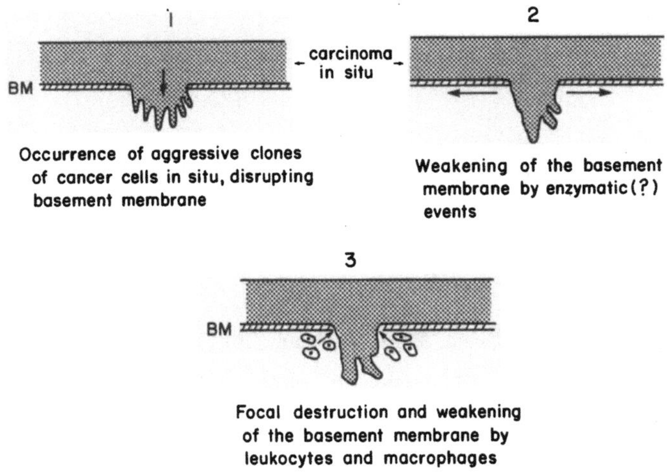

Fig. 1. Possible mechanisms of formation of minimal neoplasia

rounding tissue, may actually weaken the basement membrane and facilitate the invasive process.
4. A number of these possibilities may occur in a synchronous or metachronous manner, leading to invasive cancer.

It must be stressed that for some organs such as the breast the international definition of minimal carcinoma includes ductal and lobular carcinomas in situ, still further blurring the concept of minimal neoplasia (Ackerman and Katzenstein 1977).

Detection Systems

The discovery of minimal carcinoma is either incidental to the search for precursor stages of cancer, for example, during cytologic screening for precursors of carcinoma of the uterine cervix, or as a consequence of biopsies of visible lesions, for example, colonic polyps. In general minimal cancers are asymptomatic, unless they occur within space-occupying lesions, such as polyps or papillary lesions of the bladder. The means of detection of these early cancers and their clinical significance vary from organ to organ.

Table 1 summarizes the cancer detection methods that may lead to the discovery of minimal carcinoma in some organs. A few comments on the various organs and organ systems are in order.

Uterine Cervix. As will be discussed later on by Dr. Fu, the cervical smear is the instrument of discovery of minimal or microinvasive carcinoma of the uterine cervix. Although some of my colleagues believe that the makeup of the smear is of value in distinguishing a carcinoma in situ from microinvasive carcinoma, I am personally not persuaded that this is the case (Koss 1979a). In my experience, most early invasive carcinomas mascarade cytologically as either carcinomas in situ or morphologically less persuasive lesions, sometimes still called dysplasia, but best included with carcinoma in situ in the group of diseases known as cervical intraepithelial neoplasia, or CIN (Koss 1979a). The actual identification of early invasion usually occurs in biopsy material,

Table 1. Means of detection of minimal neoplasia in selected organs

Cervix	Cervical smear, colposcopy
Endometrium	*Symptomatic* - preceeded by hyperplasia biopsy or curettage *Asymptomatic* - hyperplasia absent or trivial, direct cytologic sampling
Urinary bladder	*Low-grade tumors* - cystoscopy *High-grade tumors* - cytology of voided urine, multiple biopsies of selected areas
Lung	*X-ray negative: central bronchi* - sputum followed by endoscopic biopsies *X-ray positive: transcutaneous aspiration,* surgical biopsy
Colon	Fiberoptic endoscopy
Breast	Mammography followed by transcutaneous aspiration or surgical biopsy

although some colposcopists claim that they can visually identify early invasion. Carcinomas of the endocervical glands may also be discovered by cervical smears. Such lesions may occur either as a primary lesion or simultanously with epidermoid carcinomas. The definition of a minimal invasive carcinoma of the endocervical glands is extremely difficult because the depth of distribution of normal glands varies from patient to patient. Thus the early invasive cancer of one observer may be still an endocervical carcinoma in situ of another observer (Koss 1979a).

Endometrium. A few words about the endometrium, an organ to be discussed later on by Dr. Stoddard. It is an axiom that women with endometrial carcinoma are identified because of abnormal vaginal bleeding or spotting. Most such women show evidence of endometrial hyperplasia adjacent to carcinoma. In a recently concluded study of over 2500 asymptomatic women age 45 years or older we observed by direct endometrial sampling that nearly 7/1000 of these women harbored occult endometrial carcinoma. Nearly one-half of the lesions were invasive, some rather deeply into the myometrium (Koss et al. 1984a). This study clearly suggested that there are two families of endometrial cancer: those lesions associated with hyperplasia, occurring in symptomatic, younger women, and those not associated with hyperplasia, occurring in older women, that may remain occult for many years.

Urinary Bladder. The urinary bladder represents yet another challenge in the recognition of minimal cancer. This is the first organ where measurements of DNA content of the tumours have proven to be of value in clarifying the nature of morphologic events. Much credit for pioneering this new knowledge goes to Tribukait (1984) from Stockholm. Briefly, significant evidence is at hand that there are two separate although sometimes overlapping pathways of neoplasia in the lower urinary tract, best defined as the diploid pattern and the aneuploid pattern. The papillary tumors of grade I are usually diploid. These tumors may extend into the lamina propria and may produce multiple

Table 2. Differences between low-grade papillary and nonpapillary tumors of the bladder

Feature	Low-grade papillary	Nonpapillary and high-grade papillary derived therefrom
Epithelial changes at origin	Hyperplasia	Carcinoma in situ and related atypias
Invasive potential	Low	High
DNA pattern	Predominantly diploid	Predominantly aneuploid
Density of nuclear pores	Normal	Increased
Reactivity with Cal antibody	Low	High
Blood group antigen expression	Present	Absent

recurrent tumors but per se rarely lead to invasion. Papillary tumors grade III are usually associated with peripheral nonpapillary carcinoma in situ. These tumors, and the carcinoma in situ, are nearly always aneuploid. The intermediate grade II tumors are in part diploid and in part aneuploid. There is excellent evidence at hand that most invasive cancers of the bladder are derived directly from carcinoma in situ (Koss 1979b). It has been shown by mapping studies of the bladder that invasive cancer occurring in patients with papillary disease is also derived from carcinomas in situ and related lesions (Koss 1979b). A summary of these observations is shown in Table 2.

Thus when one speaks of minimal carcinoma of the urinary bladder it does not suffice to state that the tumor extends into the lamina propria. This extension has a very different significance for the low-grade diploid tumors, where it is usually of little clinical importance and for the high-grade aneuploid tumors where it is of major prognostic value. Also the means of detection of these two families of tumors varies greatly (Koss 1985). Voided urine cytology is an indispensable and sensitive tool in the detection of the aneuploid, usually high grade tumors. The method is nearly worthless in the detection of low-grade diploid tumors (Koss et al. 1985). The latter must be diagnosed by cytoscopic biopsies because tumor cells cannot be recognized in the urinary sediment.

Lung. The detection of minimal lung cancer also represents a major challenge, the success of which depends greatly on the anatomic location and histologic type of lesion. About 30 years ago I observed patients with chronic cough, negative chest roentgenograms, and sputum that contained cancer cells, usually of the squamous type. In a small group of these original patients, who were seen before the era of fiberoptic bronchoscopy, carcinoma in situ of one or more of the principal bronchi was observed, sometimes with extension into the submucosa, this fulfilling the requirements of minimal bronchogenic carcinoma (Koss 1979a). It is of interest that none of these patients died of cancer. In a more recent major national study conducted in the United States by the Mayo Clinic, the Johns Hopkins Medical School, and the Memorial-Sloan Kettering Institutions, many more such cases were discovered but they constituted less than one-third of all cancers discovered in the study. The remaining two-thirds of patients with early cancer had peripheral tumors diagnosed by X-ray (Wollner et al. 1981). With the increase of the use of cigarette filters and even more so with the cessation of cigarette smoking, the classical pattern of squamous carcinoma of the main bronchi is becoming less and less common and the conclusion of the very costly study was that the search for these lesions in asymptomatic cigarette smokers by sputum cytology is not cost effective.

The peripheral lung lesions discovered by routine chest X-ray may now be diagnosed by thin needle aspiration biopsy (Koss et al. 1984b). The definition of minimal cancer for these often small lesions is very difficult because all of them have progressed beyond their site of primary origin. A further complicating factor is that a proportion of these tumors, varying from 20% to 30%, are of the small cell type and may have produced metastases at the time of their discovery. Thus for the lung, the prospects of detection of curable minimal carcinomas has paradoxically diminished with the changing smoking habits.

Colon. The colon is the site of a numerically very important group of malignant tumors: for the two sexes combined, this is the most frequent neoplastic disease in the United States. In this organ as well, a distinction must be made between polypoid and flat cancers. This issue will be discussed at length during the latter part of this symposium. What is a minimal polypoid carcinoma of the colon? It is a lesion that has extended into the submucosa, hence fulfills the criteria of Dukes' stage A lesion. In a small proportion of these lesions lymph node metastases may be observed at the time of discovery (Spratt and Ackerman 1962; Lefall and Chung 1974).

Flat neoplastic colonic lesions are uncommonly seen except in patients with ulcerative colitis or Crohn's disease (Cook and Goligher 1975). The lesions may be discovered by fiberoptic instruments and confirmed by biopsy. For some strange reason the pathologists working in this area prefer to name these neoplastic lesions dysplasia rather than carcinoma in situ. Still, some of these lesions lead to invasive cancer unless treated. In some of them the invasion is still confined to the submucosa of the colon and hence the lesions deserve the term carcinoma. There is little comfort in the identification of such lesions because they are often multiple. Lately an effort has been made to measure DNA in such lesions to determine the probability of invasion (Cuvelier et al. 1987). The results are not conclusive at this time.

Breast. Finally, a few words about mammary cancer, a topic to be discussed at length by Dr. Page. This organ has received a high share of attention in reference to minimal carcinoma.

Small breast cancers may be discovered by mammography, xerography, palpation, or as an incidental finding in biopsies for benign disease. It is beyond my competence to discuss the achievements and failures of mammography but a substantial proportion of cancers ranging anywhere from 5% to 20% will not be found by radiologic techniques. On the other hand the introduction of mammographic screening has also led to a significant number of breast biopsies for benign disease, at a substantial cost to society and to the patients (Hall 1986). So far there is no persuasive evidence that screening for breast cancer has resulted in better survival rates because breast cancer must be considered a systemic disease. All of us who had large experience with frozen sections recall with dismay the very small carcinomas which have produced lymph node metastases at the time of diagnosis.

It is of interest to mention that Nordenstrøm of Stockholm described with his colleagues a stereotaxic apparatus for thin needle aspiration biopsies of small breast lesions discovered by mammography (Bolmgren et al. 1977).

The method requires the use of a special needle, called the screw needle (Nordenstrøm 1976). The aspiration biopsy may be combined with injection of a tracer substance, such a carbon dust, that facilitates subsequent surgical removal of the lesion. It is of signal interest that measuring DNA in smears from these clinically occult minimal carcinomas, as was done by Fallenius et al. (1984), disclosed that many of the smallest lesions were in the diploid tetraploid range. Fallenius suggested, therefore, that minimal carcinomas of the breast represent those breast cancers that are less likely to progress when compared with the aneuploid lesions.

Clinical Significance

Table 3 summarizes comments on the clinical significance of minimal carcinoma of the organs that were discussed. It may be noted that for the uterus the clinical significance of the superficial invasive cancers is very small. In the urinary bladder there is little significance in reference to the low-grade papillary lesions, but the presence of high-grade lesions, mainly nonpapillary carcinoma in situ with early invasion, carries with it poor prognosis unless treated. A somewhat similar situation prevails in the lung where, unfortunately, there are no "good" cancers. The rare minimal carcinomas of the bronchus may offer a better prognosis than the peripheral cancers, but they are difficult to find and even more difficult to treat. The smaller peripheral lung tumors of large cell type are

Table 3. Clinical significance of minimal neoplasia

Cervix	*Focal invasion* - almost no chance of metastatic cancer 1:1000 *Diffuse invasion* - equivalent of invasive carcinoma stage 1 A
Endometrium	Carcinoma confined to endometrium - no invasion confined to less than 1 cm - no invasion confined to inner one-third of myometrium - chance of metastases, 5%-10% (may be DNA dependent)
Urinary bladder	Tumor type and DNA-dependent *low-grade tumors* (usually diploid) - invasion of lamina propria - no clinical significance *high-grade tumors* (usually aneuploid) - not treated, chance of progression to fully invasive carcinoma, 60%-70% Treated locally: chance of progression to fully invasive carcinoma, 30%-40% Cystectomy: usually cure
Lung	*Central bronchus tumors* - invasion of submucosa - no clinical significance invasion beyond submucosa - clinical stage I *Peripheral tumors* - tumors < 1 cm in diameter - nearly 100% cure tumors > 1 cm in diameter - clinical stage I
Colon	*Cancer confined to polyp* - nearly 100% cure *Cancer in submucosa* - Duke's stage A - capable of metastases
Breast	*Tumors < 1 cm in diameter* - nearly 100% cure with exceptions *Tumors > 1 cm in diameter* - clinical stage I (may be DNA dependent)

often sometimes curable but even there the unpleasant surprises in the form of lymph node metastases occur with disconcerting frequency. For the colon, only carcinomas confined to polyps offer a secure chance for a cure. Once the tumor is in the submucosa metastases may occur. Finally in reference to the breast, minimal carcinomas less than 0.5 cm in diameter offer a fair chance for a cure but one always has to be prepared for incidental metastases.

Thus the clinical outlook for minimal carcinoma is not necessarily favorable and is clearly organ- and tumor-type dependent. It is one of the mysteries of cancer why malignant changes still confined to the tissue of origin, hence still in situ, have such an excellent prognosis, whereas tumors that have progressed even minimally into the adjacent tissues may display a highly aggressive behavior pattern. Obviously there is still much work to be done to understand these differences in human cancer.

References

Ackerman LV, Katzenstein AL (1977) The concept of minimal breast cancer and the pathologist's role in the diagnosis of carcinoma. Cancer 39: 2755–2763

Bolmgren J, Jacobson B, Nordenstrøm B (1977) Stereotaxic instrument for needle biopsy of the mamma. AJR 129: 121–125

Burghardt E, Holzer E (eds) (1982) Minimal invasive cancer (microcarcinoma). Saunders, London (Clinics in oncology, vol 1/2)

Cook MG, Goligher JC (1975) Carcinoma and epithelial dysplasia complicating ulcerative colitis. Gastroenterology 68: 1127–1136

Cuvelier CA, Morson BC, Roels HJ (1987) The DNA content in cancer and dysplasia in chronic ulcerative colitis. Cancer (in press)

Fallenius AG, Skoog LK, Svane GE, Auer GU (1984) Cytophotometrical and biochemical characterization of nonpalpable, mammographically detected mammary adenocarcinoma. Cytometry 5: 426–429

Hall FM (1986) Screening mammography-potential problems on the horizon. N Engl J Med 314: 53–55

Henson DE, Albores-Saavedra J (eds) (1986) Pathology of incipient neoplasia. Saunders, Philadelphia

Koss LG (1979a) Diagnostic cytology and its histopathologic bases, 3rd edn. Lippincott, Philadelphia

Koss LG (1979b) Mapping of the urinary bladder: its impact on concepts of bladder cancer. Hum Pathol 10: 533–548

Koss LG (1985) Tumors of the urinary bladder. Armed Forces Institute of Pathology, Washington (Atlas of tumor pathology, fasc 11, 2nd ser, suppl)

Koss LG, Schreiber K, Oberlander SG, Moussouris HF, Lesser M (1984a) Detection of endometrial carcinoma and hyperplasia in asymptomatic women. J Obstet Gynecol 64: 1–11

Koss LG, Woyke S, Olszewski W (1984b) Aspiration biopsy: cytologic interpretations and histopathologic bases. Igaku-Shoin, New York

Koss LG, Deitch D, Ramanathan R, Sherman AB (1985) Diagnostic value of cytology of voided urine. Acta Cytol (Baltimore) 29: 810–816

Lefall LD, Chung EB (1974) Surgical management of colorectal polyps. Cancer 34: 940–947

Liotta LA, Rao NC, Barsky SH, Bryant G (1984) The laminin receptor and basement membrane dissolution: role in tumour metastasis. Ciba Found Symp 108: 146–162

Madri JA, Pratt BM, Yurchenco PD, Furthmayr H (1984) The ultrastructural organization and architecture of basement membranes. Ciba Found Symp 108: 6–24

Nordenstrøm B (1976) New instruments for biopsy. Radiology 117: 474–475

Porter R, Whelan J (eds) (1984) Basement membranes and cell movement. Ciba Found Symp 108

Spratt JS Jr, Ackerman LV (1962) Small primary adenocarcinomas of the colon and rectum. JAMA 179: 337–346

Tribukait B (1984) Flow cytometry in surgical pathology and cytology of tumors of the genito-urinary tract. In: Koss LG, Coleman DV (eds) Advances in clinical cytology, vol 2. Masson, New York, pp 165-189

Vracko R, Benditt EP (1972) Basal lamina: the scaffold for early cell replacement. J Cell Biol 55: 406-419

Woolner LB, Fontana RS, Sanderson DR, et al. (1981) Mayo lung project: evaluation of lung cancer screening through December, 1979. Mayo Clin Proc 56: 544-555

Morphology of Minimal Invasion

P. Sträuli

Abteilung für Krebsforschung, Institut für Pathologie, Universitätsspital, Birchstraße 95, 8050 Zürich, Switzerland

A Look at Local Spread of Cancer with an Attempt to Define Minimal Invasion

It is an inescapable consequence of neoplastic growth that all tumors have an inherent propensity to extend the area they occupy in the organism. The general term for this behavior, unbiased by reflections on malignancy, is spread. Most tumors in their earliest stage and the benign ones during their whole life spread by expansion. In most instances, expansive growth does not cross the natural borders of the tissue in which the tumor has originated. These borders, however, can be displaced. Both features are best recognized in epithelial tumors whose home tissue is confined by basement membrane. An example of early expansive growth with displacement of the natural tissue border is "bulky outgrowth" *(plumpes Vorwuchern)* of cervical carcinoma in situ.

In local spread of mesenchymal tumors natural tissue borders play a less prominent role. A small sarcoma, for instance, is, in most localizations, not restrained by a preexisting anatomical border, but by the capsule gradually built up during the period of expansive growth. Sooner or later, sarcoma elements pass across this border, thereby indicating the transition from expansive to invasive spread.

On the basis of these preliminaries, we can tentatively define invasion as spread beyond natural or newly formed anatomical borders. Recognition of this frontier passage is a matter of microscopic scrutiny. As such, it raises the problem of dimensions. Often, the first ominous alteration is the projection of a cellular extension - or of many such extensions - across the border. If only used as probes, such extensions are eventually retracted. But they can also develop into - or be replaced by - mechanical devices for manipulating more of the cell body and finally the whole cell through the boundary. For this purpose, the projections contain cytoskeletal arrays purportedly providing these devices with rigidity and motility. Of course our electron micrographs cannot tell us unequivocally whether we are indeed dealing with a preparatory invasion step (with "preminimal invasion", so to say). For practical purposes, it is necessary to postulate that a least one entire cancer cell - irrespective of its being an isolated element or a brick of a cohesive structure - be found beyond the border.

The two phases - extension of pseudopod-like projections across the tissue border and initiation of clear-cut minimal invasion - are shown in Figs. 1 and 2.

Recent Results in Cancer Research, Vol. 106

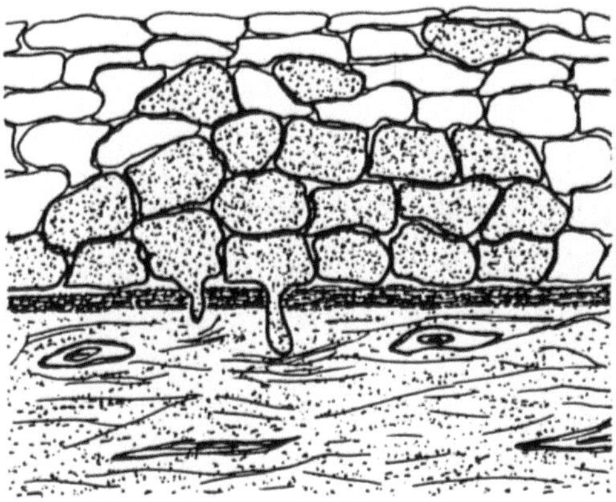

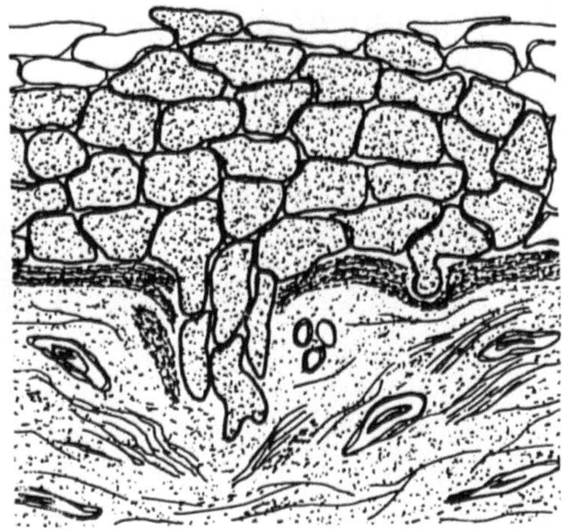

Fig. 1 *(left)*. Extension of cytoplasmic projections (probes) from basal cells of an intraepithelial carcinoma with perforation of the basement membrane can - but most not - be the first morphological manifestation of incipient minimal invasion

Fig. 2 *(right)*. The beginning of clear-cut minimal invasion is characterized by the passage of at least one entire cancer cell across the level of the basement membrane

Preinvasive Spread as Basis of Minimal Invasion

It is a widely accepted doctrine that cancer begins with a noninvasive or in situ stage. Before considering what happens in this stage we should have a look at possible exceptions to the rule. Such exceptions have been claimed for minimal carcinomas, and the term *"carcinoma invasivo d'emblé"* coined by Sirtori (1954) indicates the chief property of these tumors: a tiny cancer focus - for instance one that has not even attained full epithelial thickness in the cervix and is therefore not recognizable by colposcopy and cytology - has already infiltrated the stroma.

Figure 3 shows the principle of invasiveness ab initio. It corresponds to the tumor described by Schiller et al. (1953) as spray carcinoma. The figure also indicates a compulsory feature, the heavy reaction of the stroma. According to the concept of "early stromal erosion" (Fettig 1969), inflammatory alterations of the basement membrane can induce neoplastic cells in the basal epithelial layers to start infiltrating.

All this is, at best, an exception. No tumor of the spray type is represented in the large histological material of Hamperl (1966), Burghardt (1972), Lohe (1978), and others. And yet, it may be wise not to discard completely the possibility of a very early onset of invasion.

In most instances, however, spread of minimal carcinoma is confined first to the epithelium. Extension of cervical carcinoma in situ into the cervical glands (with a kind of lifting off of the columnar epithelium), on the portio vaginalis and vagina, and up into the endometrial cavity and even the tubes can be impressive. Richart (1967) has termed this process "intraepithelial invasion." It is obvious that this designation does not fit at all into my definition of invasion. But are we dealing with spread at all? I must raise this question because an alternative interpretation does exist, the field concept, which is supported, among others, by Hamperl (1966) and Burghardt (1972, 1984). It assumes that

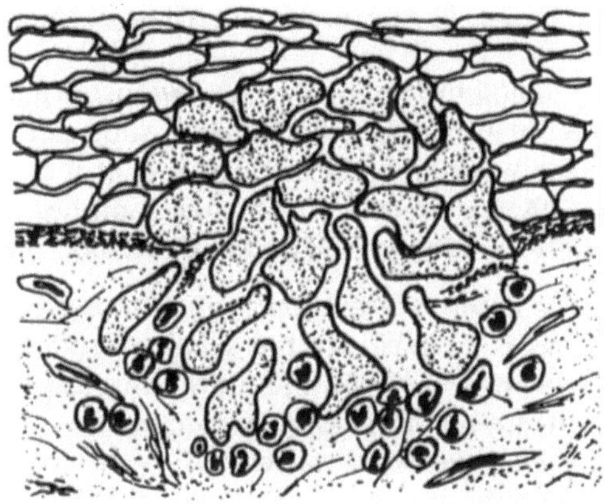

Fig. 3. Graphic reconstruction of the spray type of minimal invasion. Although the tumor focus has not yet attained full epithelial thickness, its basal cells already infiltrate the stroma. The latter is characterized by an intense inflammatory reaction

lateral extension is accomplished by apposition of whole segments or fields of new neoplastic epithelium. Both mechanisms - spread and apposition - are compatible with the fact that cervical carcinoma in situ extends predominantly as a cohesive structure. Single cells are hardly involved. This feature is maintained when passage across the epithelial border is initiated. Although the cells change their character, they maintain their cohesion. Thus, the first cancer elements extending into the stroma are solid bud-like formations. In a way, this phase, "early stromal invasion," represents the "official" beginning of cervical microinvasive carcinoma. With continuing invasion a more complex but still largely cohesive structure is created. Yet, an occasional single cell may now appear. It is remarkable that this event has been described as "the ultimate in microinvasion" by Christopherson and Parker (1964). Compared with the cautious formulation of these authors, the metaphorical rhetoric about cells that dribble off and infiltrate dropwise sounds somewhat unrealistic.

In contrast to cervical carcinoma, single cells play a considerable role in preinvasive spread and minimal invasion of mammary carcinomas. Not in all types, however. Intraductal carcinoma preferentially extends in cohesive configuration above the basement membrane, often with full preservation of the myoepithelial layer. Invasion is initiated by protrusion of buds resembling those of cervical carcinoma. On the other hand, nodular carcinoma has a propensity for dissociated (pagetoid) extension within the epithelium and maintains this mode of spread well into the invasive stage. The results are the characteristic arrangements of individual cells known as Indian files and targetoid patterns (Ozzello 1983).

Preinvasive and invasive spread in dissociated form is also displayed by an epithelium-associated tumor, malignant melanoma of the skin. The in situ stage is characterized by an increasing number of neoplastic melanocytes which extend, singly or in nests, above the dermal-epidermal junction and sometimes at every level of the epidermis. Although direct visualization of this process is not possible, it is reasonable to assume that it is due, in an almost paradigmatic manner, to the combined action of cell division and cell translocation. Sooner or later, a component of limited vertical spread is added to the horizontal (or radial) component. Horizontal spread, however, continues to prevail - at least in the most frequent tumor variety, superficial spreading melanoma. The tumor is now - and often remains for a long time - in its stage of minimal invasion, until an ill-understood change of behavior initiates the definite vertical growth phase (Kerl et al. 1982).

The Basement Membrane and Minimal Invasion

Throughout the period of preinvasive extension - and not only with the onset of invasion - the basement membrane is subject to various alterations. A rather complex border situation is thus created which may or may not influence the course of subsequent invasion. A few aspects of the interaction between tumor and basement membrane will be briefly mentioned (for further discussion see Porter and Whelan 1984).

1. *The extent of the contact area between cancer and basement membrane is determined.* This is the basis for the localization of transmembrane passage. A large area creates the possibility of a multifocal onset of minimal invasion, which is a particularly frequent event in mammary carcinoma.
2. *The equipment of cancer cells for basement membrane adhesion is modified.* The main modifications are disintegration of hemidesmosomes and reduction of receptors for type IV collagen, laminin, and other intrinsic membrane constituents. All this reflects an overal trend for disconnecting cells from the membrane.
3. *The turnover of basement membrane components is affected.* Synthesis of membrane molecules by cancer cells can continue, or can be reduced in quantitative and qualitative terms, or can cease altogether. Accordingly, the membrane persists, becomes defective, or vanishes.
4. *Lytic action is exerted on the basement membrane.* Sources of lytic enzymes are, on one side (the "upper" side of the membrane), cancer cells, on the other side (the "under" side) host cells (granulocytes, lymphocytes, macrophages, possibly also capillary endothelial cells) attracted by tumor-derived molecular messengers diffusing through the membrane.

All these conditions combine in various ways. This explains why in most instances the basement membrane abutting on to preinvasive cancer elements is abnormal. In straight morphological terms it is thicker, thinner, or focally lacking. The presence of gaps, however, is not automatically associated with transgression of the membrane level by cancer elements. It is an instructive observation made by Ozzello (1983) in intraductal mammary carcinoma that "absence of basal laminae does not necessarily alter the contour of a duct, the tumor cells retaining their original position even though no boundary separates them from the surrounding stroma."

Maybe such cancer cells are not yet ready for invasion. And this possibility tempts me into a concluding speculation:

After all, passage across basement membranes cannot be difficult - leukocytes show this incessantly. For cancer cells, membrane transgression may not primarily be a mechanical problem, but more a matter of their sensory world. They might lose what I should like to call "boundary perception." Once this loss has occurred, they go through irrespective of the presence or absence of a membrane demarcating the boundary.

References

Burghardt E (1972) Histologische Frühdiagnose des Zervixkrebses. Thieme, Stuttgart

Burghardt E (1984) Kolposkopie. Spezielle Zervixpathologie. Textbuch und Atlas. Thieme, Stuttgart

Christopherson WM, Parker JE (1964) Microinvasive carcinoma of the uterine cervix. Cancer 17: 1123-1131

Fettig O (1969) Zur Morphologie des Mikro-Karzinoms. Mitteilungsdienst der Gesellschaft zur Bekämpfung der Krebskrankheiten Nordrhein-Westfalen 5: 454-463
Hamperl H (1966) Über das infiltrierende (invasive) Tumorwachstum. Virchows Arch [Pathol Anat] 340: 185-205
Kerl H, Hödl S, Kresbach H, Stettner H (1982) Diagnosis and prognosis of the early stages of cutaneous malignant melanoma. In: Burghardt E, Holzer E (eds) Minimal invasive câncer (microcarcinoma). Saunders, London, pp 433-453
Lohe KY (1978) Early squamous carcinoma of the uterine cervix. Gynec Oncol 6: 10-30
Ozzello L (1983) Intraepithelial carcinomas of the breast. In: Hollmann KH, Verley JM (eds) New frontiers in mammary pathology, vol 2. Plenum, New York, pp 147-164
Porter R, Whelan J (eds) (1984) Basement membranes and cell movement. Ciba Found Symp 108
Richart RM (1967) Natural history of cervical intraepithelial neoplasia. Clin Obstet Gynecol 10: 748
Schiller W, Daro AF, Gollin HA, Primiano NP (1953) Small preulcerative invasive carcinoma of the cervix: the spray carcinoma. Am J Obstet Gynecol 65: 1088-1098
Sirtori C (1954) Il cancro in situ nella patologia umana esperimentale, con particolare riguardo al significato della membrana basale. Tumori 40: 42-53

Molecular Biology of Minimal Invasion

M. Mareel[1], F. van Roy[2], E. Bruyneel[1], J. Bolscher[3], D. Schallier[3], and M. de Mets[1]

[1] Department of Radiotherapy and Nuclear Medicine, Laboratory for Experimental Cancerology, University Hospital, De Pintelaan 185, 9000 Ghent, Belgium
[2] Laboratory of Molecular Biology, State University of Ghent, 9000 Ghent, Belgium
[3] Division of Cell Biology, The Netherlands Cancer Institute, Amsterdam, The Netherlands

Introduction

Invasion, uncontrolled proliferation, and often metastasis characterize malignant tumors. Benign tumors grow, but do not invade and do not metastasize. Research on the biology of minimal invasion tries to answer three questions: When do tumor cells start to invade? Which genetic alterations lead to acquisition of invasiveness? How do tumor cells invade?

The most widely accepted idea about the sequence of events during carcinogenesis is that of a multistep process: initiation, promotion, loss of growth control, invasion, and metastasis (Foulds 1969). In this concept, the acquisition of invasiveness is situated after loss of growth control. This is supported by the occurrence of carcinoma in situ and by numerous observations of incipient focal invasion in otherwise benign tumors. The possibility that invasion is acquired before or together with loss of growth control is suggested by tumors originating from invasive stem cells (e.g., choriocarcinoma, reticulum

Table 1. Separate genes for growth, invasion, and metastasis

Phenotype[a]	Examples	
	Natural	Experimental
G^+,I^-,M^-	Benign tumors	Inhibitors of invasion, permissive for growth[b]
G^+,I^+,M^-	Basocellular epithelioma Primary brain tumors	
G^+,I^+,M^+	Many malignant tumors	
G^-,I^+,M^-	Cholesteatoma	Inhibitors of growth, permissive for invasion[b]
G^-,I^+,M^+	Trophoblast, granulocytes, macrophages	

[a] *G*, tumorigenic (loss of growth control); *I*, invasive; *M*, metastatic; +, phenotype expressed; –, phenotype not expressed.
[b] See Mareel et al. (1982).

Recent Results in Cancer Research, Vol. 106

cell sarcoma) and by the invasive character of many malignant tumors without well-documented benign precursors.

The discovery of immortalizing and transforming oncogenes, shown to be implicated in growth control (Land et al. 1983; Heldin and Westermark 1984; Sporn and Roberts 1985), has suggested that oncogenes are involved also in invasion (invasogenes) and metastasis (Mareel and van Roy 1986). Circumstantial evidence in favor of the idea that invasogenes may be different from oncogenes, implicated in growth, is provided by the natural occurrence of various phenotypic combinations (Table 1). Cellular activities of invading tumor cells are: homotypic de-adhesion, adhesion to alien substrata, locomotion, secretion of lytic enzymes, and phagocytosis (reviewed by Mareel 1983). It is clear that none of these activities is specific for invasive cells. An attractive hypothesis, therefore, is that the phenotypic acquisition of invasion results from the loss of control of the above-mentioned activities.

Research of the molecular changes that are at the basis of tumor invasion may follow a number or strategies: (1) transfection of noninvasive cell lines with DNA from invasive cells, (2) transient suppression of the invasive phenotype, and (3) induced expression of the invasive phenotype.

In the experiments discussed here we tested invasion in vitro using fragments of embryonic chick heart in confrontation with cells in organ culture (Mareel et al. 1979; for discussion of this assay see Mareel 1983). Invasion in vivo was tested through s.c. or i.p. inoculation of cells in syngeneic animals or in nude mice.

Transfection of Invasogenes

We have first examined the role in invasion of oncogenes that were known to score positive in tests for growth transformation (dense focus formation, colony formation in soft agar, tumorigenicity). The results obtained with primary cell cultures or with cell lines showed that invasive cell populations can be obtained from noninvasive ones through transfection with plasmids containing transforming oncogenes (Table 2). One interpretation of these results might be that the expression of the oncogene product (a mutated p21 *ras*-protein, the polyoma virus middle-T antigen, a *gag-fos-fox* fusion protein, or an unidentified papilloma virus antigen) leads to invasion. However, a number of observations seriously question this interpretation.

Invasion may emerge in cultured cell populations in an apparently spontaneous way without expression of the above-mentioned oncogene products under one of the following circumstances. (1) Routine passage of cell lines in vitro frequently led to invasive cell populations with or without a transformed growth pattern. This has been shown, e.g., for rat (van Roy et al. 1987) and mouse embryo (Mareel et al. 1975; Greig et al. 1985) cell lines. (2) The transfection procedure per se including exposure of cells to calcium phosphate precipitated normal carrier DNA, isolation of transfectants with or without selection medium, and cloning has resulted in transformation with regard to invasion. For example, noninvasive (in vitro) Rat 2 cells became invasive after cotransfection with carrier DNA from primary cultures of syngeneic embryo cells plus a plasmid containing the thymidine kinase genes (unpublished results). Invasiveness (in vitro) was observed in immortalized rat kidney cells after cloning (Mareel and van Roy 1986). (3) Invasiveness may be acquired through a single passage of cells in a syngeneic animal or a nude mouse. For example, Rat 2 cells were not invasive in vitro and produced invasive tumors with long latency periods when injected s.c. in syngeneic Fischer rats. A cell line derived

Table 2. Acquisition of invasion in cell cultures after transfection with oncogenes

Acceptor cell type	Transfection		Invasion assay[a]	Reference
	Origin of DNA	Oncogene		
C127	pPyB1	Entire Py	In vitro	Rautmann et al. (1982) and [b]
	pV69	69% BPV1	In vitro	Meneguzzi et al. (1984) and [b]
LTRAT1	pPyMT1	PyMT	In vitro	Rassoulzadegan et al. (1983) and [b]
	pHSG272/pT24	c-Ha-*ras*	In vitro	[b]
MDCK	pT24	c-Ha-*ras*	In vivo	[b]
NIH/3T3	Leukemia	N-*ras*	In vitro	Thorgeirsson et al. (1985)
NMuMG	pSV2neo/p-*ras*H	c-Ha-*ras*	In vivo	Hynes et al. (1985)
REF	pSV2gpt/pEJ6.6	c-Ha-*ras*	In vitro	Van Roy et al. (1986)
Rat2	pT24	C-Ha-*ras*	In vitro	Van Roy et al. (1986)
	pMOL503	v-*fos*	In vitro	Michiels et al. (1986) and [b]

[a] By which transition from noninvasive to invasive was demonstrated. *C127* and *NIH/3T3*, continuous mouse cell lines; *LTRAT1*, continuous cell line derived from rat embryo cells *(REF)* after transfection with a plasmid encoding the polyoma virus large-T antigen; *MDCK*, continuous epithelial cell line from canine kidney; *NMuMG*, mouse mammary epithelial cell line; *Rat2*, thymidine kinase-deficient continuous Fischer rat cell line. Plasmids used for transfection encode all three polyoma virus tumor antigens *(pPyB1)*, polyoma middle-T antigen *(pPyMT)*, a mutated human Harvey-*ras*-1 gene product (*pT24, p-rasH*, or *pEJ6.6*), and an activated v-FBR-*gag-fos-fox* gene product *(pMOL503)*, or contain an 69% transforming fragment of the bovine papilloma virus genome *(pV69)*. Cotransfection for selection was with *pSV2neo* or *pHSG272* (resistance to geneticin), or with *pSV2gpt* (resistance to mycophenolic acid).
[b] Our unpublished results.

from such an s.c. tumor proved to be readily invasive in vitro (van Roy et al. 1986). Whether or not an endogenous oncogene was activated in this tumor-derived cell line, as suggested by Collard et al. (1985), remains to be checked. MDCK cells expressing the mutated c-Harvey-*ras* protein at high level after transfection became clearly invasive in vitro only after passage through a nude mouse (unpublished result). Whether cells acquire invasiveness through interaction with host cells, or the environment in vivo selects for a minor invasive subpopulation, is subject to debate. Further problems with the interpretation of invasion in terms of oncogene product activities remain to be solved. Why is the expression of oncogene products (for example, the mutated p21 in transformed MDCK cells) heterogeneous in invasive cell populations? Why is invasiveness conserved when the oncogene sequences (for example, bovine papilloma virus DNA) are lost (P. Coopman, personal communication)? How are the known oncogene products mechanistically related to the regulation of cellular activities that are implicated in invasion?

Transient Suppression of Invasion

Invasion of MO_4-transformed mouse cells into embryonic chick heart in organ culture was completely arrested for at least 10 days by lowering the temperature of incubation to 28 °C (Mareel et al. 1984). This temperature was premissive for proliferation of the MO_4 cells. Although the temperature remained at 28 °C, invasion started after day 10 and progressed at approximately the same rate as was observed between day 1 and day 4 in control cultures at 37 °C (Fig. 1).

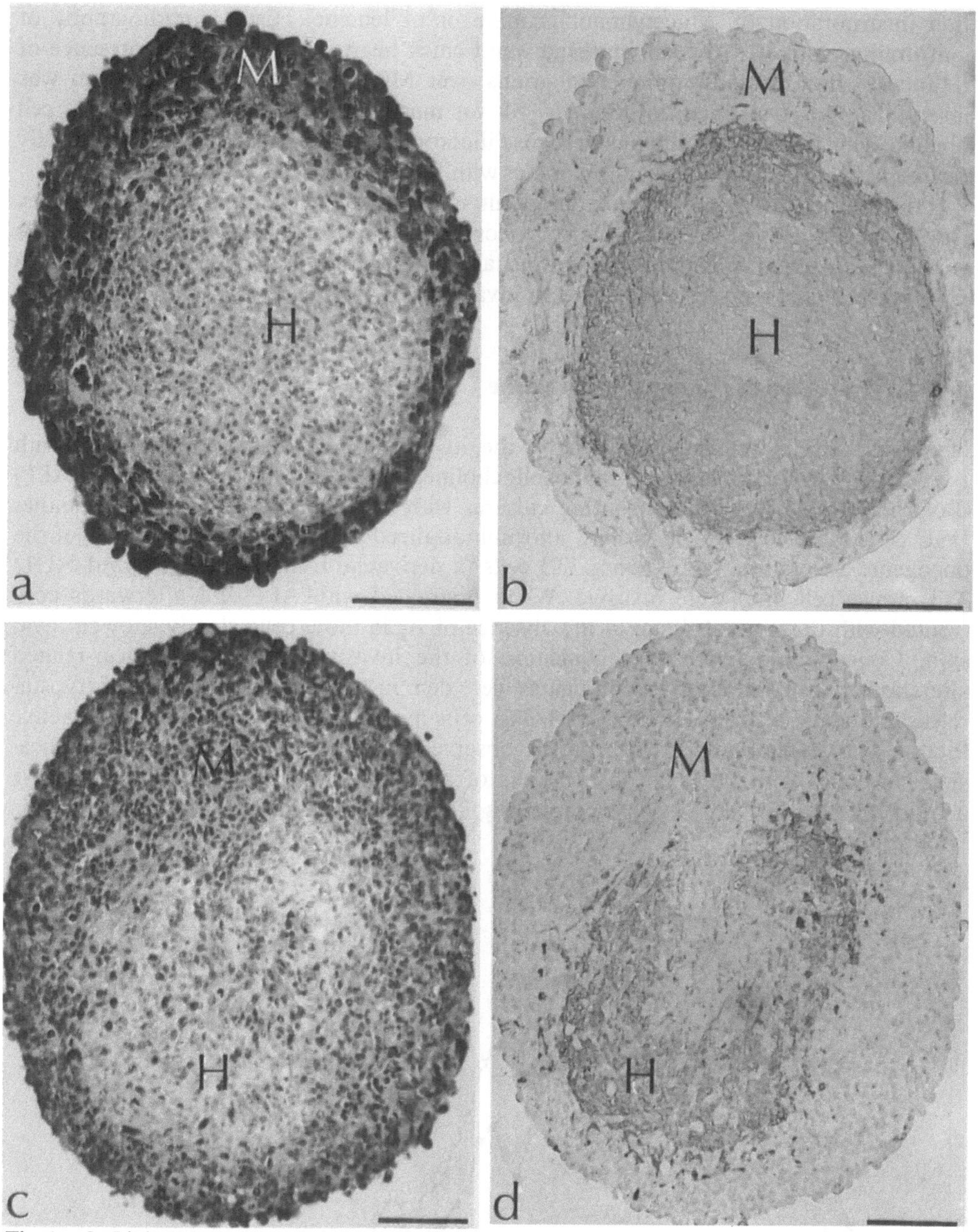

Fig. 1 a–d. Light micrographs of consecutive sections from confronting cultures between MO_4 cells *(M)* and embryonic chick heart *(H)* incubated at 28 °C and fixed after 10 days (**a, b**) or after 14 days (**c, d**). Staining was with hematoxylin and eosin (**a, c**) or with an antiserum against chick heart (**b, d**). *Scale bars,* 100 µm

Similar transitions were not observed for growth or for directional migration. In MO_4 cell cultures on artificial substrate the expression of fucosylated glycoconjugates at the cell surface was abolished when the temperature was lowered to 28 °C. In such cultures, incorporation of fucose into total cell glycoconjugates was reduced to a larger extent than incorporation of *N*-acetylmannosamine or of leucine. Histoautoradiography of confronting pairs of MO_4 cell aggregates and chick heart incubated in the presence of [^{3}H]fucose showed a low number of grains over MO_4 cells as long as invasion was absent. The onset of invasion after day 10 was marked by a net increase in MO_4 cell labeling. This increase in radioactive fucose incorporation was most obvious in centrally located MO_4 cells that had been in contact with the heart tissue.

Lowering of the temperature certainly alters other steps in the metabolic pathways, as well. Nevertheless, the coincidence of fucose incorporation and invasion by MO_4 cells in a time-dependent transition that is unusual for other cellular activities suggests a role for tumor cell surface glycoconjugates in invasion.

Induced Expression of the Invasive Phenotype

Noninvasive cells acquired temporarily the invasive phenotype after treatment with 1-0-octadecyl-2-0-methylglycero-3-phosphocholine, an alkyllysophospholipid (ALP) (Bolscher et al. 1986). In confronting cultures with fragments of normal tissue neither HSU cells (derived from rat kidney, and immortalized with a genomic fragment of the oncogenic adenovirus type 12) nor 3T3 cells (a derivative from an immortalized NIH/3T3 mouse cell line) were invasive. When pretreated with ALP and afterwards confronted with the normal tissue in the absence of ALP, these cells clearly showed invasion. Concomitantly with the acquisition of the invasive phenotype, cancer-related alterations in cell surface glycoconjugates were demonstrated by gel filtration of trypsin-releasable material from HSU or NIH/3T3 cells metabolically labeled with radioactive fucose. This shift in gel-filtration profile observed upon phenotypic induction of invasion correlates with previous observations of profile shifts accompanying constitutive acquisition of invasiveness (for example, Fig. 2). This correlation suggests a mechanistic

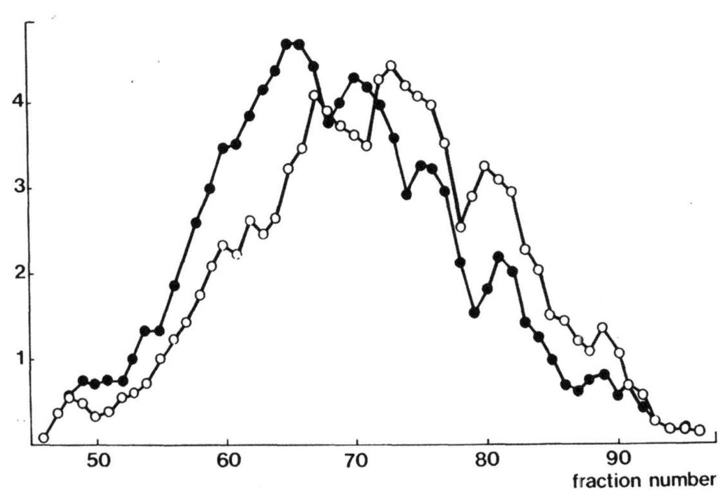

Fig. 2. Gel-filtration profiles (percentage radioactivity) of cell surface glycopeptides derived from noninvasive mouse M0 cells *(open symbols)* and from their invasive counterpart MO_4 *(closed symbols)*. Cells were metabolically labeled with [^{3}H]- or [^{14}C]fucose for 16 h. Glycopeptides were isolated from the cell surface by trypsinization followed by pronase digestion and cochromatographed on a Bio-Gel P-10: Sephadex G-50 (2:1, w/w) column

role of cell surface glycoconjugates in invasion, at least in vitro. Remarkably, the same ALP that made noninvasive cells invasive was able to inhibit the invasion of well-documented invasive cells (Storme et al. 1985). In the latter experiments, however, ALP was present in the culture medium during the invasion assay. This means that both the invasive cells and the normal tissue were affected at the same time, resulting in the confrontation of a constitutively invasive cell population with a cell population that presumably showed a drug-dependent invasive phenotype. This interpretation is supported by the finding that pretreatment of the normal tissue with ALP was sufficient to inhibit invasion of the confronting invasive cells (Schallier et al. 1987).

The experiments with ALP indicate that invasion depends on the interaction between glycoconjugates of both the tumor and the normal tissue. Among the molecules presumed to be involved in the perception of signals regulating cellular activities, cell surface glycoconjugates are interesting candidates because of their documented recognition function (Gabriel 1982).

Conclusion

We cannot say when, why, and how tumor cells invade because the molecular mechanisms of invasion are not yet understood. Experiments done so far leave space for various concepts: (1) A single gene change causes a discrete molecular alteration that permits cells to invade. For example, one can imagine that alteration of a receptor at the cell surface leads to loss of control on cellular activities implicated in invasion. (2) A single gene change may result in a cascade of molecular events affecting a number of cellular activities. Such cascades are well known in proteolysis. (3) Multiple molecular changes resulting from multiple gene alterations are needed to turn a noninvasive cell into an invasive one. Today, at least, we dispose of a number of experimental tools to refine our analysis of the molecular biology of minimal invasion.

Acknowledgments. F. V. R. is a Research Associate of the Belgian N. F. W. O. Work in the authors's laboratories is supported by grants from the Nationaal Fonds voor Wetenschappelijk Onderzoek (20093 and 3.000.584), the Kankerfonds van de Algemene Spaar- en Lijfrentekas, the Sport Vereniging tegen Kanker, Brussels, Belgium, and the Netherlands Cancer Foundation (NKI, KWF 84-16), Amsterdam, the Netherlands.

The authors thank Jean Roels van Kerckvoorde for preparing the illustrations and G. Matthys-De Smet for typing the manuscript.

References

Bolscher JGM, Schallier DCC, Smets LA, van Rooy H, Collard JG, Bruyneel EA, Mareel MMK (1986) Effect of cancer-related and drug-induced alterations in surface carbohydrates on the invasive capacity of mouse and rat cells. Cancer Res 46: 4080-4086

Collard JG, van Beek WP, Janssen JWG, Schijven JF (1985) Transfection by human oncogenes: concomitant induction of tumorigenicity and tumor-associated membrane alterations. Int J Cancer 35: 207-214

Foulds L (1969) Neoplastic development, vol 1. Academic Press, New York

Gabriel O (1982) Carbohydrates and receptor recognition. In: Kahn LD (ed) Hormone receptors. Wiley and Sons, New York, pp 137-156

Greig RG, Koestler TP, Trainer DL, Corwin SP, Miles L, Kline T, Sweet R, Yokoyama S, Poste G (1985) Tumorigenic and metastatic properties of "normal" and ras-transfected NIH/3T3 cells. Proc Natl Acad Sci USA 82: 3698-3701

Heldin C-H, Westermark B (1984) Growth factors: mechanism of action and relation to oncogenes. Cell 37: 9-20

Hynes NE, Jaggi R, Kozma SC, Ball R, Muellener D, Wetherall NT, Davis BW, Groner B (1985) New acceptor cell for transfected genomic DNA: oncogene transfer into a mouse mammary epithelial cell line. Mol Cell Biol 5: 268-272

Land H, Parada LF, Weinberg RA (1983) Cellular oncogenes and multistep carcinogenesis. Science 222: 771-778

Mareel MM (1983) Invasion in vitro: methods of analysis. Cancer Metastasis Rev 2: 201-218

Mareel MM, van Roy FM (1986) Are oncogenes involved in invasion and metastasis? Anticancer Res 6: 419-436

Mareel MM, de Ridder L, de Brabander M, Vakaet L (1975) Characterization of spontaneous, chemical, and viral transformants of a C3H/3T3-type mouse cell line by transplantation into young chick blastoderms. JNCI 54: 923-929

Mareel MM, Kint J, Meyvisch C (1979) Methods of study of the invasion of malignant C3H mouse fibroblasts into embryonic chick heart in vitro. Virchows Arch [Cell Pathol] 30: 95-111

Mareel MM, Bruyneel EA, de Bruyne GK, Dragonetti CH, van Cauwenberge RM-L (1982) Growth and invasion: separate activities of malignant MO_4 cell populations in vitro. In: Galeotti T, et al. (eds) Membranes in tumour growth. Elsevier, Amsterdam, pp 223-232

Mareel MM, Bruyneel EA, Dragonetti CH, de Bruyne GK, van Cauwenberge RM-L, Smets LA, van Rooy H (1984) Effect of temperature on invasion of MO_4 mouse fibrosarcoma cells in organ culture. Clin Exp Metastasis 2: 107-125

Meneguzzi G, Binétruy B, Grisoni M, Cuzin F (1984) Plasmidial maintenance in rodent fibroblasts of a BPV1-pBR322 shuttle vector without immediately apparent oncogenic transformation of the recipient cells. EMBO J 3: 365-371

Michiels L, van Roy FM, de Saint-Georges L, Mergaert J (1986) Genome organization of the FBR-osteosarcoma virus complex: identification of a subgenomic *fos*-specific message. Virus Res 5: 11-26

Rassoulzadegan M, Naghashfar Z, Cowie A, Carr A, Grisoni M, Kamen R, Cuzin F (1983) Expression of the large T protein of polyoma virus promotes the establishment in culture of "normal" rodent fibroblast cell lines. Proc Natl Acad Sci USA 80: 4354-4358

Rautmann G, Glaichenhaus N, Nahgashfar Z, Breathnach R, Rassoulzadegan M (1982) Complementation of a tsa mutant and replication of a recombinant DNA carrying the viral ori region in mouse cells transformed by polyoma virus. Virology 122: 306-317

Schallier D, Bolscher J, van Rooy H, Storme G, Smets L (1987) Modification of cell surface carbohydrates and invasive behavior by an alkyllysophospholipid. To be published

Sporn MB, Roberts AB (1985) Autocrine growth factors and cancer. Nature 313: 745-747

Storme GA, Berdel WE, van Blitterswijk WJ, Bruyneel EA, de Bruyne GK, Mareel MM (1985) Antiinvasive effect of racemic 1-0-octadecyl-2-0-methyl glycero-3-phosphocholine (ET-18-OCH_3) on MO_4 mouse fibrosarcoma cells in vitro. Cancer Res 45: 351-357

Thorgeirsson UP, Turpeenniemi-Hujanen T, Williams JE, Westin EH, Heilman CA, Talmadge JE, Liotta LA (1985) NIH/3T3 cells transfected with human tumor DNA containing activated ras oncogenes express the metastatic phenotype in nude mice. Mol Cell Biol 5: 259-262

Van Roy FM, Messiaen L, Liebaut G, Jin G, Dragonetti CH, Fiers WC, Mareel MM (1986) Invasiveness and metastatic capability of rat fibroblast-like cells before and after transfection with immortalizing and transforming genes. Cancer Res 46: 4787-4795

Minimal Neoplasias in Experimental Liver Carcinogenesis

H. M. Rabes

Pathologisches Institut, Universität München, Thalkirchner Straße 36, 8000 München 2, FRG

The rodent liver provides a unique opportunity to study the early stages of chemical carcinogenesis. If a rat or a mouse is exposed for a long period to a hepatocarcinogen, hepatocellular carcinomas develop which invade and replace part of the normal liver, and sometimes tumor cells disseminate to give rise to lung metastasis. Long before this final stage is reached cellular changes can be observed in the liver parenchyma. Foci of altered hepatocytes appear which show an aberration from the enzymatic pattern of normal hepatocytes. These foci can best be demonstrated in enzyme histochemical preparations in cryostat sections prepared from the liver at early stages of carcinogen exposure. Small islands of hepatocytes are then seen which show a deficiency of glucose-6-phosphatase as described in a preliminary report first in 1964 by the Friedrich-Freksa group (Gössner and Friedrich-Freksa 1964). In the same year, Bannasch and Müller reported that during hepatocarcinogenesis foci of glycogen-storing cells can be observed and they related their occurrence to the previous exposure to a hepatocarcinogen. Interestingly, it was in 1961 that Grundmann pointed out that basophilic foci occur in the liver after carcinogen exposure and he suggested that these subpopulations in the liver might represent precursor lesions in hepatocarcinogenesis.

In the meantime these foci of altered hepatocytes have been studied thoroughly with respect to various enzymatic aberrations (see Farber 1980; Pitot and Sirica 1980; Williams 1980; Scherer 1984; Bannasch 1986). It became evident that these foci were not only deficient of certain enzymes as demonstrated by histochemistry, but at the same time showed an over- or neoexpression of other enzymes, for instance, glucose-6-phosphate dehydrogenase or alphafetoprotein. Table 1 gives a summary of aberrations, as based on data from the literature. It is difficult to follow the thread with all these aberrations. It has been postulated that they represent a switch from glycolytic processes in the cells to the pentose phosphate pathway, further, that the occurrence of alphafetoprotein is a sign of reactivation of the fetal enzymatic phenotype. Other aberrations such as the changes of enzymes of the adenylate cyclase system were interpreted to represent changes of the second messenger system which transduces external signals to the functional cellular compartment. At the moment, however, it is not yet possible to prove that each enzymatic aberration as found in the foci bears the same essential implications for the process of carcinogenesis and we still wait for the unifying concept which takes into account all the diverse aberrations.

However, several observations during recent years strongly support the assumption that these enzyme-aberrant foci in the liver represent preneoplastic and early neoplastic

Recent Results in Cancer Research, Vol. 106

Table 1. Markers of carcinogen-induced preneoplastic hepatocellular subpopulations. (Compiled from Farber 1980; Scherer 1984; Bannasch 1986)

Negative markers	*Positive* markers
Glucose-6-phosphatase	Glucose-6-phosphate dehydrogenase
Adenosine triphosphatase	Epoxid hydrolase
β-Glucoronidase	Glutathione transferase
Serine dehydratase	UDP-glucuronyl transferase
Glycogen phosphorylase	Gammaglutamyl transpeptidase
Acid and alkaline nucleases	Glycogen accumulation
Microsomal monooxygenase	Increased glutathion content
NADPH-cytochrome P-450 reductase	Alphafetoprotein
Adenylate cyclase	
Resistance to iron accumulation	
Loss of lipid peroxidation	

lesions. Some observations gave indirect proof: Kunz et al. (1978) showed in a dose-time plot that there is a highly significant correlation between the number and size of ATPase-deficient foci in the liver after continuous carcinogen exposure and the frequency of later occurring hepatocellular carcinomas. Kaufmann et al. (1985) calculated the risk of an enzyme-aberrant focus and hepatoma development to range between 1 and 10^3 or 10^4 depending on the mode of treatment after carcinogen exposure. A high frequency of hepatomas was observed after additional phenobarbital exposure, which acts as a promotor of liver carcinogenesis (see Pitot and Sirica 1980).

Up to now the only direct evidence for the minimal neoplastic nature of these enzyme-aberrant foci comes from experiments which were performed to prove or disprove that these foci originate by clonal growth or a single initiated cell. If so, one could assume their neoplastic nature, if not, these foci could not be characterized as minimal neoplasias in a strict sense.

For this experiment mice of a specific strain were used which expresses a mutant phosphoglycerate kinase. The enzyme is coded on the X chromosome. Mating of a wild-type phosphoglycerate kinase PGK-1B female mouse with a PGK-1A mutant male mouse gives rise to an offspring with the females being heterozygous for PGK. Due to early embryonic lyonization, the random inactivation of either the paternal or the maternal X chromosome, the heterozygous female mouse consists of a mosaic of PGK 1A and PGK 1B cells. In such mice, enzyme-aberrant ATPase-deficient foci were induced by 2-acetylaminofluorene feeding. In cryostat sections ATPase-deficient loci were localized, and in the subsequent unstained thick section the respective area was punched out and compared with normal liver tissue. The microelectrophoretic pattern disclosed unequivocally a consistent coexpression of PGK type A and B in normal tissue, but in almost all samples taken from ATPase-deficient foci a selective expression of either PGK-1A or PGK-1B was observed. It can be concluded that ATPase-deficient foci develop in all probability by clonal growth from a single initiated cell (Rabes et al. 1982a). In the meantime this finding was confirmed by other groups using histochemical methods (Howell et al. 1985).

This implies that these foci result from abnormal growth of hepatocytes at the background of the quiescent, nonproliferating adult rodent liver. Thus it can be concluded that enzyme-aberrant foci in the liver are in a peculiar very early stage of neoplastic development. They appear to be endowed with an increased growth potential as compared with normal adult hepatocytes. However, to use the term "minimal neoplasia" may be misleading. Because of the very early stage of development, we prefer still to use the term "preneoplastic lesions" to avoid the misinterpretation that from the beginning these lesions are in a state of rapid neoplastic progression. This is not the case. Nevertheless, in our mind the essential for the early neoplastic nature of the foci is this change of the proliferative pattern (Rabes 1983). Therefore I shall focus on the role of cell proliferation during initiation and progression of preneoplastic foci in the liver.

Clonal origin of preneoplastic foci implies specific target cells for the initiating action of a carcinogen. Proliferation has an important impact on initiation of liver carcinogenesis. What do we know about the characteristics of a target cell with respect to cell proliferation? Fifteen years ago, Warwick (1971) was among the first to demonstrate that liver tumors can be induced by a single dose of a chemical hepatocarcinogen after partial hepatectomy, when hepatocytes are triggered into the cell cycle. A single exposure to a hepatocarcinogen effectively induces hepatomas either if given in a very high, hepatotoxic dose which is followed by liver cell necrosis and subsequent regeneration, or when partial hepatectomy and feeding of a low dose of 2-acetylaminofluorene follows, the Solt-Farber model (Solt and Farber 1976). The same effect can be achieved by partial hepatectomy, a moderate carcinogen dose, and subsequent phenobarbital feeding as introduced for instance by Pitot (Pitot and Sirica 1980), or by exposing newborn rats or mice to a carcinogen when liver cell proliferation continues for a few postnatal days, as shown by Vesselinovitch et al. (1984).

A closer view of the relation between time of carcinogen exposure and cell proliferation reveals that it is not proliferation per se which renders a cell capable of undergoing the initiation process. The most sensitive period for carcinogen action appears to be the first day after partial hepatectomy, as already reviewed by Craddock (1976). Kaufmann et al. (1981) demonstrated a close relation between initiation sensitivity and DNA synthesis in hydrocortisone-synchronized hepatocytes. With the use of hydroxyurea as a synchronizing agent in regenerating rat liver we were able to show that initiation sensitivity of hepatocytes increases in late G_1 of the cell cycle and reaches a peak in early S phase, followed by a steep decline in middle and late S phase. Maximum initiation sensitivity is clearly related to early S phase exposure (Rabes et al. 1986).

It has been argued that this high initiation sensitivity in early S phase might have been biased by the preceding hydroxyurea treatment. Therefore we tested the hypothesis of early S phase transformation sensitivity in unsynchronized regenerating rat liver after partial hepatectomy. At 2-h intervals the tritiated thymidine-labeling index of hepatocytes was determined. It shows a steep increase between 16 and 18 h and a plateau between 20 and 24 h after partial hepatectomy. Because duration of DNA synthesis has been determined to last 7 h, one can calculate the G_1-S transit rate or the fraction of cells in early S phase as a function of time after partial hepatectomy. The calculation reveals a high G_1-S transit rate between 16 and 18 h, with a decline thereafter and an additional increase between 22 and 24 h.

After a single exposure to methylnitrosourea at different intervals after partial hepatectomy, ATPase-deficient preneoplastic foci occur in a frequency which appears to be closely related to the G_1-S transit rate; a rapid decline is observed when cells are carcinogen exposed in the middle or late S phase. Although the tritiated thymidine labeling index is still high, the initiation sensitivity is lower than before. However, an exception from high early S phase sensitivity is observed after carcinogen exposure at 22 h when a large percentage of cells is at the G_1-S boundary or early S phase, but these cells do not respond with an increased transformation sensitivity. A careful autoradiographic analysis shows that these cells in early S phase at 22 h after partial hepatectomy are located in the intermediary and perivenous part of the liver lobule, in contrast to the cells in early S phase at 16 or 18 h after partial hepatectomy which are preferentially located in periportal areas of the liver lobule (Maguire and Rabes 1987).

We suggest that the peculiar target cell for the initiating action of a carcinogen is a cell at the G_1-S boundary or early S phase. However, clonogenic potential appears an additional, essential target cell characteristic. Those cells located in intermediary or perivenous parts of the liver lobule which respond rather slowly to the proliferative stimulus apparently lack clonogenic potential and, although carcinogen exposed in the most sensitive early S phase, fail to form a clonal progeny of initiated hepatocytes, the minimal neoplastic focus.

Because all these experiments about cell cycle-related carcinogen sensitivity were performed with alkylating nitroso compounds the question arises whether this early S phase transformation sensitivity is related to increased alkylation and/or decreased repair of promutagenic DNA base adducts in this phase. However, the results of a large series of experiments do not support this assumption. With dimethylnitrosamine given during G_1 phase, 12 h after partial hepatectomy, or 24 h after the operation when 30% hepatocytes are in S phase or during the hydroxyurea-synchronized S phase with 80% cells in S phase, the molar fraction of the main alkylation product 7-methylguanine becomes lower with an increasing number of cells in S phase, and so does the molar fraction of the promutagenic 0^6-methylguanine (Rabes et al. 1979, 1982b). If the ratio of 0^6-methylguanine/7-methylguanine is plotted against the number of cells in S phase, a steep decrease is observed with an increasing size of the S phase fraction. In contrast, the 3-methyladenine/7-methylguanine ratio remains largely constant irrespective of the number of S phase cells (Rabes et al. 1984).

Quantitative data obtained with an 0^6-methylguanine-DNA transferase assay using liver extracts at various intervals after partial hepatectomy and hydroxyurea show that this enzyme increases in regenerating rat liver in late G_1, early S, and decreases later in the cell cycle (Schuster et al. 1985). One has to recall in this context, however, that this methyl-transferase is expended during the reaction and does not prevent, once it is consumed in the cell, persistence of 0^6-alkylguanine in the DNA. This base adduct may then lead to base mispairing and point mutation when the DNA is replicated.

With this in mind, one could interprete the high transformation sensitivity of hepatocytes in early S phase as the result of persisting promutagenic lesions which lead to point mutations in those transformation-related genes which replicate in the early phase of DNA synthesis.

The race between DNA repair and start of DNA synthesis appears to be critical for the initiation probability of a hepatocyte. The outcome of this race is determined partly by the length of the interval between carcinogen exposure and start of DNA synthesis, and partly by the repair potential of a cell. The longer the interval is between carcinogen exposure and start of DNA synthesis, the lower is the probability of transformation. An inherent cellular deficiency to repair promutagenic DNA lesions like 0^6-alkylguanine or 0^4-alkylthymine, on the other hand, would increase the transformation probability. A possible repair aberration of hepatocytes cannot be studied in the putative target cells, but only with the progeny of such initiated cells, the altered hepatic focus.

Recently, experiments were performed in collaboration with Rajewsky and Adamkiewicz to test the possibility that these foci might show an aberrant DNA repair. A fluorescent-labeled monoclonal antibody against 0^6-ethyldeoxyguanosine was used to determine the persistence of this base adduct after the pulse of ethylnitrosourea in normal liver and in preneoplastic foci. 0^6-ethyldeoxyguanosine as determined by binding of the monoclonal antibody showed an almost identical decay in normal hepatocytes and in preneoplastic foci (Adamkiewicz, Rabes, and Rajewsky, in preparation).

It can be concluded that an impaired repair of the promutagenic 0^6-alkylguanine does not belong to the characteristics of the target cell for liver carcinogenesis, but that the proximity of early S phase might indeed be a critical determinant of the transformation probility of hepatocytes.

An essential prerequisite for the expression of the transformed phenotype is proliferative potential. Initiated hepatocytes are endowed with a proliferative advantage over normal hepatocytes. This leads to the formation of clones of enzyme-aberrant cells in the liver. The proliferative advantage becomes evident in particular when a carcinogen is continuously administered. After continuous feeding of diethylnitrosamine the relative frequency of cells with a short cell cycle time increases with prolongation of the carcinogen feeding. The cell cycle distribution curves show only a small percentage of rapidly cycling cells after 20 days of carcinogen exposure, but a large fraction with a t_c of about 20 h after 118 days of carcinogen feeding. Selective counting of the labeling index after a single dose of tritiated thymidine showed an increase concomitantly with enlargement of the foci, a decrease in the duration of DNA synthesis, and a shortening of the potential population doubling time t_{pot} (Rabes and Szymkowiak 1979). On the cellular level, it is evident from studies performed in collaboration with Bannasch and Zerban that clear and acidophilic cells show a rather low labeling index which increases in populations of mixed and basophilic cells to reach a maximum in hepatocellular carcinomas (Zerban, Rabes, and Bannasch, in preparation).

A sequence can be postulated which starts with the clonal expansion of cells with a moderately enhanced proliferation. This can be increased by the action of tumor promotors like phenobarbital as has been shown by Schulte-Hermann et al. (1981). However, during further development the population does not remain a homogeneous clone but shows diversification with regard to phenotypic expression as well as proliferative activity.

Evidence for this sequence from a homogeneous clone to a heterogeneous neoplastic population comes from DNA measurements in ATPase-deficient foci (Sarafoff et al. 1986). Single cell cytophotometry in a large variety of ATPase-deficient foci at different intervals after a single dose of methylnitrosourea shows clones which are composed almost selectively of diploid hepatocytes, but tetraploid preneoplastic clones are also observed, though less frequently. The third group of foci consists of hepatocytes with a heterogeneous ploidy pattern. Di-, tetra-, and octoploid cells are present with S phase cells in between, indicating a higher fraction of proliferating cells. This is confirmed by determination of the size of the foci. Whereas purely di- or tetraploid foci are small, heterogeneous foci are significantly larger, indicating a more rapid mode of proliferation. It seems that clonal homogeneity is preserved as long as the mode of proliferation is slow. With the occurrence of more rapidly proliferating hepatocytes in the frame of a preneoplastic focus the homogeneity appears to be lost.

At present it cannot be proven in vivo that further development again yields clones of cells which might take the lead in the process until hepatomas arise. However, in vitro studies with preneoplastic cells indicate that this might be true. Rats were fed continuously with diethylnitrosamine in the drinking water at a dose of 5 mg/kg per day for about 2 months. Hepatocytes were obtained by collagenase perfusion of the liver and the cells were kept in vitro in primary cultures for 8 weeks. After this time interval, foci or proliferating epithelial cells developed and were subcultured. After a few passages the cells grew in soft agar and in suspension. After transplantation to nude mice hepatocellular carcinomas developed (Kerler and Rabes 1986). The chromosomal pattern indicates that this cell line is clonally derived from the preneoplastic cells cultured in vitro after diethylnitrosamine-feeding in vivo. All cells of the hyperdiploid line show a quadruplication of chromosome 3, and the chromosomes 7 and 12 are present in tri- or quadruplicates (Holecek and Rabes 1986). Consistent translocations and deletions in several other chromosomes are further in support of the assumption that the cell line is a tumorigenic hepatocellular clone which had originated by clonal selection from preneoplastic cells.

This clone shows aberrations from the normal hepatocellular genotype: DNA of the tumorigenic cell line contains an increased number of copies of the H-*ras* gene, most of them forming a separate band in the Southern blot, indicating a translocation to another part of the genome. The pattern of DNA hybridization in the tumorigenic cell line was similar to that of the methylnitrosourea-induced hepatoma, but different from normal and fetal liver. This indicates that in this rapidly proliferating clone in vitro some of the essential genomic aberration might be overexpressed. Clonal selection would then pertain to those cells which represent the fraction of preneoplastic cells most capable of autonomous growth (Suchy, Kerler and Rabes, unpublished observations).

Preneoplastic foci arise in the liver by clonal growth of a single hepatocyte initiated preferentially during early DNA synthesis. A change in the regulation of proliferation leads to a growth advantage over normal hepatocytes. Alteration of metabolic pathways in combination with an increased rate of proliferation might be essential prerequisites for a genetic or at least phenotypic instability (Nowell 1976), which might pave the way to the generation of new aberrant clones in the frame of a preneoplastic focus. A few of these newly developing subpopulations or even only a single one might finally give rise to an autonomously growing hepatocellular carcinoma.

References

Bannasch P (1986) Preneoplastic lesions as end points in carcinogenicity testing: I. Hepatic preneoplasia. Carcinogenesis 7: 689-695

Bannasch P, Müller HA (1964) Lichtmikroskopische Untersuchungen über die Wirkung von *N*-Nitrosomorpholin auf die Leber von Ratte und Maus. Arzneimittelforsch 14: 805-814

Bannasch P, Mayer D, Hacker HJ (1980) Hepatocellular glycogenosis and hepatocarcinogenesis. Biochim Biophys Acta 605: 217-245

Craddock VM (1976) Cell proliferation and experimental liver cancer. In: Cameron D, Linsell A, Warwick GP (eds) Liver cell cancer. Elsevier, Amsterdam, pp 153-201

Farber E (1980) The sequential analysis of liver cancer induction. Biochim Biophys Acta 605: 149-166

Gössner W, Friedrich-Freksa H (1964) Histochemische Untersuchungen über die Glucose-6-Phosphatase in der Rattenleber während der Cancerisierung durch Nitrosamine. Z Naturforsch [B] 19: 862-864

Grundmann E (1961) Die Zytogenese des Krebses. Dtsch Med Wochenschr 86: 1077-1084

Holecek B, Rabes HM (1986) Cytogenetic analyses of normal and diethylnitrosamine-initiated preneoplastic hepatocytes. J Cancer Res Clin Oncol 111: S95

Howell S, Wareham KA, Williams ED (1985) Clonal origin of mouse liver cell tumors. Am J Pathol 121: 426-432

Kaufmann WK, Kaufman DG, Rice JM, Wenk ML (1981) Reversible inhibition of rat hepatocyte proliferation by hydrocortisone and its effect on cell cycle-dependent hepatocarcinogenesis by *N*-methyl-*N*-nitrosourea. Cancer Res 41: 4653-4660

Kaufmann WK, Mackenzie SA, Kaufman DG (1985) Quantitative relationship between hepatocytic neoplasms and islands of cellular alteration during hepatocarcinogenesis in male F344 rat. Am J Pathol 119: 171-174

Kerler R, Rabes HM (1986) In vitro propagation of preneoplastic hepatocytes initiated in vivo by diethylnitrosamine. J Cancer Res Clin Oncol 111: S46

Kunz W, Appel KE, Rickart R, Schwarz M, Stöckle G (1978) Enhancement and inhibition of carcinogenic effectiveness of nitrosamines. In: Remmer H, Bolt HM, Bannasch P, Popper H (eds) Primary liver tumors. MTP Press, Lancaster, pp 261-283

Maguire S, Rabes HM (1987) Transformation sensitivity in early S-phase and clonogenic potential are target-cell characteristics in liver carcinogenesis by N-methyl-N-nitrosourea. Int J Cancer 39: 385-389

Nowell PC (1976) The clonal evolution of tumour cell populations. Science 194: 23-28

Pitot HC, Sirica AE (1980) The stages of initiation and promotion in hepatocarcinogenesis. Biochim Biophys Acta 605: 191-215

Rabes HM (1983) Development and growth of early preneoplastic lesions induced in the liver by chemical carcinogens. J Cancer Res Clin Oncol 106: 85-92

Rabes HM, Szymkowiak W (1979) Cell kinetics of hepatocytes during the preneoplastic period of diethylnitrosamine-induced liver carcinogenesis. Cancer Res 39: 1298-1304

Rabes HM, Kerler R, Wilhelm R, Rode G, Riess H (1979) Alkylation of DNA and RNA by (^{14}C) dimethylnitrosamine in hydroxyurea-synchronized regenerating rat liver. Cancer Res 39: 4228-4236

Rabes HM, Bücher T, Hartmann A, Linke I, Dünnwald M (1982a) Clonal growth of carcinogen-induced enzyme-deficient preneoplastic cell populations in mouse liver. Cancer Res 42: 3220-3227

Rabes HM, Wilhelm K, Kerler R, Rode G (1982b) Dose- and cell cycle-dependent 0^6-methylguanine elimination from DNA in regenerating rat liver after (^{14}C)dimethylnitrosamine injection. Cancer Res 42: 3814-3821

Rabes HM, Kerler R, Rode G, Schuster C, Wilhelm R (1984) 0^6-Methylguanine repair in liver cells in vivo: comparison between G_1- and S-phase of the cell cycle. J Cancer Res Clin Oncol 108: 36-45

Rabes HM, Müller L, Hartmann A, Kerler R, Schuster CH (1986) Cell-cycle dependent initiation of ATPase-deficient populations in adult rat liver by a single dose of *N*-methyl-*N*-nitrosourea. Cancer Res 46: 645-650

Sarafoff, Rabes HM, Dörmer P (1986) Correlations between ploidy and initiation probability determined by DNA cytophotometry in individual altered hepatic foci. Carcinogenesis 7: 1191-1196

Scherer E (1984) Neoplastic progression in experimental hepatocarcinogenesis. Biochim Biophys Acta 738: 219-236

Schulte-Hermann R, Ohde G, Schuppler J, Timmermann-Trosiener I (1981) Enhanced proliferation of putative preneoplastic cells in rat liver following treatment with the tumor promoters phenobarbital, hexachlorocyclohexane, steroid compounds and nafenopin. Cancer Res 41: 2556-2562

Schuster C, Rode G, Rabes HM (1985) 0^6-Methylguanine repair of methylated DNA in vitro: cell cycle-dependence of rat liver methyltransferase activity. J Cancer Res Clin Oncol 110: 98-102

Solt D, Farber E (1976) New principle for the analysis of chemical carcinogenesis. Nature 263: 702-703

Vesselinovitch SD, Koka M, Mihailovich N, Rao KVN (1984) Carcinogenicity of diethylnitrosamine in newborn, infant and adult mice. J Cancer Res Clin Oncol 108: 60-65

Warwick GP (1971) Effect of the cell cycle on carcinogenesis. Fed Proc 30: 1760-1765

Williams GM (1980) The pathogenesis of rat liver cancer caused by chemical carcinogens. Biochim Biophys Acta 605: 167-189

Pathology and Therapy

Minimal Endometrial Carcinoma

L. D. Stoddard

Department of Pathology, Medical College of Georgia, Augusta, GA 30912, USA

Before examining the question of minimal carcinoma of the endometrium, we need to have accurate concepts of what a carcinoma is. Carcinomas are not to be understood in terms of what cells look like. Carcinomas have to be understood as disturbed societal relationships among populations of cells. Carcinomas, themselves, are made up of organized populations of cells (Pierce 1974), and the disturbances have to do with the carcinoma's relationships to normal, organized populations of cells (Leighton and Tchao 1984). Such pathological relationships are well known. The local abnormalities are carcinomatous infiltration of normal tissues and reorganization of vascular and stromal structure. Meantime, as the carcinoma advances, it reorganizes its own structure. With time, its cell populations change by differentiation. Such differentiation probably is a consequence of rearrangement of the genome (transpositions), as Barbara McClintock's work has made us aware (Fedoroff 1984). Stem cells often increase at the expense of postmitotic differentiated cells. Distant pathological disturbances depend upon circumstances that allow critical masses of cells of the carcinoma to gain entrance to neighboring veins, to embolize, to set up viable transplants in capillaries, to extend through the capillary walls, and then to repeat more or less the infiltrating growth and development of the spreading primary tumor. "Minimal carcinoma" would seem to be the least advanced lesion that has high, almost absolute, predictive value for the biopathological progression outlined.

The critical event in the life history of a carcinoma is beginning infiltration, or invasion. It compares with birth in the life history of a human being. Of course, many events go on before invasion or before birth. There always have been, as there are today, arguments about when a human being becomes a person, but there is little reason to dispute the fact that a human being becomes a member of society and begins societal relationships at birth, hardly before. Similarly, there are arguments about when in the course of carcinogenesis populations of cells become a carcinoma. Nevertheless, it is with beginning invasion that one can reasonably say an abnormal societal relationship has developed between populations of cells, not before. It is the beginning of the abnormal relationship that we understand as carcinoma.

We have stated that carcinomas are not to be understood in terms of what cells look like. However, problems arise because microinvasion seldom occurs in fields of otherwise normal-appearing epithelium. Historical perspective as regards cervical carcinoma highlights the problems best. When I began to study cervical carcinogenesis in 1947, the main difficulty was semantic. Surface fields of abnormal squamous epithelium looking

Recent Results in Cancer Research, Vol. 106

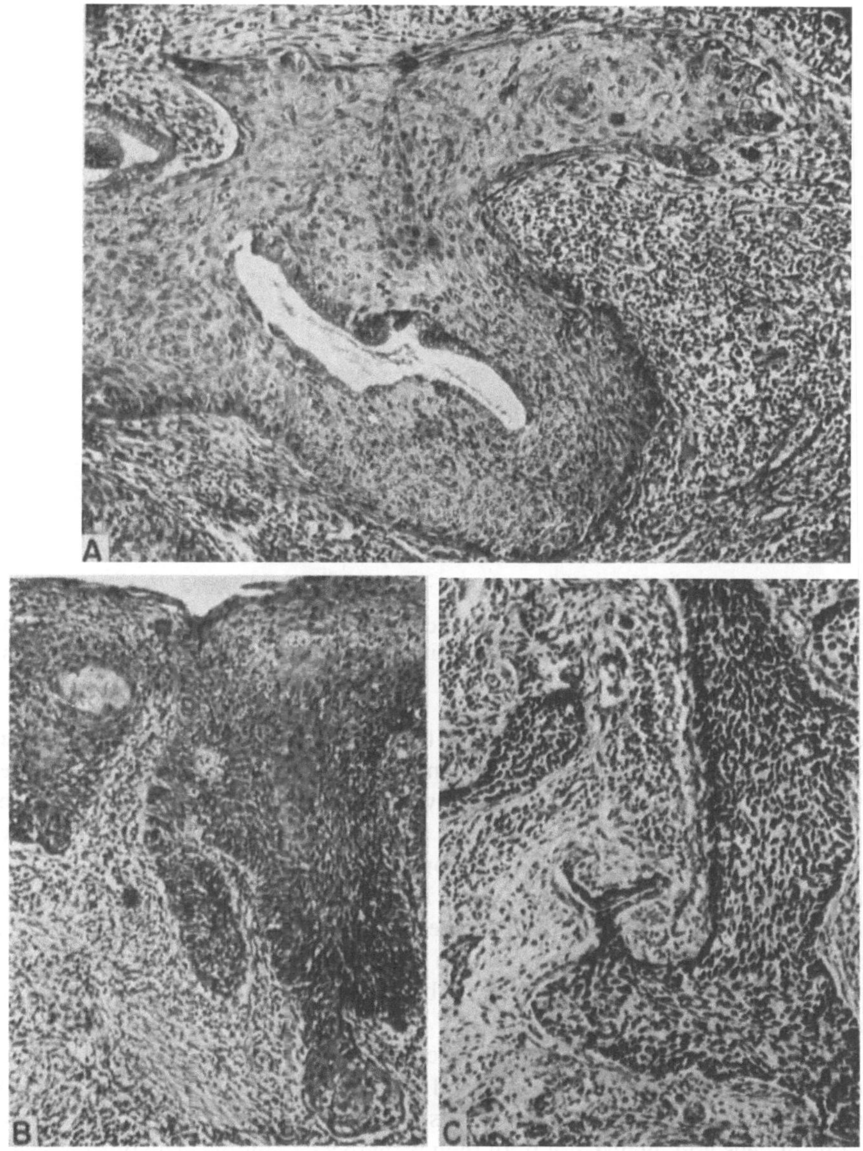

Fig. 1 A–C. Microscopic invasive buds. **A** Carcinoma in situ arising from reserve cell proliferation beneath the columnar epithelium of a gland; *above right:* a better-differentiated invasive bud irregularly invading loose stroma; *above left:* possible invasion. **B** Carcinoma in situ of the portio; *lower right:* a better-differentiated invasive bud; *left:* a noninvasive intraepithelial pseudopearl. **C** *Right:* carcinoma in situ filling a gland; *left:* an undifferentiated, forked invasive bud projecting upward and clusters of invasive carcinoma. (Stoddard 1952b, p. 235)

much like carcinoma had been reported already many years before. No matter what names were given to such surface fields, some persons contended that they looked so much like carcinoma that they should be called carcinoma. But others said that since there was no evidence of invasion, they were not carcinomas and, therefore, should not be called carcinoma. I began serially sectioning such lesions in the hope that some

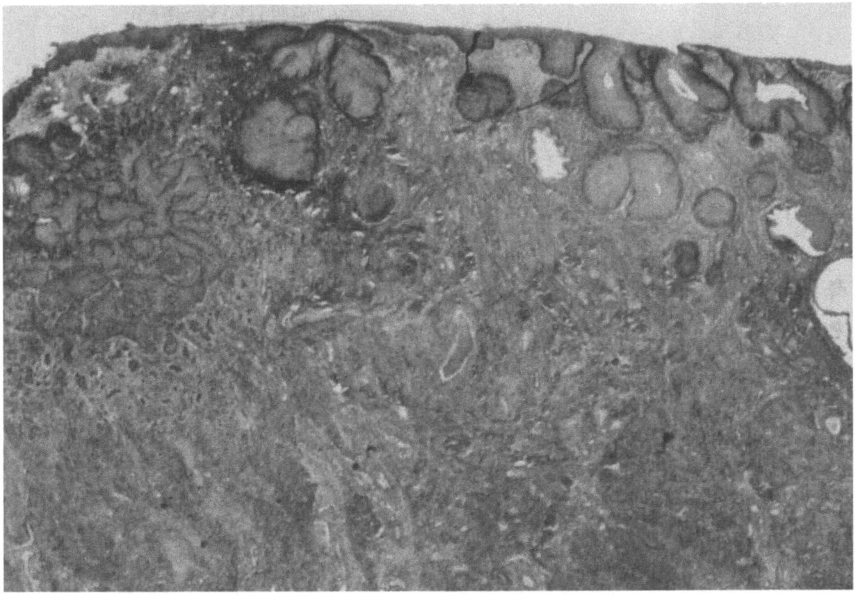

Fig. 2. An aggregation of microinvasive buds in a locus *(upper left)* has produced a miniature, invasive carcinoma. A large field of carcinoma-in-situ occupies glands higher in the endocervical canal

observation might be made to bridge the gap between the surface lesions and invasive carcinomas and put an end to the semantic confusion. I did not have expectations of what the observations might be but was lucky enough to find what I reported then (Stoddard 1952a, b) and still refer to as microinvasive buds (Fig. 1). However, the discovery that microinvasive buds developed in surface fields of carcinoma-in-situ did not reveal how often they develop. That has never been determined, nor how often they aggregate in a small locus and become what I call a miniature carcinoma (Fig. 2), probably like those Mestwerdt reported in 1947. And so, what is the predictive value of all the cytological abnormalities that can be found in surface fields of cervial carcinoma-in-situ? It is unknown.

Up to this point we have established three concepts. The first is that carcinomas are to be understood in terms of disturbed societal relationships of populations of cells. The second is that not until invasion occurs is there a disturbed relationship between populations of cells and, hence, not until then is there a carcinoma. The third is that carcinomas are not to be understood in terms of what cells look like.

For a moment let us consider what the predictive value of invasion would be if half of invasive carcinomas progressed and half either became stationary or regressed. In that case, invasion would not be a watershed biopathological event, and finding an invasive carcinoma in a biopsy would have no predictive value. There would be an equal chance that the tumor would progress or that it would not. Invasion would still remain an interesting biopathological phenomenon but would have no bearing on prognosis. However, as things are, it has high predictive value. If left untreated, the lesion will be progressive. Therefore, it seems to me that identifying a lesion to be called "minimal carcinoma" should depend upon identifying beginning invasion.

Unfortunately, stromal invasion developing in glandular fields of endometrial hyperplasia is not so easy to recognize as it is in surface fields of abnormal epithelium in the cervix. More to the point, beginning invasion cannot be recognized in the endometrium with the same assurance that it can be recognized in the gut. The counterpart of infiltration of the lamina propria of the gut is rarely encountered by invasion of the endometrial stroma. What is called stromal invasion usually is only a closely packed group of hyperplastic glands. There are still other difficulties. In the gut, the lamina muscularis mucosae is interposed between the mucosa and the submucosa, and one can tell whether or not that boundary layer has been breached. There is no such boundary between endometrium and myometrium, and, to make matters even more difficult, the basalis of the endometrium undulates above the myometrium. While a fairly shallow biopsy sample of the gut includes the muscularis mucosae, endometrial biopsies usually do not extend deeply into the myometrium.

Largely denied the possibility of using microinvasion, as in the cervix uteri, to define minimal carcinoma of the endometrium, pathologists turned their attention to precursor lesions: endometrial hyperplasia with varying degrees of glandular and cytological atypicality. The lesions range from simple hyperplasia, associated with anovulatory cycles or persistent anovulation, to adenomatous hyperplasia and atypical adenomatous hyperplasia.

Anovulatory hyperplastic endometrium is characterized by large proliferative glands lined by closely set, tall epithelial cells having pseudostratified nuclei (Fig. 7). Mitoses can be found, sometimes in large numbers (6-20/20 cross-sections of glands) but usually less frequently. Uniformly, the stroma is made up of large round cells having recognizable cytoplasm, identical to the stroma of normal, hypothetical postovulatory day 5-7. It is amazing that this reliably diagnostic stroma in the presence of proliferative glands goes unmentioned in standard descriptions of anovulatory hyperplasia even though accompanying photomicrographs, if of good quality, depict it. Irregularly distributed, small subnuclear vacuoles often can be found.

Adenomatous hyperplasia carries a wide range of variable histopathological features depending upon the investigator reporting. It can be no more than anovulatory hyperplasia with a few isolated glands marked by outpouching, budding, or branching. Other illustrations show a microadenoma of closely set glands often owing, I think, to hyperconvolution of one, or a few glands. Dysplasia, or atypical hyperplasia should connote somewhat larger microscopic lesions characterized by evidently abnormal conformation of closely set glands lined by abnormal cells. However, such lesions sometimes are labeled adenomatous hyperplasia. Severe dysplasia, or atypical adenomatous hyperplasia, exhibits greater cellular and glandular atypicality. The term carcinoma-in-situ is applied to various lesions; some forego the term altogether.

Lack of consensus about the histological definition of these diagnostic terms reminds me of some problems in general semantics discussed by Korzybski (1948). He cautioned that we get into trouble if we do not realize that "the word is not the thing" and "the map is not the territory." I have paraphrased those dicta for pathologists as follows: "The name is not the lesion" and "the disease is not biopathological reality" (Fig. 3). The

THE WORD IS NOT THE THING
THE NAME IS NOT THE LESION

THE MAP IS NOT THE TERRITORY
THE DISEASE IS NOT THE REALITY

Fig. 3. With apologies to Korzybski (1948)

same name may be applied to different lesions, and different names may be applied to similar lesions. Because the same name does not necessarily mean the same lesion to everyone, photomicrographs should accompany references to various kinds of endometrial hyperplasia. What amounts to a small histological atlas of endometrial lesions was published by Sommers (1982). The photomicrographs are at standard magnifications and are accompanied by legends and an explanatory text. The pathologist can use Sommers' article as a guide to follow or a means to clarify his own histopathological criteria in this troublesome area.

To avoid trouble we also must remember that disease maps are not the pathological territory. Disease maps are abstractions and can be changed while reality has not changed at all. For example, Gusberg and Kaplan (1963) by fiat changed the designation "adenomatous hyperplasia" in a group of patients under prospective study to "stage 0 cancer" because 12% of 68 cases which were followed from more than 1 year but not beyond the 10th year subsequently developed carcinoma. Their data can be handled in different ways, but the maximum cumulative risk of carcinoma at the beginning of the 10th year was 30% compared with no appreciable risk for control groups.

Let us recall that we are concerned with the predictive value of precursor glandular hyperplasia as regards biopathological progression. In the instance of Gusberg and Kaplan (1963), changing the name of the lesion changed the disease map from adenomatous hyperplasia to cancer but did not change the pathological territory: the cumulative risk of progression in up to 10 years was 30%, whichever name you choose.

Another careful study of precursor lesions was done by Abell (1982) on adenocarcinoma in situ of the endometrium. He reported 111 cases of lesions having various histological patterns. Eighty-nine were treated by hysterectomy within 12 months of initial biopsy diagnosis: 11 of them had no gland atypia, 6 had adenomatous hyperplasia, and, on the other hand, 11 had stromal invasion and 5 had superficial myometrial invasion. It can be concluded that as many lesions disappeared or regressed as progressed in up to 1 year.

In studies with Greenblatt et al. (1982; Greenblatt and Stoddard 1978) we have found that some precursor hyperplasias are reversible by cyclical progestogen therapy. Vellios (1974) came to the same conclusion, which is now widely held. In one of our

Fig. 4 *(upper left).* Atypical adenomatous hyperplasia with focal squamous metaplasia in two of ▷ seven tissue fragments. Frequent mitoses found in the microadenoma illustrated and in remaining hyperestrogenic endometrium (not illustrated). H & E, × 10 objective, × 60

Fig. 5 *(upper right).* Reproduced from Gore (1973, Fig. 3, p. 259). "An atypical glandular pattern ... very suggestive of well differentiated adenocarcinoma." Published magnification 150, reduced 1/5

Fig. 6 *(lower left).* Biopsy after progestogen treatment, 6 months following the biopsy illustrated in Fig. 4. One microadenoma *(left, lower corner)* in 13 tissue fragments. Some subnuclear secretion vacuoles but no mitoses seen in microadenoma or in small, tubular, endometrial glands. H & E, × 4 objective, × 25

Fig. 7 *(lower right).* Anovulatory endometrium. Biopsy 4 years following that illustrated in Fig. 6. Ovulatory cycles resulted in a twin pregnancy. Subsequently, menstrual irregularities characteristic of anovulation. Large proliferative glands, tall epithelial cells, pseudostratified nuclei, frequent mitoses; large, round stromal cells identical to those of a normal postovulatory day 5–7, infiltrated with smaller red blood cells. Abundant curettements had no trace of adenomatous hyperplasia or atypicality. H & E, × 10 objective, × 235

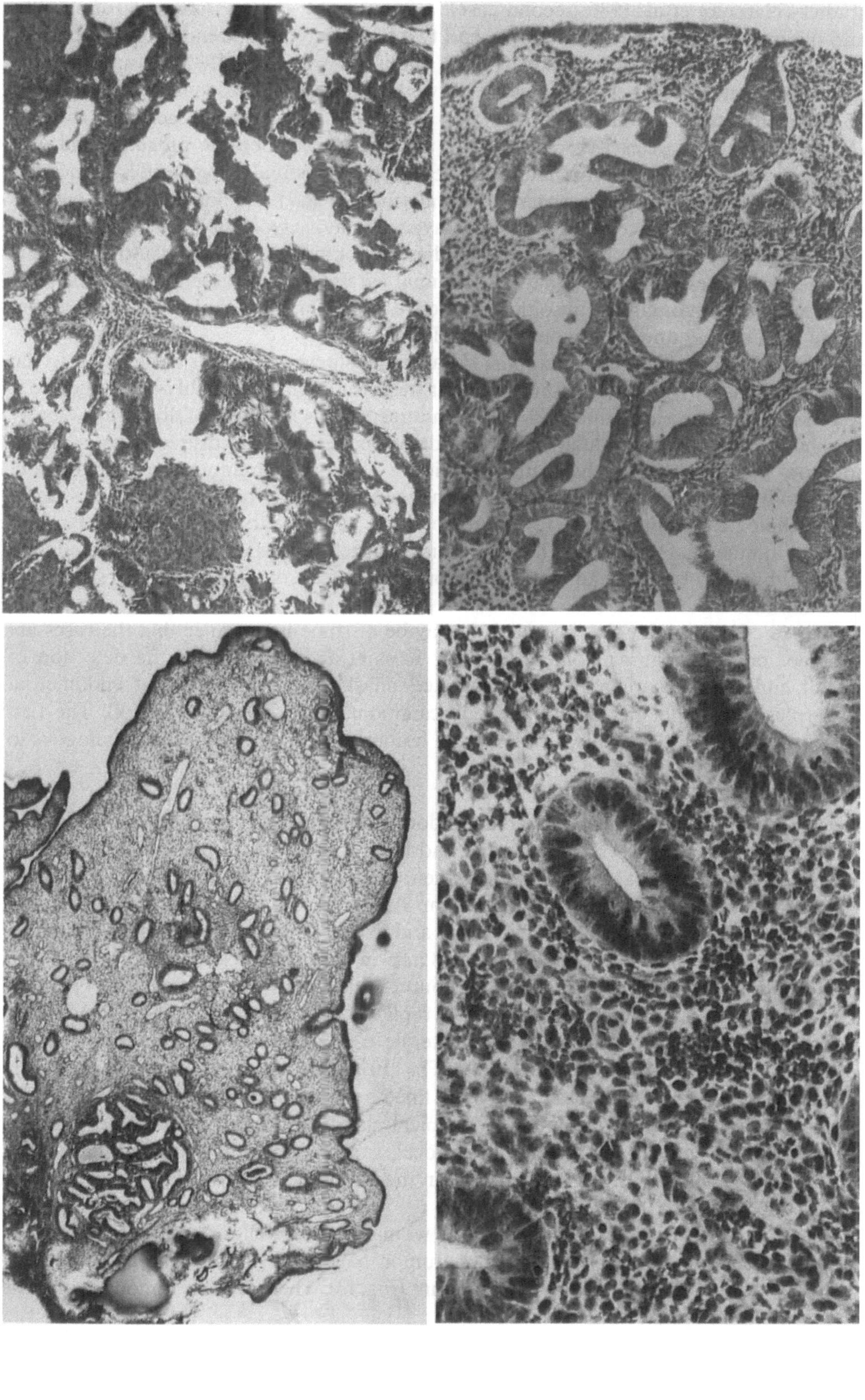

studies (Natrajan et al. 1986, second case), a 25-year-old woman was seen for sterility and oligomenorrhea. The initial biopsy had two foci of atypical adenomatous hyperplasia (Fig. 4) comparable to a lesion (Fig. 5) published by Gore (1973) as an "atypical glandular pattern ... very suggestive of well differentiated adenocarcinoma" in a 26-year-old patient. In our case, there was a response to cyclical progestogen therapy (Fig. 6). Ovulatory cycles were established, and the patient became pregnant and was delivered of twins. Four years later, she developed menstrual irregularities associated with an anovulatory hyperestrogenic endometrium (Fig. 7). In the abundant curettements, there was no trace of adenomatous hyperplasia or atypicality.

We have to conclude that follow-up studies do not make precursor glandular hyperplasias candidates for the designation "minimal carcinoma" of the endometrium. They do not have a high, almost absolute, predictive value for biopathological progression. Some even regress under hormonal manipulation.

It may be that "minimal carcinoma" is an unsatisfactory term for application to the endometrium. However, let me propose that the term might reasonably be applied to a lesion in which the entire thickness of the endometrium is made up of abnormal, closely packed, proliferative, glandular or nonglandular epithelium. The disease map is drawn to show that such lesions have high predictive value for carcinomatous progression. There may not be enough checkpoints on the map to be sure that it precisely represents the pathological territory, but I venture to think its predictive value would be high enough to make it a good map. The reason is that such lesions often are associated with larger fungating, typical, exophytic carcinomas that may or may not show suggestive invasion as well.

Three cases in point are presented. It may be of some importance that the cases are those of postmenopausal women. In 1984, Koss et al. published on the detection of occult endometrial carcinoma and suggested on statistical grounds that endometrial hyperplasia does not necessarily precede carcinoma in women past age 50. The first case, presented (P. R.) has focal endometrial lesions that may be somewhat analogous to cervical carcinoma-in-situ.

Case P. R. A 70-year-old woman had an endometrial biopsy after spotting for 1 week. A hysterectomy was done 9 days later. She had had no hormonal replacement therapy or bleeding for the previous 7 years. Before then, she had taken Premarin 0.625 mg q. o. d. for about 4 years. The uterus was 6.5 × 4 cm. An exophytic, polypoid mass 3 × 2 cm in size covered half the anterior endometrium and extended along the left lateral endometrial surface. The myometrium was only 8 mm in greatest thickness. No lesions that could potentially produce estrogens were found in the small, atrophic ovaries. Figures 8 and 9 show a thin endometrium completely replaced by atypical, closely set glands from which a polypoid mass projects into the uterine cavity. Adjacent endometrium, a little more distal from the mass, is pictured in Figs. 10 and 11. Although not grossly hyperplastic, it is atypical. Small basal glands are lined by hyperplastic epithelium of endosalpingian type. They are surmounted by atypical glands that might be considered carcinoma-in-situ. Figure 12 is a focus of equivocal, superficial myometrial invasion. There was no tumor found beyond the uterus or in the lymph nodes sampled.

Case C. H. A 59-year-old postmenopausal woman had a well-differentiated, secretory tumor. The endometrium was thick. A tumor having a gland-within-gland pattern appeared to be pushing into the myometrium (Fig. 13). There was no tumor beyond the uterus or in the lymph nodes or omentum.

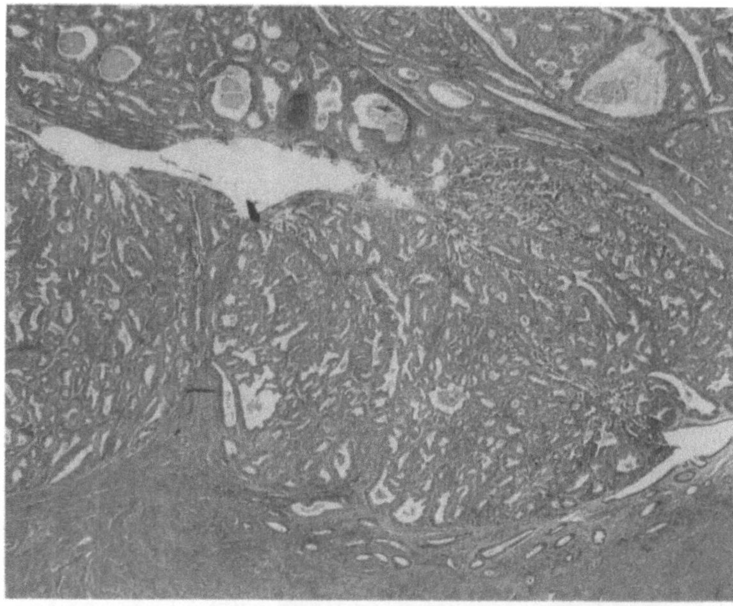

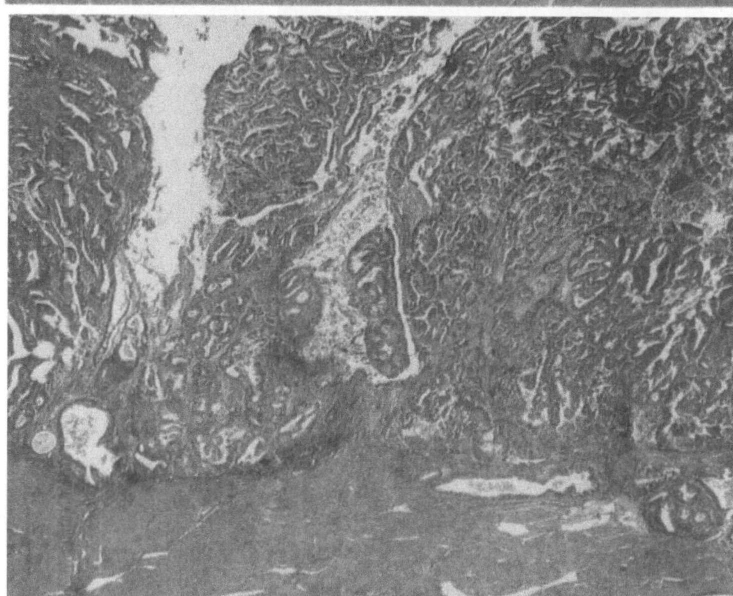

Fig. 8 *(above)*. Case P. R. A thin endometrium seen *at the right* becomes completely replaced by atypical, closely set glands from which a polypoid mass projects into the uterine cavity. H & E, × 1 objective, × 20

Fig. 9 *(below)*. Case P. R. Similar to Fig. 8 except that the thin endometrium persists only as a few isolated glands *at the right*. As in Fig. 8, tangled masses of glands in the polypoid tumor are lined by tall cells having large nuclei frequently in mitosis. H & E, × 1 objective, × 20

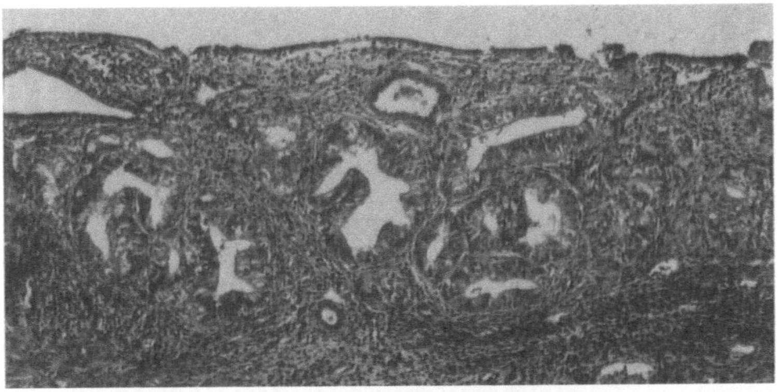

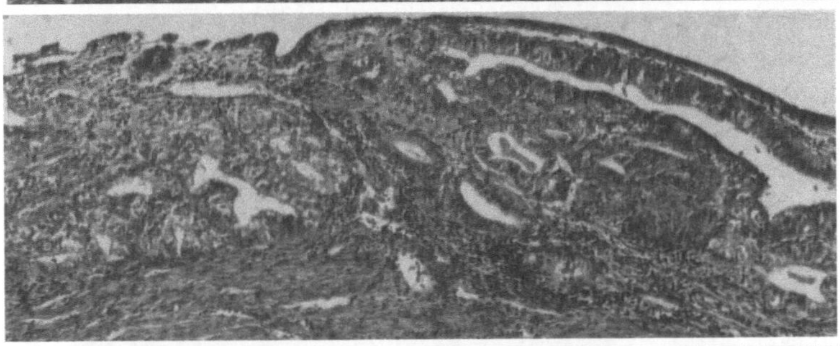

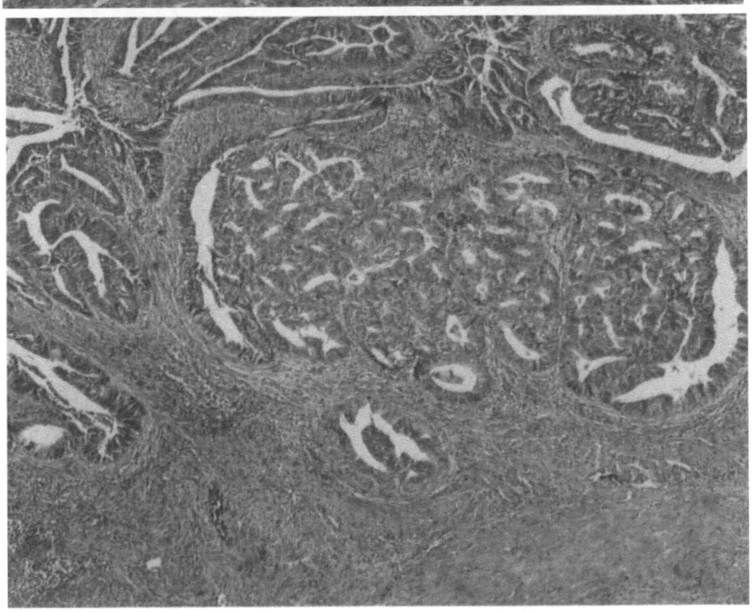

Figs. 10 *(above)*, **11** *(middle)*. Case P. R. Contiguous fields in a strip of thin abnormal endometrium bordering a "minimal carcinoma." No normal glands; a few basilar glands of endosalpingian type; remainder, atypical configurations, lined by tall, pale cells with large vesicular nuclei and small nucleoli. H & E, × 4 objective, × 80

Fig. 12 *(below)*. Case P. R. A focus of equivocal, superficial, myometrial invasion. H & E, × 2.5 objective, × 50

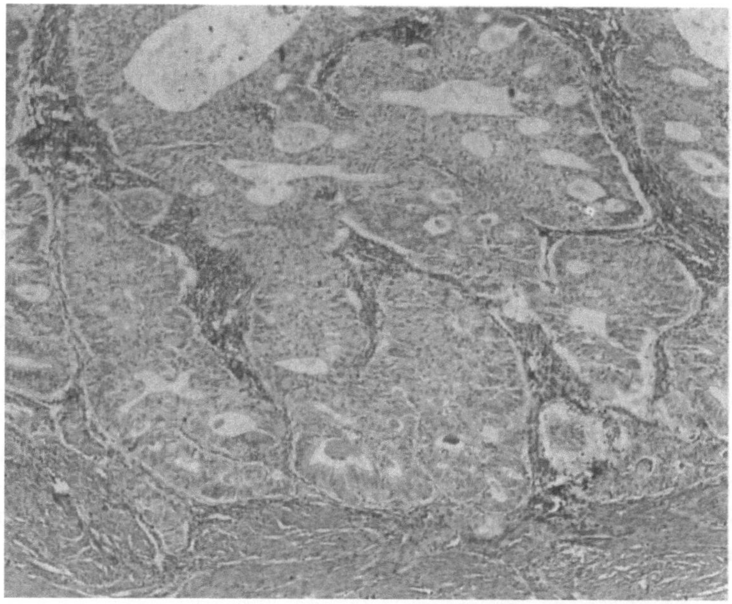

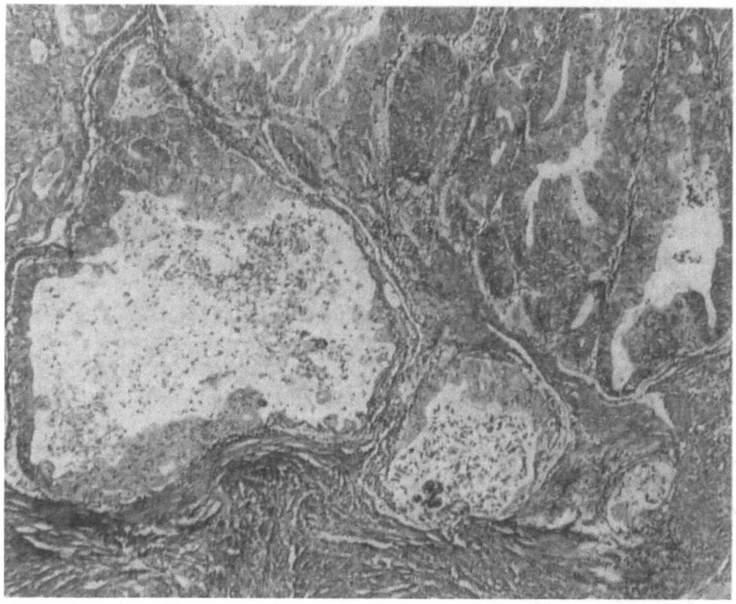

Fig. 13 *(above)*. Patient C.H. A pale cell, secretory tumor having a gland-within-gland pattern. Endometrium thickened and a pushing boundary with the myometrium. H & E, × 2.5 objective, × 50

Fig. 14 *(below)*. Patient M.R. A tumor similar to that in Fig. 13 but incomplete glands at the advancing margin with the myometrium indicating early infiltration. H & E, × 2.5 objective, × 50

Case M.R. The patient, 70 years old, had a well-differentiated tumor confined to the uterus. It appeared to push against the myometrium, but unlike the previous case, there were incomplete glands at the advancing margin (Fig. 14), much like some instances of beginning invasion of colonic tumors.

Conclusion

Carcinomas are identified by disturbed societal relationships between populations of cells, not by histological appearances and attributes of individual cells. The identifying disturbances are infiltration and local invasion followed by distant spread and dissemination. "Minimal carcinoma" might be defined as the least advanced lesion that has high, almost absolute, predictive value for biopathological progression. In squamous carcinoma of the cervix uteri, the lesion is a concentration of microinvasive buds arising in a small locus of abnormal surface epithelium. In adenocarcinoma of the gut, it is invasion of the lamina propria and adjacent lamina muscularis mucosae. Comparable definition of "minimal carcinoma" of the endometrium is very difficult because normal tissue boundaries are indistrinct and early infiltration is often equivocal. Precursor endometrial hyperplasias do not have high predictive value as regards carcinomatous progression, and some even regress after progestogen treatment. "Minimal carcinoma" of the endometrium might be used for lesions in which the entire thickness is made up of abnormal, closely packed, proliferative, glandular or nonglandular epithelium. The endometrium usually is thick and accompanied by intracavitary polypoid growth. Such "minimal carcinomas" may be found particularly in postmenopausal women.

References

Abell MR (1982) Adenocarcinoma (gland-cell carcinoma) in situ of endometrium. Pathol Res Pract 174: 221-236

Fedoroff NV (1984) Transposable genetic elements in maize. (The mobile genes Barbara McClintock discovered 40 years ago have since been identified in bacteria, other plants, and animals.) Sci Am 250: 85-98

Gore H (1973) Hyperplasia of the endometrium. Monogr Pathol 14: 255-275

Greenblatt RB, Stoddard LD (1978) The estrogen-cancer controversy. J Am Geriatr Soc 26: 1-8

Greenblatt RB, Gambrell RD Jr, Stoddard LD (1982) The protective role of progesterone in the prevention of endometrial cancer. Pathol Res Pract 174: 297-318

Gusberg SB, Kaplan AL (1963) Precursors of corpus cancer. IV. Adenomatous hyperplasia as stage 0 carcinoma of the endometrium. Am J Obstet Gynecol 87: 662-678

Korzybski A (1948) Selections from science and sanity. The International Non-Aristotelian Library Publishing Company, Institute of General Semantics, Distributors, Lakeville

Koss LG, et al. (1984) Detection of endometrial carcinoma and hyperplasia in asymptomatic women. Obstet Gynecol 64: 1-11

Leighton J, Tchao R (1984) The propagation of cancer, a process of tissue remodeling. Studies in histophysiologic gradient culture. Cancer Metastasis Rev 3: 81-97

Mestwerdt G (1947) Die Frühdiagnose des Kollumkarzinoms. Zentralbl Gynakol 69: 198-205

Natrajan PK, Greenblatt RB, Stoddard LD (1986) Traitement des atypies endométriales chez des femmes jeunes présentant des cycles anovulatoires. Gynecologie 37: 41-44

Pierce GB (1974) Neoplasms, differentiations and mutations. Am J Pathol 76: 103-114

Sommers SC (1982) Defining the pathology of endometrial hyperplasia, dysplasia and carcinoma. Pathol Res Pract 174: 175-197

Stoddard LD (1952a) Studies in the histogenesis of intraepithelial carcinoma and early invasive carcinoma of the cervix uteri. Acta Unio Int Contra Cancrum 8 (1): 117-119

Stoddard LD (1952b) The problem of carcinoma in situ with reference to the human cervix uteri. In: McManus JFA (ed) Progress in fundamental medicine. Lea and Febiger, Philadelphia, pp 203-260

Vellios F (1974) Endometrial hyperplasia and carcinoma-in-situ. Gynecol Oncol 2: 152-161

Therapeutic Procedure for Minimal Endometrial Cancer

J. Baltzer

I. Universitätsfrauenklinik München, Maistraße 11, 8000 München 2, FRG

The therapeutic consequences of minimal endometrial neoplasias require that a reliable pretherapeutic diagnosis be made. It is therefore important to review the problems involved in diagnosis before discussing treatment. Definition of minimal neoplasia is based on prognostic and therapeutic considerations. Excellent survival rates in case of such lesions justify the concept of a limited therapy. There is, however, no standard description and nomenclature for minimal endometrial neoplasia, since the information available regarding the expression and/or extension of minimal cancer is highly variable. Measurement of the greatest depth of invasion has been suggested as parameter to achieve a better comparison of lesions with minimal invasion. In spite of it being possible to perform exact measurements, there is no agreement on how these particular measurements are to be carried out.

Figure 1, for instance, shows the measurement of the depth of invasion in early invasive cancer of the vulva. Three different procedures are depicted (Wilkinson et al. 1982). Method A measures the depth of invasion starting from the basement membrane of the most superficially lying dermal papilla; method B determines the tumor thickness; and method C is based on the measurement of the depth of invasion from the tip of the longest normal rete peg.

For those tumors which can be recorded three dimensionally, tumor volume, consisting of tumor length, height, and width may be calculated in addition to the depth of invasion (Burghardt et al. 1973; Lohe 1978; Lohe et al. 1978). For microcarcinoma of the cervix, for example, a tumor volume of 500 mm^3 has been reported. However, it has been demonstrated that this tumor volume is not applicable to the so-called microcarcinoma of the vulva (Friedrich and Wilkinson 1986). Another problem derives from the fact that the above-mentioned measurements do not consider whether the tumor grew uni- or multifocally. Thus, a multifocal tumor growth was observed in 34.5% of cases of

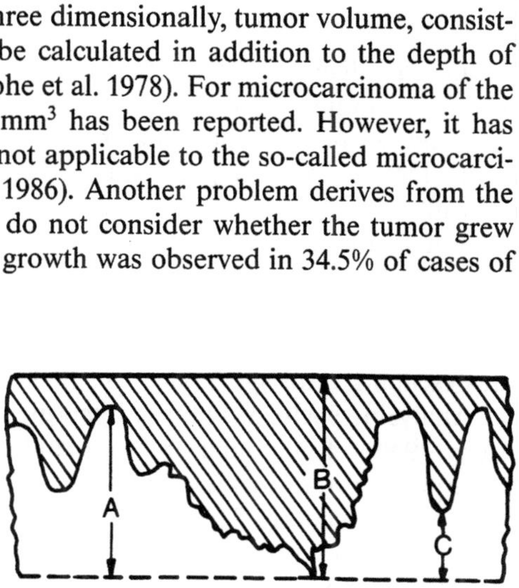

Fig. 1. Depth of invasion should be measured from *A*, the top of the most dermal papilla, rather than *B*, the inconstant surface, or *C*, the deepest ridge

Recent Results in Cancer Research, Vol. 106

early invasive vulva carcinoma (Woodruff 1982). Such aspects clearly demonstrate how deficient are standard definition and nomenclature of minimal neoplasias of the female genital tract. These problems are particularly evident in the case of minimal endometrial neoplasias.

No standard definition, description, and nomenclature are available in the literature for these neoplasias. Both the severe hyperplasia forms as well as those carcinomas limited to the endometrium and/or with minimal invasion are included in this group of lesions (Demopoulos 1977; Hendrickson and Kempson 1980; Dallenbach-Hellweg 1981; Stoddard 1982; Pickel and Girardi 1982; Dallenbach-Hellweg and Schmidt-Matthiesen 1984). To what extent a diagnosis is possible in the case of minimal endometrial cancer should be analyzed, even though the lesions are not totally visible after pretherapeutic diagnosis. The appropriate therapeutic procedure should be based on this diagnosis.

Exact pretherapeutic diagnosis, including the above-mentioned tumor measurements, is possible in the case of the cervix. In spite of the numerous methods tested to date for the early detection of endometrial neoplasias in symptom-free patients, the well-known success gynecologists have enjoyed for many years in the case of early detection of cancer of the cervix has unfortunately not been achieved.

Cytological and histological methods of analysis have been applied (Soost and Baur 1980; Koss et al. 1981; Soost 1982; Mestwerdt 1983; Mestwerdt and Kranzfelder 1983; Schneider 1985). Cytological analysis is performed on cell material obtained using different instruments either as contact smear (Schneider and Czekelius 1983) or as rinse cytology (Gravlee 1969).

Histological analysis is performed on material obtained, for instance, with the Vabra suction curettage, which permits extraction of histologically evaluable endometrium (Jensen 1970; Baltzer et al. 1974).

Reasons for the unsatisfactory reliability of existing early detection procedures are both methodical and morphological:

1. Cervical canal not passable
2. Risk of intrauterine operation
3. Basal localization of hyperplasia
4. Lack of cytodiagnostic criteria

Intrauterine diagnosis can be performed in only two-thirds of all cases due to the cervical canal preventing the introduction of the instrument in older women. All procedures share the risk of an intrauterine operation. Also the two morphological aspects (3 and 4) for the localization of hyperplasias and for the evaluation of the cellular material are significant.

Systematic analysis of the localization of endometrial hyperplasias in the surgical specimen has demonstrated that only 8.6% of glandular and/or glandular-cystic hyperplasias are located in the superficial endometrium, 30.5% are located in superficial and deep segments of the endometrium, and 8.6% are located in deep endometrial regions, thus escaping cytological diagnosis (Schneider 1986).

Analyzing exclusively those hyperplasia forms located in deep areas of the endometrium, 39.9% of glandular and/or glandular-cystic hyperplasias, 27.8% of adenomatous hyperplasias, and 14.4% of atypical adenomatous hyperplasias were found in these endometrial sections. This localization renders it impossible to perform a reliable cytological survey (Schneider 1986). Cytological analysis of precancerous endometrial hyperplasia was problematic in 22.5% of cases, where there was no nucleus enlargement, in

14.3% of cases, where there was no chromatin alteration, and in 8.6% of cases, where no nucleus alteration whatsoever was observed (Schneider 1985).

Comparison of endometrial cytology and histology clearly showed up the difficulties involved in pretherapeutic diagnosis in symptom-free patients. A satisfactory cytological diagnosis was made in only 74.4% of cases.

These data clearly demonstrate that, in contrast to the early detection of minimal neoplasias of the cervix, early diagnosis of endometrial lesions in symptom-free women is problematic. Critical considerations have therefore led most authors to avoid applying the existing procedures for intrauterine diagnosis as a general screening method; rather they have implemented them only for very particular medical indications and/or for high-risk patients.

In the case of pathological bleeding, the chosen method of diagnosis is fractioned curettage, in which cervix and uterine corpus curettage are performed separately. The first important aspect for reliable histological processing is how the curettage material was extracted and collected. Even the most experienced histologist cannot guarantee a reliable analysis when handling inadequately collected material. Nonetheless, even with carefully collected curettage material, the diagnosis of a minimal endometrial neoplasia cannot be made with absolute certainty. This difficulty is again due to methodical and morphological reasons. Even a carefully performed curettage does not guarantee 100% extraction of the corpus mucosa. It must be borne in mind that pathologically altered fractions of mucosa might remain uncollected.

Morphologically, and unlike the case of lesions of the cervix, the disadvantage in this case is that the lesion is not surveyed in its overall extension on the curettage material. Parallel to the diagnosed minimal neoplasia undiscovered fragments of a carcinoma may exist which by far exceed this alteration. Curettage only reveals the minimal alteration. The full extent of the lesion is only detectable on the surgical specimen of the uterus. In contrast to bioptic diagnosis of the cervix in the case of endometrial neoplasias, metric determinations are impossible to perform pretherapeutically on the curettage material.

In order to improve pretherapeutic diagnosis additional procedures were introduced, namely hysterography (Anderson et al. 1976) and hysteroscopy (Lindemann 1980).

Hysteroscopy permits the removal, under visual display, of suspicious tissue from the uterine cavity. Hysterography provides information on the site, size, and degree of expansion of the tumor by determining wall and/or content defects. Based on the hysterographic picture of mucosal defects, Anderson (1982) has even been able to establish the preoperative diagnosis of an endometrial microcarcinoma.

To date, the use of both examination procedures has not led to diagnostic certainty in terms of expansion and size determination of minimal endometrial neoplasias, as compared with the cervical diagnosis.

In spite of the above-mentioned problems related to pretherapeutic diagnosis, the question concerning a limited treatment is still valid, also for patients with minimal endometrial neoplasia. The following considerations, which have proved reliable for the treatment of cervical neoplasias (Zander et al. 1981), are the basis for such an individualized treatment.

Clinical and histological primary findings establish the hypothesis. A complete histological examination permits the current proof of this hypothesis. The report of survival rates makes a final proof of this hypothesis possible. This analysis of the decision-making process may be applied to the treatment of other malignomas:

1. Clinical staging, histological findings → primary hypothesis
2. Complete histological investigation of the surgical specimen → examination of the primary hypothesis
3. Exact data on the survival rates → final evaluation of the hypothesis

Considering the different age distributions of patients with cervical and endometrial neoplasias, the question concerning the necessity of a limited treatment arises. Cervical lesions are mainly observed in women of childbearing age, in which case an organ-preserving treatment is highly desirable. On the contrary, minimal endometrial neoplasia arises mainly in older patients already beyond their reproductive age. In most of these cases, the question of preservation of their childbearing capacity becomes superfluous.

In the past few years, however, endometrial cancer has also been observed to occur with increasing incidence in younger patients (Fig. 2) (Population Reports 1977). According to these incidence rates the chances of occurrence of minimal endometrial neoplasias also in younger patients are increasing. Thus, the question of a possibility of organ preservation again becomes of current interest. Treatment procedures by means of

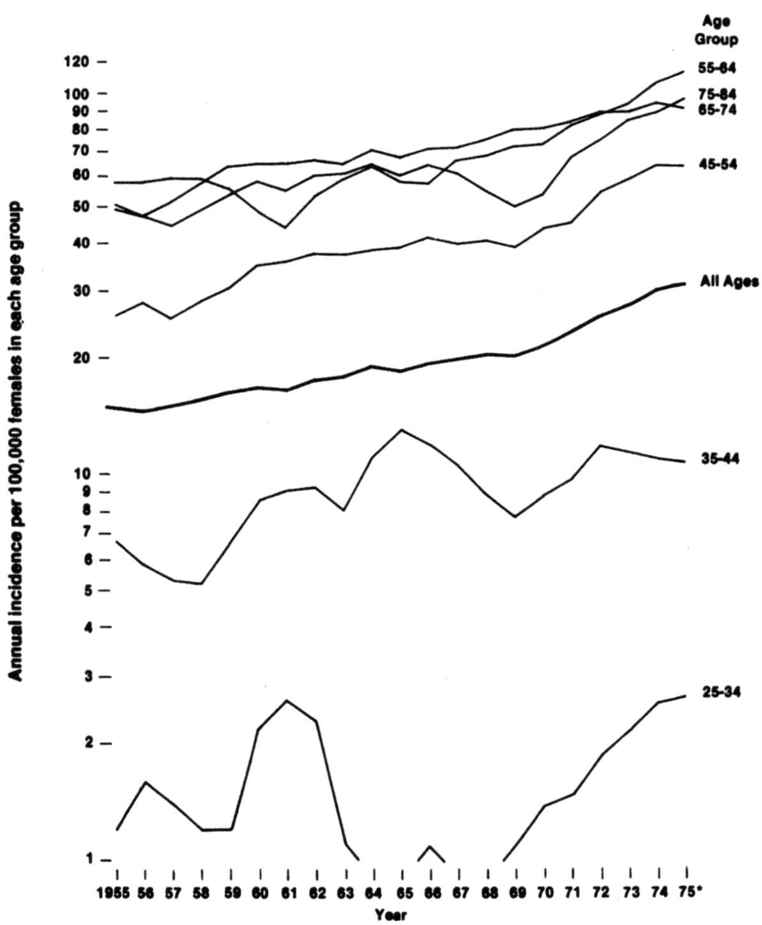

Fig. 2. Incidence rates in patients with endometrial carcinoma, age 25–84 years, by 10-year age groups, using 3-year moving averages, Connecticut, 1955–1975. (Population Reports 1977)

which surgical intervention may be avoided are also worth being taken into consideration in the case of elderly patients in a poor general condition and thus presenting a high-risk for surgery (Baltzer and Lohe 1986). Thus, the correct therapeutic strategy depends on the severity of the histologically determined lesion and the age of the patient (Kistner 1982; Greenblatt et al. 1982).

In the case of younger patients who wish to have children, the first step is to try to induce ovulatory cycles (Table 1). In the case of adenomatous hyperplasia grade II and III a gestagen treatment is undertaken. A control curettage is necessary after 2–3 months. Premenopausic women, or those who do not want to have children, may be submitted to a gestagen treatment with subsequent control curettage, in the case of grade I hyperplasia. In the case of grade II hyperplasia, an autonomous growth might be suspected. This lesion can also be treated initially with gestagens, treatment which requires performing a control curettage. Indication for hysterectomy is then established, when the lesion persists. Grade III hyperplasias generally require extirpation of the uterus. Since curettage cannot rule out with absolute certainty the common incidence of hyperplasia and endometrial carcinoma, removal of the uterine adnexa, as in patients with endometrial cancer, has to be taken into consideration.

For women in postmenopause with grade I hyperplasia, a preliminary gestagen treatment with control curettage is possible. In the case of persistent hyperplasia, or grade II and III hyperplasia, hysterectomy is advisable. Considering the more advanced age of those patients with fading ovarian function, extirpation of the uterus is thus combined with removal of the adnexae.

In some selected cases of elderly patients with grade III hyperplasia who present a high-risk for surgery, gestagen treatment may also be justified.

An organ-preserving individualized treatment requires a close follow-up and reliable cooperation between gynecologist, pathologist, and the patient. Only under such conditions is it possible to prevent a deficient therapy with the increased risk of an inadequately treated endometrial lesion and excessive therapy with the risk of an unnecessary operation (Zander and Baltzer 1986).

In most cases of women with cervix neoplasias, it is quite possible to carry out an organ-preserving treatment and a close posttherapeutic follow-up to control the treatment results, including cytological checkups.

Monitoring of organ-preserving therapy is difficult to perform in patients with minimal endometrial neoplasia. The already mentioned methodical reasons render cytology insufficient for the posttherapeutic screening of the endometrium. Extraction of histologically evaluable material is unavoidable. Only on endometrial tissue is the diagnosis

Table 1. Therapeutic procedure in patients with endometrial hyperplasia

Endometrium	Young infertile patient	Premenopause, no desire of pregnancy		Postmenopause
Hyperplasia I	Stimulation of ovulation	Gestagen therapy, control curettage		Gestagen therapy, control curettage
Hyperplasia II	Gestagen therapy, control curettage	(Gestagen therapy) (control curettage)	Extirpation of the uterus	Extirpation of the uterus with adnexae
Hyperplasia III	Gestagen therapy, control curettage	Uterus extirpation (with adnexae)		

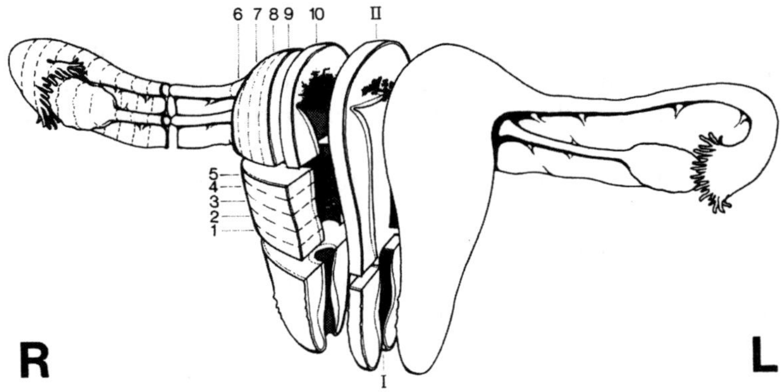

Fig. 3. Technique of sectioning the surgical specimen

of more basally located endometrial sections possible. Suction or fractioned curettage are the methods available for such a diagnosis. The advantage of suction curettage is that it can be performed without anesthesia when the cervical canal is passable.

If the uterus is removed as a consequence of diagnosis of an endometrial lesion on the curettage material, the next step is to perform a systematic histological examination of the surgical specimen. The following histological procedure has proved successful in our department (Lohe et al. 1976; Baltzer and Lohe 1981, Fig. 3). This standardized examination serves to judge the size of the lesion and to rule out an invasive carcinoma. In the case of an invasive tumor, it is possible to determine the depth of invasion in relation to the myometrial thickness. A tumor growth which is limited to the mucosa or carcinoma with minimal depth of invasion needs no subsequent treatment.

This histological procedure enables a mosaic-like evaluation of the endometrial lesion to be carried out. The prognostic significance of morphological tumor criteria is known (Baltzer et al. 1983). For minimal endometrial neoplasia there is a lack of further defined morphological prognostic criteria. It has been observed in the case of microcarcinoma of the cervix that not only the tumor volume, but also other criteria such as tumor invasion in blood vessels are significant for further therapeutic decisions and/or the survival rates of the patients (Burghardt 1982).

Also in the case of minimal endometrial neoplasia it is conceivable that additional factors might be of significance for their prognostic evaluation and the initiation of treatment. It is also conceivable that the term "minimal endometrial neoplasia" summarizes a range of lesions with very different prognostic significance.

Concluding Comments

Contrarily to the case of minimal cervix neoplasia, no standard definition and/or nomenclature exists for the minimal endometrium neoplasia. A range of very different lesions are summarized under the term "minimal endometrium cancer".

Diagnosis on symptom-free patients is difficult since no sufficient screening program has been achieved for lesions for the endometrium comparable in certainty to the cervix diagnosis. Fractioned curettage performed for pretherapeutic diagnosis of patients with menstrual disorders can only reveal the minimal lesion. The maximum of the endometrial alteration can only be determined on the surgical specimen.

Age of the patient and severity of the minimal endometrium neoplasia are taken into consideration when deciding on the treatment. An organ preserving individualized treatment requires close follow-up and a reliable cooperation between gynaecologists, pathologists and the patient.

Contrarily to the follow-up of patients after organ preserving treatment of minimal cervix neoplasia, the monitoring of results after organ-preserving treatment of women with minimal endometrium neoplasia is complicated due to methodical and morphological aspects. A reliable clinical and cytological control is possible for patients with minimal cervical neoplasia. For women with minimal endometrium neoplasia, the clinical and cytological control is insufficient. In the case of these patients, an enhanced histological endometrium diagnosis is unavoidable.

References

Anderson B (1982) The relationship of tumour volume to prognosis in endometrial cancer. In: Burghardt E, Holzer E (eds) Minimal invasive cancer (microcarcinoma). Saunders, London (Clinics in oncology)

Anderson B, Marchant DJ, Munzenrieder JE, Moore JP, Mitchell GW (1976) Routine non invasive hysterography in the evaluation and treatment of endometrial carcinoma. Gynecol Oncol 4: 354-367

Baltzer J, Lohe K-J (1981) Maligne Tumoren des Corpus uteri. In: Hermanek P (ed) Kompendium der Klinischen Tumorpathologie 3. Witzstrock, Baden-Baden

Baltzer J, Lohe K-J (1986) Präneoplasien und Karzinome des Endometriums. In: Schmidt-Matthiesen H (ed) Spezielle gynäkologische Onkologie I. Urban and Schwarzenberg, Munich

Baltzer J, Wolf W, Lohe K-J (1974) Die diagnostische Saugcurettage des Uterus. Frauenarzt 3: 194-195

Baltzer J, Lohe K-J, Kürzl R, Scheer KP, Zander J (1983) Prognostic criteria in patients with endometrial cancer. Arch Gynecol 234: 121-129

Burghardt E (1982) Diagnostic and prognostic criteria in cervical microcarcinoma. In: Burghardt E, Holzer E (eds) Minimal invasive cancer (microcarcinoma). Saunders, London (Clinics in oncology)

Burghardt E, Mestwerdt G, Ober KG (1973) Der Unterschied zwischen der Einstufung Zervixkrebs des Stadium Ia und dem Begriff "Mikrokarzinom". Geburtshilfe Frauenheilkd 33: 168-172

Dallenbach-Hellweg G (1981) Endometrium, 2. Aufl. Springer, Berlin Heidelberg New York

Dallenbach-Hellweg G, Schmidt-Matthiesen H (1984) Nomenklaturdiskussion. Hyperplasien, Präkanzerosen und Karzinome des Endometriums. Pathologe 5: 58-59

Demopoulos RJ (1977) Endometrial hyperplasia, carcinoma of the endometrium. In: Blaustein A (ed) Pathology of the female genital tract. Springer, Berlin Heidelberg New York

Friedrich EG, Wilkinson EJ (1986) Das mikroinvasive Karzinom der Vulva. In: Zander J, Baltzer J (eds) Erkrankungen der Vulva. Urban and Schwarzenberg, Munich

Gravlee LC (1969) Jet-irrigation method for the diagnosis of endometrial adenocarcinoma, its principle and accuracy. Obstet Gynecol 34: 168-172

Greenblatt RB, Don Gambrell R, Stoddard LD (1982) The protective role of progesterone in the prevention of endometrial cancer. Pathol Res Pract 174: 297-318

Hendrickson MR, Kempson RL (1980) Surgical pathology of the uterine corpus. Saunders, Philadelphia

Jensen JG (1970) Vacuum curettage. Out-patient curettage without anaesthesia. A report of 350 cases. Dan Med Bull 17: 199-202

Kistner RW (1982) Treatment of hyperplasia and carcinoma in situ of the endometrium. Clin Obstet Gynecol 25: 63-74

Koss LG, Schreiber K, Oberlander SG, Moukhtar M, Levine HS, Moussouris HF (1981) Screening of asymptomatic women for endometrial cancer. Obstet Gynecol 57: 681-691

Lindemann HJ (1980) Atlas der Hysteroskopie. Fischer, Stuttgart
Lohe K-J (1978) Early squamous cell carcinoma of the uterine cervix. Definition and histology. Gynecol Oncol 6: 10-30
Lohe K-J, Baltzer J, Zander J (1976) Histologische Diagnose und individuelle Krebsbehandlung in der Gynäkologie. MMW 118: 1373-1378
Lohe K-J, Burghardt E, Hillemanns HG, Kaufmann C, Ober KG, Zander J (1978) Early squamous cell carcinoma of the uterine cervix. Clinical results of a cooperative study in the management of 419 patients with early stromal invasion and microcarcinoma. Gynecol Oncol 6: 31-50
Mestwerdt W (1983) Früherkennung des Endometriumkarzinoms. Arch Gynecol 235: 173-181
Mestwerdt W, Kranzfelder D (1983) Neue diagnostische Möglichkeiten beim Endometriumkarzinom und seinen Vorstufen. Gynaekologe 16: 87-92
Pickel H, Girardi E (1982) The diagnosis of endometrial microinvasive adenocarcinoma. In: Burghardt E, Holzer E (eds) Minimal invasive cancer (microcarcinoma). Saunders, London (Clinics in oncology)
Population Reports (1977) Supplement to series A, no 4. The John's Hopkins University population information program, Baltimore
Schneider ML (1985) Untersuchung zur Effektivität eines gezielten zytologischen Früherkennungsprogramms beim Endometriumkarzinom. *Habilitationsschrift,* University of Erlangen/Nürnberg
Schneider ML (1986) Die Lokalisation der Endometriumhyperplasien und ihre Kernmorphologie. Geburtshilfe Frauenheilkd 46: 381-387
Schneider ML, Czekelius P (1983) Die diagnostische Treffsicherheit der intrakavitären Entnahme-Techniken mit Prävical und Accurette. Arch Gynecol 235: 190-191
Soost HJ (1982) Möglichkeiten der Früherkennung des Endometriumkarzinoms. Geburtshilfe Frauenheilkd 42: 899-902
Soost HJ, Baur S (1980) Gynäkologische Zytodiagnostik. Thieme, Stuttgart
Stoddard LD (1982) Endometrial carcinomas. Pathol Res Pract 174: 169-174
Wilkinson EJ, Rico MJ, Pierson KK (1982) Microinvasive carcinoma of the vulva. Int J Gynecol Pathol 1: 29-39
Woodruff JD (1982) Early invasive carcinoma of the vulva. In: Burghardt E, Holzer E (eds) Minimal invasive cancer (microcarcinoma). Saunders, London (Clinics in oncology)
Zander J, Baltzer J (1986) Die Individualisierung der Behandlung gynäkologischer Krebse. In: Melchert F, Beck L, Hepp H, Knappstein PG, Kreieinberg R (eds) Aktuelle Geburtshilfe und Gynäkologie. Springer, Berlin Heidelberg New York
Zander J, Baltzer J, Lohe K-J, Ober KG, Kaufmann C (1981) Carcinoma of the cervix: an attempt to individualize treatment. Am J Obstet Gynecol 139: 752-759

Minimal Cervical Cancer: Definition and Histology[*]

Y.S. Fu and J.S. Berek

Department of Pathology, UCLA Medical Center, Los Angeles, CA 90024-1732, USA

The concept of a prognostically favorable, early cervical cancer was first proposed by Mestwerdt (1947) as "microcarcinoma," which he defined as a lesion that invades less than 5 mm into the cervical stroma measured from the basement membrane. Since then, many investigators have applied different terms and criteria in an effort to define an intermediate stage of development between an intraepithelial neoplasia and frankly invasive carcinoma. These include early stromal invasion (Stoddard 1952; Burghardt and Holzer 1977), borderline microinvasive carcinoma (Friedell et al. 1958; Wilkinson and Komorowski 1978), microinvasive carcinoma (Christopherson and Parker 1964; Ng and Reagan 1969), and stage IA cervical cancer (American Joint Committee 1978).

With an increasing number of early cervical cancers detected by the current use of cytologic screening, colposcopy, and biopsies, and the desire to provide an optimal treatment, it has become a clinical necessity to define better their malignant potential. In this report, we will review the available data and define a subset within the spectrum of early cervical cancer, which has a minimal risk of spread beyond the cervix. The proposed morphologic criteria should ideally be reproducible in most of the routine histology laboratories. For the convenience of discussion, the term early cervical cancer, unless otherwise specified, includes the earliest microscopic carcinoma to that fulfilling the criteria for FIGO stage IA cancer.

Frequency

Most early cervical cancers are seen in asymptomatic women, detected initially in cytologic smears, and confirmed subsequently by punch biopsies, conization, or hysterectomy specimens. Early invasive carcinomas 5 mm or less in depth are found in 7.1% of specimens excised for in situ carcinoma (Savage 1972), in 8.4% of all invasive cervical cancers (Ng and Reagan 1969), and in 12% of clinical stage I cervical cancers (Rubio et al. 1974). Over the period of 2 decades, the relative frequency of early cancers has increased from 1.2% in the 1940s to 20.9% of all cervical cancers in the 1960s, an increase attributed to the effective cytologic detection (Ng and Reagan 1969).

* The study is supported by a USPHS grant, number CA 34870, awarded by the National Cancer Institute, DHHS.

Recent Results in Cancer Research, Vol. 106

Histopathologic Findings in Early Cervical Cancers

In the earliest invasion, a focus of well-differentiated cells with abundant eosinophilic cytoplasm and prominent nucleoli projects at the base of an intraepithelial neoplasm into the underlying stroma. This focus elongates to form a tongue-like process, from which additional isolated nests develop (Fig. 1). Progressively, multiple foci of invasion arise from the mucosa and endocervical glands. The tumor increases in dimensions vertically and laterally. The stroma responds by a band-like lymphoplasmacytic infiltration, desmoplastic reaction, granulomatous formation to the necrotic tumor cells and keratin debris, and dilatation of capillary and lymphatic spaces.

Among the early cervical cancers, which measure 5 mm or less in depth, 56% involve the anterior lip, 33% both the anterior and posterior lips, and 11% the posterior lip alone

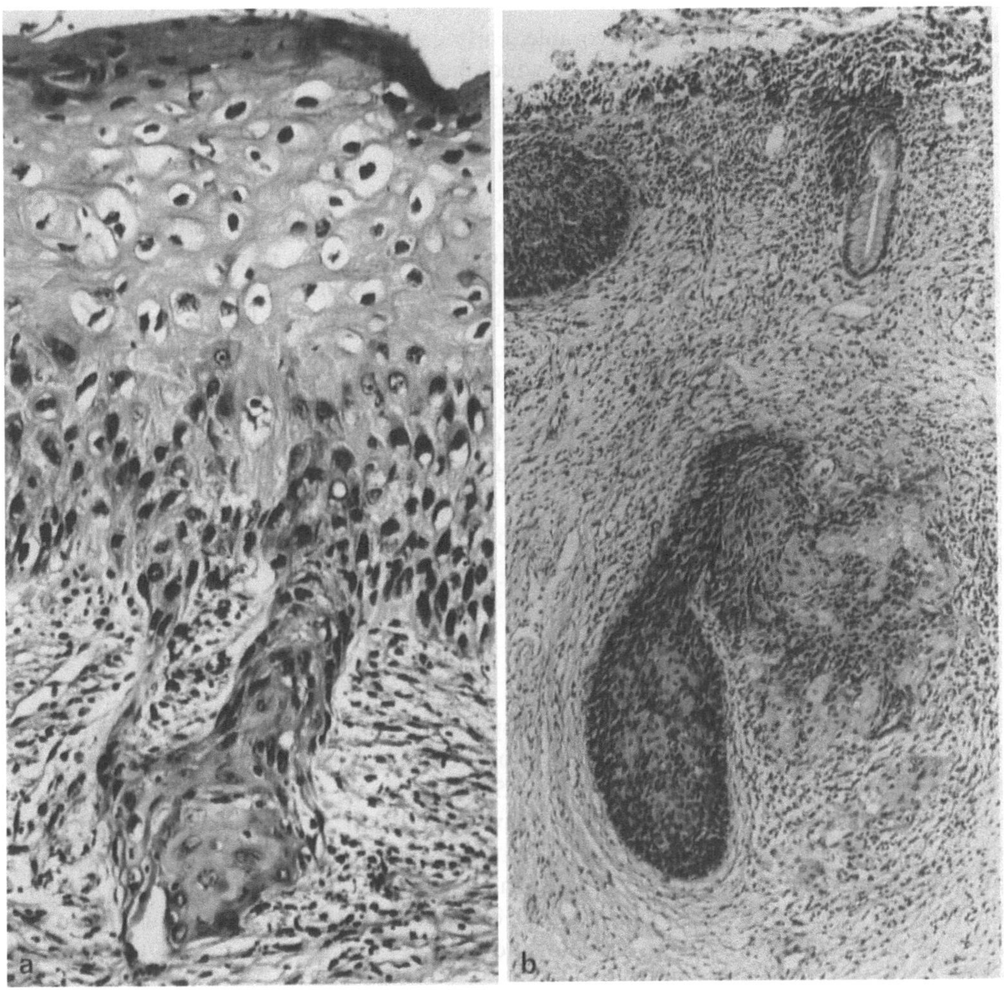

Fig. 1. **a** A focus of earliest invasion arising from the base of a mild dysplasia with a tongue-like projection. **b** A focus of invasion arising in an endocervical gland. Clusters of well-differentiated cells break through the basement membrane and give rise to isolated tumor aggregates in the stroma. H & E, **a** ×200, **b** ×80

(Ng and Reagan 1969). The invasive foci are mostly multicentric (92%). The epithelia overlying the invasive carcinoma resemble carcinoma in situ in 68%, dysplasia in 5%, indeterminate in 14%, normal in 2%, and ulcerated in the remaining cases (Ng and Reagan 1969). Islands of well-differentiated squamous cells occur in 60% of the intraepithelial neoplasms (Ng and Reagan 1969). Such features are also found at the point of invasion in 85% of microinvasive carcinomas 5 mm or less in depth (Sedlis et al. 1979).

Early cervical cancers grow in different patterns. Some infiltrate in finger-like processes or form networks of invasive cords with confluence. Infrequently, the tumors invade diffusely in small clusters or infiltrate by bulky solid sheets. The confluent pattern is generally defined as a lesion in which anastomosing tongues of tumor with pushing borders are present (Seski et al. 1977; Sedlis et al. 1979; van Nagell et al. 1983). Creasman et al. (1985) define confluent pattern as a tumor mass occupying at least 1 mm^2.

While the prognostic value of growth patterns in early cervical cancer has remained unsettled, there is evidence to support that the confluent pattern is a function of the depth of invasion. When the studies of Sedlis et al. (1979) and Creasman et al. (1985) are combined, the confluent pattern is associated with 3% (2/75) of tumors less than 1 mm in depth, 27% (30/111) of neoplasms between 1 and 3 mm, and 43% (18/42) of tumors between 3 and 5 mm in depth ($P=0.000$).

The histologic cell type of early invasive carcinomas is large cell nonkeratinizing type in 76%-88%, while 9%-18% are the keratinizing type, and 3%-6% are the small cell type (Larsson et al. 1983; van Nagell et al. 1983).

Comparison of the DNA stem cell modal values in the surface neoplasia and the underlying invasive carcinoma suggests the evolution of new stem cell lines with increasing depth. The stem cell lines in the surface neoplasia and the invasive carcinoma retain comparable DNA modal values in three of four tumors, which are less than 2.5 mm in depth. However, the stem cell lines in five of eight invasive carcinomas between 2.5 and 5.0 mm in depth have a significantly higher level of DNA content than those present in the surface neoplasia (Fu et al. 1980). This difference corresponds to a greater degree of nuclear pleomorphism in the invasive carcinoma, when compared with the surface neoplasia.

Tumor cells gain access to the vascular lymphatic channels early in their invasion. Because a distinction between capillary and lymphatic spaces is impossible in routine histologic preparations, invasion of such spaces is generally considered together as capillary-lymphatic invasion (C-L invasion). The reported frequency of C-L invasion varies from 8% (Ng and Reagan 1969) to 57% (Roche and Norris 1975). Such a divergence can be explained by the morphologic criteria, the type of histologic preparation, and the depth of invasion. Clear spaces around the periphery of tumor nests caused by fixation artifact may be confused with C-L invasion (Fig. 2). To identify C-L invasion, one needs to visualize clearly the endothelial cells, which are preferably associated with blood, serum, or fibrin thrombi (Fig. 2). Roche and Norris (1975) have demonstrated that by step section of conization specimens, the frequency of C-L invasion is increased from 30% to 57%. Finally, C-L invasion and the depth of invasion are closely related. By combining the series of Sedlis et al. (1979) and Creasman et al. (1985), C-L invasion occurs in 8% (6/75) of tumors less than 1 mm, 22% (24/111) of neoplasms between 1 and 3 mm, and 38% of tumors between 3 and 5 mm in depth ($P=0.0004$).

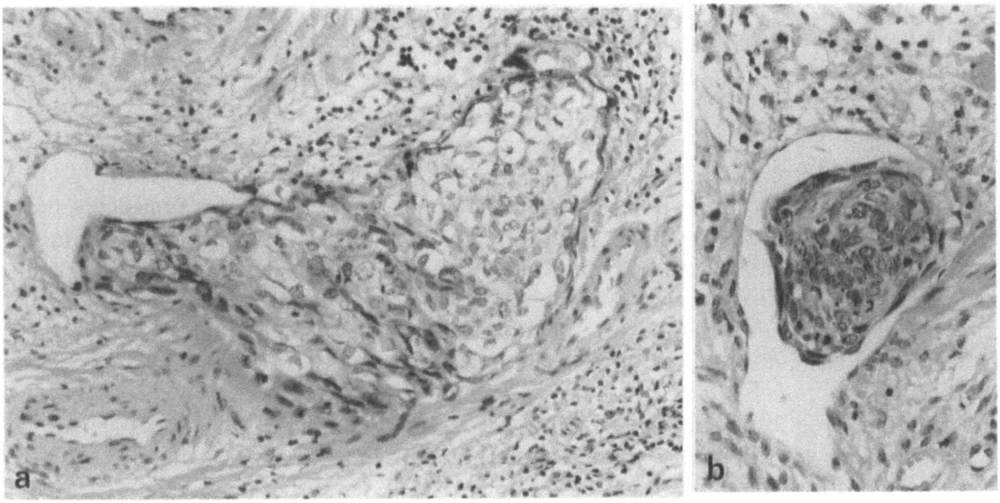

Fig. 2. **a** A shrinkage artifact simulating capillary-lymphatic invasion. Note the lack of endothelial lining. **b** A true capillary-lymphatic invasion. The space is lined by endothelial cells and contains serum-like material between the endothelium and tumor cells. H & E, **a** ×200, **b** ×250

Depth of Invasion in Early Cervical Cancers

Of all the pathologic parameters, the depth of invasion has been most extensively studied. The depth of invasion should be measured by a calibrated ocular micrometer. Although all investigators agree that the deepest focus of invasion is the end point of measurement; some prefer to measure from the tumor surface (Rubio et al. 1974; Roche and Norris 1975; Leman et al. 1976; Sedlis et al. 1979), while the majority measure from the point of invasion or the adjacent basement membrane (Averette et al. 1976; van Nagell et al. 1983; Creasman et al. 1985). The difference between the two is estimated at 0.3 mm, the average thickness of cervical squamous mucosa.

Of early carcinomas measuring 5 mm or less in depth, the combined series of Sedlis et al. (1979) and Hasumi et al. (1980) reveal that 41% measure 1 mm or less, 40% are between 1.1 and 3.0 mm, and 19% are between 3.1 and 5.0 mm. Among the FIGO stage IA carcinomas 9 mm or less in depth, 24% are 1 mm or less, 45% are between 1 and 3 mm, 21% are between 3 and 5 mm, and only 10% are deeper than 5 mm (combined series of Creasman et al. 1985 and Larsson et al. 1983). Thus, 70%-80% of early cervical cancers are 3 mm or less in depth.

Diagnostic Problems of Early Cervical Cancers

In the study of Sedlis et al. (1979), 37% (99 of 265) of specimens initially submitted by the participating pathologists of the Gynecologic Oncology Group as microinvasive carcinoma are judged to be noninvasive neoplasms. In our experience, overdiagnosis of invasive carcinoma most frequently occurs in the tangential cuts of glandular extension by intraepithelial neoplasia (Fig. 3), reactive atypical squamous epithelium whose basement membrane is obscured by inflammatory cells, and entrapped dysplastic cells in the stroma following previous biopsy. If there is question as to the invasiveness, multiple

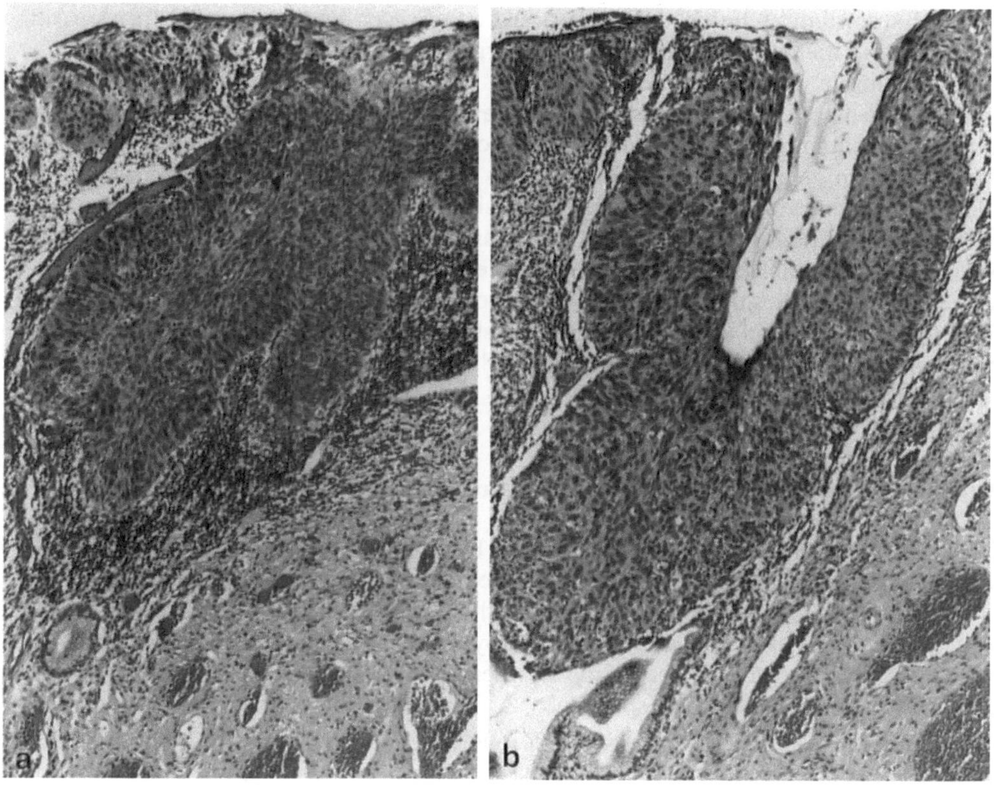

Fig. 3. **a** In the initial cut, the pattern of bulky processes extending into the stroma suggests invasion. The basement membrane is obscured by lymphocytic infiltration. Isolated tumor aggregates and desmoplastic reaction are not seen. **b** In a serial deeper cut, the questionable focus of invasion represents a glandular extension by severe dysplasia. The bulky processes correspond to the branching pattern of endocervical glands. H & E, **a, b** ×80

serial cuts should be requested (Fig. 3). Questionable foci of invasion often appear as irregular rete pegs extending into the stroma. Unless they are associated with isolated tumor nests and desmoplasia, they should be regarded as an intraepithelial abnormality. It is helpful to recall that circumscribed areas of better-differentiated cells are often observed within or adjacent to the point of invasion.

Although FIGO states that clinical stage IA cervical cancer may be diagnosed by punch biopsies, it is clear that such specimens often underestimate the depth of invasion (Larsson et al. 1983). It has been emphasized that the diagnosis of early cervical cancer requires a comprehensive histologic examination of the entire cervix, i.e., study of specimen obtained by conization, trachelectomy, or hysterectomy. It is important to handle the conization specimens appropriately allowing for accurate assessment of the depth of invasion and the surgical margins. Tangentially cut sections and excessive manipulations of the specimen, which often result in denudation and crush artifact of the neoplasm, have to be avoided.

In our laboratory, the conization specimen is received in fresh state, cut initially along the cervical canal at 12 o'clock, opened and pinned to a corkboard, and fixed in formalin for several hours. Then, the entire specimen is cut around the clock and vertically to the mucosal surface in 12–15 blocks. Tissue blocks are embedded separately or grouped according to the quadrant. This method of sectioning is adequate for assessing the depth and the length of tumor and the surgical margins.

According to the study of Creasman et al. (1985), if the surgical margins of conization specimens are clear of microinvasive carcinoma, the chance of finding residual invasive carcinoma in the subsequent hysterectomy specimens is 4% (2 of 45, both less than 0.5 mm in depth). If the surgical margins are involved by invasive carcinoma, 77% (10/13) of hysterectomy specimens contain residual invasive carcinoma (Creasman et al. 1985). More importantly, the depth of invasion in 8 of 12 hysterectomy specimens exceeds that of conization specimens (Sedlis et al. 1979). Thus, those invasive carcinomas extending to the surgical margins of the conization specimen should be disqualified from the FIGO clinical stage IA. Even if the surgical margins are involved by only dysplasia or carcinoma in situ, Larsson et al. (1983) have found this finding to be a significant risk factor for tumor recurrence.

Morphologic Criteria for Defining Early Cervical Cancer

Early cervical cancers are basically defined by tumor volume, tumor dimensions, or depth of invasion with or without additional conditions.

Burghardt and Holzer (1977) reconstruct the tumor volume from the macrosections. The fixed cervical specimen is first dissected by a median sagittal cut. The two pieces are embedded entirely for step sectioning at intervals of 100–200 μm. Usually, 60–70 sections are prepared from each specimen. A "microcarcinoma" is defined as having a tumor volume of less than 500 mm^3. Only 1 of 87 women with microcarcinoma died of tumor recurrence.

Lohe et al. (1978) define "microcarcinoma" as less than 5 mm in depth and less than 10 mm in longitudinal length and width. Only 3 (2.2%) of 134 women with microcarcinoma died of recurrent tumor. None of 285 women with early stromal invasion without confluent pattern in the tumor developed recurrence.

Measurement of the depth of invasion by an ocular micrometer is simple, widely used, and proven to be reproducible among pathologists. More importantly, the depth of invasion correlates with the longitudinal length (Ng and Reagan 1969; Sedlis et al. 1979) and circumference of the tumor (Ng and Reagan 1969). Thus, the tumor volume may be adequately represented by the depth of invasion alone.

Some investigators define early cervical cancer by a specific depth of invasion, others qualify the depth with additional parameters. For example, those tumors having a confluent pattern or capillary-lymphatic invasion or both are excluded from the microinvasive carcinoma.

Factors Affecting Pelvic Lymph Node Status in Early Cervical Cancer

In their critical review of the literature, Benson and Norris (1977) have found that most previous publications are biased in assessing the pelvic nodal status. In some studies, the depth of invasion is not confirmed histologically or is based on inadequate cone or punch biopsies. The latter often underestimate the true depth, and bias toward a higher frequency of pelvic nodal metastasis. Some studies include cases with questionable invasion or exclude those having capillary lymphatic invasion or confluent pattern, thus favoring a lower rate of pelvic nodal metastasis. Treatment modality, such as selection of more advanced tumor for lymphadenectomy and radiotherapy given prior to lymphadenectomy, may have influenced the frequency of pelvic nodal status. Using similar criteria to Benson and Norris (1977), we have included more recent reports (Tables 1-3). Only those patients treated by radical hysterectomy and pelvic lymphadenectomy are listed. Reports of Taki et al. (1979) and Yajima and Noda (1979), which exclude tumors with capillary-lymphatic invasion, are not included.

If the depth of invasion is 1 mm or less, the risk of having pelvic nodal metastasis is 0.4% (1 of 237) and that of tumor recurrence is 0% (Table 1). The only metastasis occurred in a tumor 0.7 mm in depth without capillary-lymphatic invasion.

In patients whose invasive tumor measures 0.1-3.0, 1.5% (5 of 332) of patients had pelvic lymph node metastasis. Two of these women developed tumor recurrence and died, representing an overall risk of 0.6% (Table 2).

Among the 106 tumors between 3.1 and 5.0 mm in depth, 8 (7.6%) metastasized to the pelvic lymph nodes. Tumors in three women, including one with pelvic lymph node metastasis, recurred. Two died of tumor (Table 3). This review of the literature confirms that the difference in the frequency of pelvic lymph node metastasis for tumors 0.1-3.0 mm and 3.1-5.0 mm in depth is statistically significant ($P<0.05$).

The confluent pattern, the cell type, the presence of capillary-lymphatic invasion, and the amount of lymphoplasmacytic stromal response in early cervical cancer 5 mm or less in depth have no apparent association with pelvic nodal metastasis (Roche and Norris 1975; Leman et al. 1976; Seski et al. 1977; van Nagell et al. 1983).

Table 1. Cervical squamous carcinoma up to 1 mm in depth

Authors	No. patient	LN+	Recurrence/ death
Averette et al. (1976)	162	0	0
Seski et al. (1977)	14	0	0
Hasumi et al. (1980)	61	1[a]	NA
Total	237	1 (0.4%)	0

NA, not available; *LN+*, lymph nodes affected.
[a] 0.7 mm in depth, no evidence of capillary-lymphatic invasion.

Table 2. Cervical squamous carcinoma 0.1-3.0 mm in depth

Authors	No. patients	LN+	Recurrence/ death
Foushee et al. (1969)	16	0	0
Roche and Norris (1975)	9	0	0
Leman et al. (1976)	32	0	0
Bohm et al. (1977)	56	4[a]	2/2
Seski et al. (1977)	37	0	0
Hasumi et al. (1980)	106	1[b]	NA
Van Nagell et al. (1983)	52	0	0
Creasman et al. (1985)	24	0	0
Total	332	5 (1.5%)	2/2 (0.6%)

NA, not available; *LN+*, lymph nodes affected.
[a] Two, no evidence of disease, two, recurred and died.
[b] 0.7 mm in depth.

Table 3. Cervical squamous carcinoma 3.1-5.0 mm in depth

Authors	No. patients	LN+	Recurrence/ death
Foushee et al. (1969)	13	1	0
Roche and Norris (1975)	21	0	0
Leman et al. (1976)	3	0	0
Hasumi et al. (1980)	29	4	NA
Van Nagell et al. (1983)	32	3[a]	3/2
Creasman et al. (1985)	8	0	0
Total	106	8 (7.6%)	3/2 (3%/2%)

[a] Two with no evidence of disease, one recurred and alive.

In FIGO stage IA cancers with a depth of invasion of 9 mm or less, the significant risk factors for pelvic lymph node metastasis include depth of invasion greater than 5 mm and a confluent pattern with or without capillary-lymphatic invasion (Creasman et al. 1985).

Factors Affecting Tumor Recurrence in Early Cervical Cancers

Due to the variations in the duration of follow-up and the treatment modality, the pathologic parameters affecting tumor recurrence are difficult to assess. In tumors 5 mm or less in depth, only depth of invasion greater than 3 mm and the presence of capillary-lymphatic invasion are significant risk factors for tumor recurrence (van Nagell et al. 1983). Although there is a possible relationship between capillary-lymphatic invasion and tumor recurrence in the microinvasive cancers less than 3 mm in depth (Iversen et al. 1979), the number of cases is too small to be conclusive. In the series of van Nagell et al. (1983), none of the 17 patients with capillary-lymphatic invasion in tumors less than 3 mm in depth developed recurrence. Among the 16 patients having tumors between 3.1 and 5.0 mm in depth and without capillary-lymphatic invasion, only two women developed carcinoma in situ of the vaginal apex, which was controlled by local excision or radiotherapy. However, 3 of 16 women having capillary-lymphatic invasion in tumors between 3.1 and 5.0 mm in depth developed recurrent invasive carcinoma and 2 of them died. Although the number of cases is small, the presence of capillary-lymphatic invasion in cervical carcinomas greater than 3 mm in depth suggests an increased risk for tumor recurrence.

For stage IA cervical cancers up to 9 mm in depth, an increased risk of tumor recurrence is associated with greater than 5 mm in depth and confluent pattern with or without capillary lymphatic invasion (Creasman et al. 1985).

Conclusions

The diagnosis of early cervical cancer requires a comprehensive histologic examination of the cervix. Proper specimen orientation for vertical sectioning through the mucosal surface is critical for assessing the tumor dimensions, the surgical margins, and additional pathologic features. In suitably prepared specimens with uninvolved margins, it is possible to define the risk for pelvic nodal metastasis and tumor recurrence.

We propose that early cervical cancers can be divided into the following categories: minimum-risk group for tumors measuring up to 3 mm in depth with or without capillary-lymphatic invasion, low-risk group for tumors between 3.1 and 5.0 mm in depth without capillary-lymphatic invasion, increased-risk group for tumors between 3.1 and 5 mm in depth with capillary-lymphatic invasion, and high-risk group for tumors greater than 5 mm in depth. Utilization of 3 mm as the cutoff measurement is the most accurate means of predicting the likelihood of tumor spread beyond the cervix.

References

American Joint Committee (1978) Manual for staging of cancer. Whiting, Chicago

Averette HE, Nelson JH, Ng ABP, Hoskins WJ, Boyce JG, Ford JH (1976) Diagnosis and management of microinvasive (stage IA) carcinoma of the uterine cervix. Cancer 38: 414-425

Benson WL, Norris HJ (1977) A critical review of the frequency of lymph node metastasis and death from microinvasive carcinoma of the cervix. Obstet Gynecol 49: 632-638

Bohm JW, Krupp PJ, Lee FYL, Batson HWK (1976) Lymph node metastasis in microinvasive epidermoid cancer of the cervix. Obstet Gynecol 48: 65-67

Burghardt E, Holzer E (1977) Diagnosis and treatment of microinvasive carcinoma of the cervix uteri. Obstet Gynecol 49: 641-653

Christopherson WM, Parker JE (1964) Microinvasive carcinoma of the uteerine cervix. Cancer 17: 1123-1131

Creasman WT, Fetter BF, Clarke-Pearson DL, Kaufmann L, Parker RT (1985) Management of stage IA carcinoma of the cervix. Am J Obstet Gynecol 153: 164-172

Foushee JHS, Greiss FC, Lock FR (1969) Stage IA squamous cell carcinoma of the uterine cervix. Am J Obstet Gynecol 105: 46-58

Friedell GH, Hertig AT, Younge PA (1958) The problems of early stromal invasion in carcinoma in situ of the uterine cervix. Arch Pathol 66: 494-503

Fu YS, Temmin L, Olaizola YM, Reagan JW (1980) Nuclear DNA characteristics of microinvasive squamous carcinoma of the uterine cervix. In: Fenoglio CM, Wolff MW (eds) Progress in surgical pathology, vol 1. Masson, New York, pp 398-407

Hasumi K, Sakamoto A, Sugano H (1980) Microinvasive carcinoma of the uterine cervix. Cancer 45: 928-931

Iversen T, Abeler V, Kjorstad KE (1979) Factors influencing the treatment of patients with stage I a carcinoma of the cervix. Br J Obstet Gynaecol 86: 593-597

Larsson G, Alm P, Gullberg B, Grundsell H (1983) Prognosis factors in early invasive carcinoma of the uterine cervix. A clinical, histopathologic, and statistical analysis of 343 cases. Am J Obstet Gynecol 146: 145-153

Leman MH, Benson WL, Kurman RJ, Park RC (1976) Microinvasive carcinoma of the cervix. Obstet Gynecol 48: 571-578

Lohe KJ (1978) Early squamous cell carcinoma of the uterine cervix. I. Definition and histology. Gynecol Oncol 6: 10-30

Lohe KJ, Burghardt E, Hillemanns HG, Kaufmann C, Ober KG, Zander J (1978) Early squamous cell carcinoma of the uterine cervix. II. Clinical results of a co-operative study in the management of 419 patients with early stromal invasion and microcarcinoma. Gynecol Oncol 6: 31-50

Mestwerdt G (1947) Probeexzision und Kolposkopie in der Frühdiagnose des Portiokarzinoms. Zentralbl Gynaekol 4: 326-322

Ng ABP, Reagan JW (1969) Microinvasive carcinoma of the uterine cervix. Am J Clin Pathol 52: 511-529

Roche WD, Norris HJ (1975) Microinvasive carcinoma of the cervix. The significance of lymphatic invasion and confluent patterns of stromal growth. Cancer 36: 180-186

Rubio CA, Soderberg G, Einhorn N (1974) Histological and follow-up studies in cases of microinvasive carcinoma of the uterine cervix. Acta Pathol Microbiol Scand [A] 82: 397-410

Savage EW (1972) Microinvasive carcinoma of the cervix. Am J Obstet Gynecol 113: 708-717

Sedlis A, Sol S, Tsukada Y, Park R, Mangan C, Shingleton H, Blessing J (1979) Microinvasive carcinoma of the uterine cervix: a clinical-pathologic study. Am J Obstet Gynecol 133: 64-74

Seski JC, Abell MR, Morley GW (1977) Microinvasive squamous carcinoma of the cervix - definition, histologic analysis, late results of treatment. Obstet Gynecol 50: 410-414

Stoddard L (1952) The problem of carcinoma in situ with reference to the human cervix uteri. In: McManus JFA (ed) Progress in fundamental medicine. Lea and Febiger, Philadelphia, pp 203-260

Taki I, Sugimore H, Matsuyama T, Kashimura Y, Yoshivo T (1979) Treatment of microinvasive carcinoma. Obstet Gynecol Surv 34: 839-840

Van Nagell JR, Greenwell N, Powell DF, Donaldson ES, Hanson MB, Gay EC (1983) Microinvasive carcinoma of the cervix. Am J Obstet Gynecol 145: 981-991

Wilkinson EJ, Komorowski RS (1978) Borderline microinvasive carcinoma of the cervix. Obstet Gynecol 51: 472-476

Yajima A, Noda K (1979) The results of treatment of microinvasive carcinoma (stage IA) of the uterine cervix by means of simple and extended hysterectomy. Am J Obstet Gynecol 135: 685-688

Therapy of Minimal Cervical Cancer

H. G. Bender, H.-G. Schnürch, and K. W. Degen

Frauenklinik, Medizinische Einrichtungen, Universität Düsseldorf, Moorenstraße 5,
4000 Düsseldorf 1, FRG

The term "minimal cervical cancer" provokes the impression that one is dealing with an entity for which a generally applicable therapeutic concept can be outlined. This is supported by the fact that after long discussions the FIGO classification of 1976 defined stage I a as microinvasive cancer (early stromal invasion), whereas all other cases of stage I are included in stage I b. This impression needs to be corrected. "Minimal cervical cancer" must be interpreted as a spectrum of different entities each of which deserves a special therapeutic assessment. This concept is due to the following reasons:

1. The knowledge which has accumulated concerning the different morphological pictures of minimal cervical cancer
2. The role of other factors which have to be considered for therapy planning in the individual patient

Studies on the development of cervical cancer and the role and form of its precursors and early phases date far back to Carl Ruge of Berlin (Fig. 1), who can be regarded as the pioneer of systematic morphological studies of the uterine cervix. In his book *Zur Pathologie der Vaginalportion* (Fig. 2, left) which was published in 1878, he described many phenomena of precancerous and malignant changes of the uterine cervix strongly suggesting biopsies for the evaluation of lesions at this site and basically developing the concept of conization (Fig. 3), which was rediscovered several decades later. Since those days a considerable amount of knowledge has been accumulated and from the many studies a relatively clear treatment concept for the different phases in the development of cervical cancer has been suggested. When discussing "minimal cervical cancer" the following subgroups need to be addressed specifically: microcarcinoma, early stromal invasion, and cervical intraepithelial neoplasia.

For several reasons intraepithelial neoplasia of the uterine cervix is included in the discussion though it is not cancer in the true sense. Particularly this field offers new perspectives of carcinogenesis and the challenges of an individual treatment. So we shall include these intraepithelial forms of cervical neoplasia into the discussion.

Obviously an individualized therapy is closely related to a reliable morphological examination and the treating physician should be informed about the controversies that have accompanied the evolution of the diagnosis "microinvasive cancer of the uterine cervix" (Table 1). Since Mestwerdt (1947) suggested including lesions up to a maximal invasion of 5 mm in this group, many authors have debated the 5-mm threshold and some have proposed reserving reduced therapy for lesions with a lesser degree of inva-

Recent Results in Cancer Research, Vol. 106

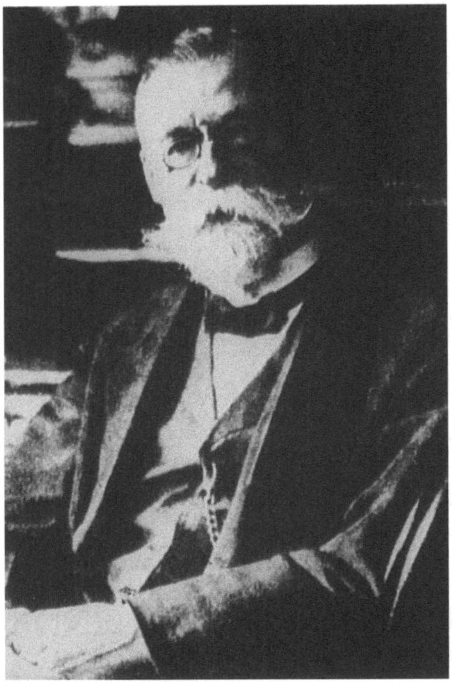

Fig. 1. Carl Ruge, Berlin (1846-1926)

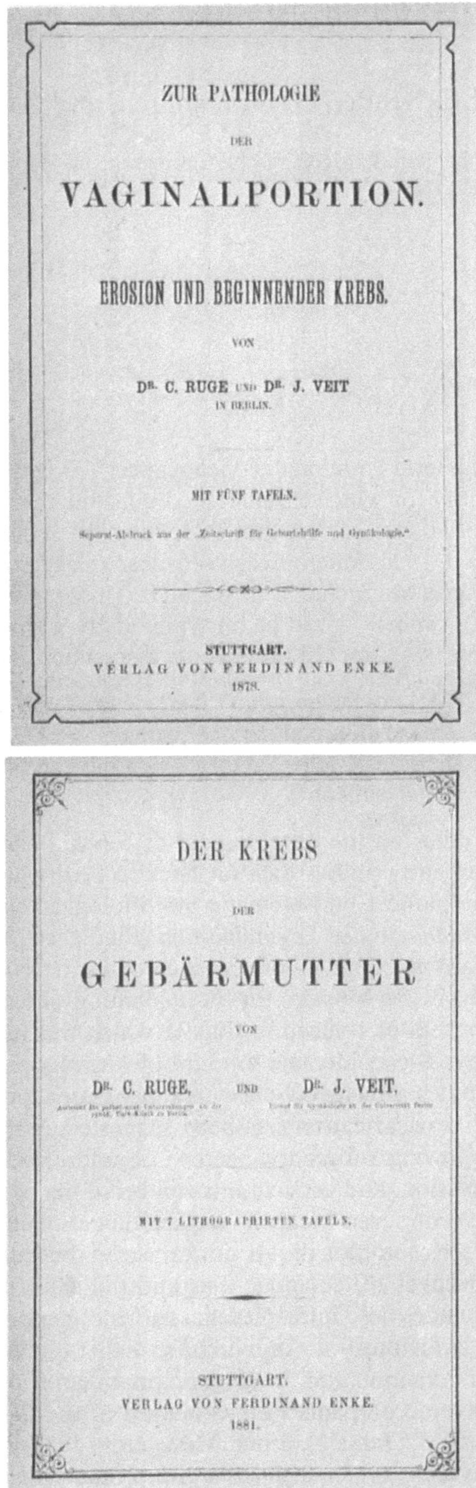

ZUR PATHOLOGIE

DER

VAGINALPORTION.

EROSION UND BEGINNENDER KREBS.

VON

DR. C. RUGE UND DR. J. VEIT

IN BERLIN.

MIT FÜNF TAFELN.

Separat-Abdruck aus der „Zeitschrift für Geburtshülfe und Gynäkologie."

STUTTGART.

VERLAG VON FERDINAND ENKE.

1878.

DER KREBS

DER

GEBÄRMUTTER

VON

DR. C. RUGE, UND DR. J. VEIT,

MIT 7 LITHOGRAPHIRTEN TAFELN.

STUTTGART.

VERLAG VON FERDINAND ENKE.

1881.

▷

Fig. 2. *Above:* Front page of Ruge's book in cooperation with J. Veit: *Zur Pathologie der Vaginalportion, Erosion und beginnender Krebs* (1878). *Below:* Front page of Ruge's book in cooperation with J. Veit: *Der Krebs der Gebärmutter* (Cancer of the Uterus) (1881)

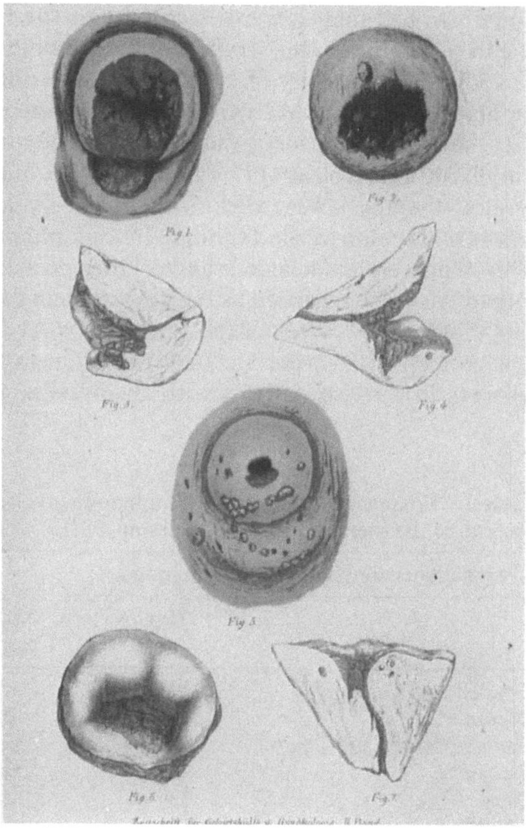

Fig. 3. Ruge's illustration of cone biopsies

Table 1. Authors and their definitions of microinvasive cancer of the uterine cervix. (Coppleson 1981)

Microinvasive carcinoma		
Author	Year	Maximum depth of invasion (mm)
Friedell and Graham	1959	1
Nelson, Averette, and Richart	1975	1
Mussey, Soule, and Welch	1969	3
Frick, Janovski, Gusberg et al.	1963	3
DiSaia, Morrow, and Townsend	1975	3
Bohm, Krupp, Lee et al.	1976	3
Duncan and Walker	1977	3
Seski, Abell, and Morley	1977	3
Ullery, Boutselis, and Botschner	1965	3-4
Margulis, Ely, and Ladd	1967	5
Kolstad	1969	5
Ng and Reagan	1969	5
Roche and Norris	1975	5
Boutselis, Ullery, and Charme	1971	5
Leman, Benson, Kurman et al.	1976	5
Mestwerdt	1947	5
Sedlis, Sall, Tsukada et al.	1979	5
Christopherson, Gray, and Parker	1976	5
Morton	1964	9

sion down to 1 mm. Nevertheless these metric figures are subject to possible inaccuracy due to difficulties in the workup of the specimen and to subjectivity in its interpretation. In addition to intensity of invasion, cellular differentiation, mitotic activity, confluency, capillary invasion, and DNA contents can be evaluated. Some European investigators have suggested replacing the parameter depth of invasion by a volume description. Burghardt and Holzer (1977) have drawn a line at 500 mm^3 up to which a less radical surgical therapy is regarded as adequate. Coppleson (1981) supplemented a histology report with colposcopic findings. In his opinion colposcopically visible lesions are the ones which are associated with a higher probability of metastatic potential. Lymphatic spread has to be regarded as the key problem for the establishment of a therapeutic concept (Table 2). A survey of the literature by Averette et al. in 1976 revealed that in a patient group with invasion up to 1 mm no metastases in the lymph nodes were detected, whereas in 3.5% of patients with an invasion depth between 1 and 5 mm lymph node

Table 2. Frequency of metastatic lymph node involvement in stage I a carcinoma of the uterine cervix. (Coppleson 1981)

Lymphadenectomy in stage I a carcinoma	Year	No. of cases	Involved nodes
Friedell and Graham	1959	40[a]	1
Moore et al.	1961	16	0
Bangle, Berger, and Levin	1963	35	0
Dockerty	1964	50 approx.	0
Gray	1964	28	1[b]
Enterline	1965	7	0
McLaren	1967	10	0
Way, Hennigan, and Wright	1968	23[c]	0
Thompson	1968	49	0
Foushee, Greiss, and Lock	1969	29	1
Kolstad	1969	38	1[d]
Mussey, Soule, and Welch	1969	53	1
Ng and Reagan	1969	10	0
Brandl, Georgiades, and Kraus	1970	69	1
Sidhu, Koss, and Barber	1970	41	2
Sall	1971	23	0
Creasman and Parker	1973	19	1
Coppleson	1974	90	1[e]
Bohm, Krupp, Lee et al.	1976	56	4
Leman, Benson, Kurman et al.	1976	47	0
Averette, Nelson, Ng et al.	1976	160	0
Kovacic, Novak, Stucin et al.	1976	122	0
Seski, Abell, and Morley	1977	37	0
Duncan and Walker	1977	42	0
Lohe	1978	66	0
Sedlis, Sall, Tsukada et al.	1979	74	0

[a] Includes overt carcinomas less than 1 cm in diameter.
[b] Actually frank invasive carcinoma of cervix on review.
[c] May include some cases of carcinoma in situ.
[d] Probably stage I b endocervical cancer.
[e] Colposcopically suspect overt carcinoma.

metastases could be demonstrated. Benson and Norris (1977) extended this survey, including another 150 cases with lymph node resection. According to their calculations the rate of metastases in regional lymph nodes is less than 2%. Lohe et al. (1978) contributed the observation that half the women who died did so despite previous radical treatment.

Once one has gone through all these discussions and selected a particular surgical procedure for the individual lesion on a theoretical basis one has to weigh the risks and drawbacks of the intervention under consideration. This includes intra- and postoperative complications and for the great number of young patients the loss of childbearing and menstrual function. This price has to be discussed with the individual patient on the basis of a general management strategy.

Simple hysterectomy is commonly suggested as standard therapy for patients with microcarcinoma of the uterine cervix. But as mentioned before patient-specific aspects may modify this basic approach. This deviation is partially influenced by treatment data and complication rates of a particular institution. So conization and a radical or modified radical hysterectomy can be considered a potential alternative in the management of this disease. Patients with lesions of a moderate volume of up to approximately 300 mm^3, reasonable cell differentiation, and no infiltration of vascular spaces are possible candidates for a reduced radical approach. That means that conization can be regarded as sufficient if the patient wants to preserve the uterus because her family planning has not yet been fulfilled or she feels that continuation of the menstrual cycle has a high value for her self-esteem. But there are two prerequisites which are of outstanding importance: The surgeon has to be absolutely sure that there is no additional invasive area with a potentially even deeper infiltration. The statement that the neoplastic alteration is surrounded by clear margins is one of the basic requirements for reduced radicality. The second requirement is that an elaborate colposcopic examination ensures that there is no discontinuous lesion on the outer surface of the uterine cervix or in the vagina. This study helps preoperatively to define the circumcision line for the conization procedure. Under these conditions conization appears to offer a satisfactory level of safety for this selected group of patients. In contrast simple hysterectomy primarily serves prophylactic aims in our opinion. The sophisticated resection procedure for conization and careful morphological investigation of the specimen should ensure that no residual tumor is left behind in the uterus. So this organ itself should not impair the prognosis of the patient except for a local recurrence after a longer interval. Nevertheless this perspective is reason enough for many patients and physicians to solve the problem definitely by removing the uterus. This decision may be facilitated in a considerable number of patients who have additional problems which can be eliminated or improved by a hysterectomy. Irregular bleeding and urinary stress incontinence are common symptoms which may strongly advocate a hysterectomy in combination with a favorable microcarcinoma. Patients presenting with less favorable lesions, i.e., a tumor volume of 400-500 mm^3, marked pleomorphism, infiltration of capillaries or lymphatic spaces, or a combination of these are definitely not candidates for treatment less radical than hysterectomy. In patients with very pronounced unfavorable factors one has to consider including the area at risk in the therapy, i.e., the lymph nodes along the iliac vessels and in the obturator fossa.

The difficult decision of whether the parametria are to be resected or not has to be taken. One has to discuss the advantages and disadvantages of simple, modified radical, and radical hysterectomy. Lohe et al. (1978) summarized that "the literature discloses not a single case in which early cervical cancer was accompanied by metastatic invasion of the parametrial lymph nodes". On the other hand, one has to take into account that lymphatic spread into the lymph node groups follows the parametrial pathways so that these also potentially harbor tumor cells. As mentioned before one has to include all the factors of a risk benefit analysis into a decision. In the experience of our institution the complication rate of radical hysterectomy is very low, transitory postoperative bladder dysfunction being one of the few problems of major practical importance. For this reason we select radical hysterectomy for the few patients with the above-defined high-risk microcarcinoma of the uterine cervix. Among the 15 patients treated so far we have seen metastatic lesions in an external iliac lymph node of one patient but no signs of tumor progression or recurrence.

In older patients we consider a simple or modified radical hysterectomy as suggested by Te Linde with or without pelvic lymphadenectomy as a reasonable therapeutic approach. We have performed three abdominal hysterectomies and two modified radical hysterectomies in combination with pelvic lymphadenectomies in three out of these five patients. There were no demonstrable lymph node metastases and no evidence of progression or recurrence after a median observation time of 21 months. After discussing our opinions concerning a stepwise therapy concept for patients with microinvasive cancer of the uterine cervix, our attitude toward therapy of early stromal invasion is more or less similar. We regard it as one of the particularly favorable forms of microinvasive cervical cancer for which conization with clear broad margins is sufficient in the majority of patients. Questionable reliability of morphology, anxiety of the patient, or additional problems related to the uterus may well contribute to a complex situation which is optimally solved by hysterectomy.

As stated at the beginning of this article, cervical intraepithelial neoplasia does not constitute a form of cervical cancer in its proper sense but is closely related to its prevention and the differential diagnosis against minimal invasive cancer. For this reason it shall be briefly discussed in this regard.

Standard therapy of CIN-grade 3 is conization in our opinion. Specific solutions have to be found for patients whose conization specimen does not show clear margins in the endocervical canal. Sixteen percent of our specimen are reported in this way. Consecutive problems may arise from invasive areas which were missed and also arise from noninvasive components that persist or develop. In patients who accept none of these risks and who desire no more children, hysterectomy is the preferable treatment. Out of 16 patients we have treated in this manner, 11 showed residual but not invasive neoplastic tissue. In 21 patients we preserved the uterus after the patients had declared that they would take the risks of a close colposcopic-cytological follow-up program to maintain the chance of pregnancy. In six patients of this group we observed persistent or recurrent abnormal cytological findings which finally resulted in hysterectomy. Nine children were born in the remaining 11 women, 4 of which had to have a cerclage for cervical incompetence. For some years we have tried to prevent incomplete resections by using endocervical contact hysteroscopy for the delineation of the upper resection line. With this assessment we have reduced the frequency of reports with suspected incomplete CIN removal to 5%. Late complications such as the above-mentioned cervical incompetence have to be considered when the indication of this procedure is discussed. During the Fifteenth Symposium of this Society we presented our calculation that approximately 35000–40000 conizations were performed in the Federal Republic of Germany in 1981 (Bender and Schnürch 1985) (Table 3). A rate of 1.4% intra- and immediate postoperative complications has been recorded. It is our feeling that both figures are unacceptably high. One must assume that a substantial number of conizations are performed

Table 3. Calculated frequency of conization in the Federal Republic of Germany in 1981. (Bender and Schnürch 1985)

Central Institute of Medical Services 1981	
275.3 million treatment documents	
0.085% conizations in outpatient services per year	24000
Estimated from the multicenter gynecological surgery complication study:	
Conizations on inpatients per year	16800
Total	35000–40000

Table 4. Distribution of HPV results in patients of a dysplasia clinic. Asymptomatic age-matched controlled and asymptomatic prostitutes

HPV 6/11	HPV 16/18	HPV 6/11 HPV 16/18	No HPV
16.2%	24.1%	12.7%	47%
Asymptomatic age-matched female population 8%		Asymptomatic prostitutes 12.5%	

in young patients with mild or moderate grade I or II CIN or even no dysplasia at all without adequate consideration of these hazards. For this reason our and some other institutions have established a dysplasia clinic which aims at a minimally destructive assessment of these alterations. Colposcopically directed biopsies and additional laser coagulation are the treatment modalities in this program. Ninety-five percent of all our patients treated in this clinic for cervical dysplasia problems and 98% of those with a cytological smear group III_D returned to normal colposcopic and cytological findings by applying this therapy concept. This result persisted after 12 months in 90% of the patients. Nine percent of the remaining 10% were again colposcopically and cytologically reversed to normal after second-line treatment.

During recent years human papilloma virus has been named as one of the cofactors contributing to the development of cancer of the uterine cervix. In our dysplasia patients we have found HPV 6/11 in 16.2% of the cases and HPV 16/18 in 24.1% of the cases, with 47% patients showing none and 12.7% patients showing both of the virus groups (Table 4). In an age-matched control-group the frequency of positive HPV results was 8%. In one of our recent studies HPV-positive results were obtained in 12.5% of colposcopically and cytologically normal prostitutes, who are at risk of developing cervical cancer according to epidemiological data.

It is fascinating that treatment of minimal cervical cancer may be transferred into another dimension so that it becomes a subject for the application of virustatic agents. Until the oncogenic role of HPV is definitely delineated and effective treatment modalities have been developed to interrupt this process we shall have to control cervical cancer by conventional strategies as far as possible.

References

Averette HE, Nelson JH Jr, Ng ABP, Hoskins WJ, Boyce JG, Ford JH Jr (1976) Diagnosis and management of microinvasive (stage I a) carcinoma of the uterine cervix. Cancer [Suppl 1] 38: 414

Bender HG, Schnürch H-G (1985) Conization data in the Federal Republic of Germany. In: Bender HG, Beck L (eds) Cancer of the uterine cervix. Fischer, Stuttgart, pp 59-66

Benson WL, Norris HJ (1977) A critical review of the frequency of lymphnode metastases and death from microinvasive carcinoma of the cervix. Obstet Gynecol 49: 632

Burghardt E, Holzer E (1977) Diagnosis and treatment of microinvasive carcinoma of the uterine cervix. Obstet Gynecol 49: 641

Coppleson M (1981) Gynecologic oncology. Livingstone Edinburgh

Lohe KJ, Burghardt E, Hillemanns HG, Kaufmann C, Ober KG, Zander J (1978) Early squamous cell carcinoma of the uterine cervix. II. Clinical results of a co-operative study in the management of 419 patients with early stromal invasion and microcarcinoma. Gynecol Oncol 6: 31

Mestwerdt G (1947) Frühdiagnose des Kollumkarzinoms. Zentralbl Gynaekol 69: 326

Ruge C, Veit J (1878) Zur Pathologie der Vaginalportion. Erosion und beginnender Krebs. Enke, Stuttgart

Ruge C, Veit J (1881) Der Krebs der Gebärmutter. Enke, Stuttgart

Anatomic Markers of Human Mammary Premalignancy and Incipient Breast Cancer

D. L. Page

Department of Pathology (C-3321), Vanderbilt University Medical Center,
1161 21st Avenue South, Nashville, TN 37232, USA

Word definitions in the broad area of incipient mammary carcinoma are as imprecise as our understanding of carcinogenetic events themselves. What is known is that the development of a malignant neoplasm having the capacity at time of detection to produce metastases and death involves a complex series of events. This series of events is complete when a population of cells is capable of invading stroma, traveling to distant parts of the body, and establishing distant colonies capable of growth with detrimental effects to the host. The identification of any stage or event in this series may not guarantee with certainty that metastatic capacity will be attained. The development of malignant capacity is a stochastic process in which our predictions rest upon percentage likelihood of attaining death-dealing capability. In the breast, unlike at sites where anatomic identification of these early stages may rest upon exfoliated cells, the performance of the biopsy itself obviously alters the process by removing cells and stroma for microscopic analysis. In summary, we must be content with identifying processes having different levels of magnitude of risk for subsequent development of carcinoma. Where or at what level of risk one might decide that such identification merits the appellation of incipient carcinoma may vary, but is usually reserved for lesions with stromal invasion. Word assignment is less important than the understanding of relevance to an individual patient, and this presentation will focus upon those anatomic changes which have relevance in assessing risk for breast carcinoma (Page 1986). We have chosen to utilize anatomic terms rather than phrases relating such changes to malignancy such as "precancerous". This has been done with the exception of lesions long accepted as carcinoma in situ. One important consequence of the risk assessment approach is that different types of carcinoma in situ should be understood with regard to their specific natural history, or at least our current knowledge thereof. Thus the natural history of each reliably identifiable histologic lesion is assessed, rather than accepting them as carcinoma or precancer because of the terminology utilized.

Many important investigations have supported the idea that epithelial proliferation within the breast is associated with the development of carcinoma. These studies have most frequently been done in a concurrent fashion, that is by the evaluation of epithelial changes within the breast at the time carcinoma is diagnosed. In the early 1940s Foote and Stewart (1945), utilizing the term papillomatosis for the most common of these proliferative changes, found them to be more frequent in cancer-associated breasts than in benign ones. The most carefully conducted of these concurrent studies (Wellings et al. 1975; Jensen et al. 1976) utilized a more complex classification system beginning with

Recent Results in Cancer Research, Vol. 106

the number *one* indicating active-appearing cells which were not increased in number and ending with the number *five* indicating carcinoma in situ. All of these alterations were more common in cancer-associated breasts than in benign ones. Black et al. (1972) using an analogous system beginning with *one* as normal and ending with *five* as carcinoma in situ demonstrated the greater association of categories three and four with carcinoma development in a retrospective case control study. The same histologic classification system utilized in a cohort study came to the same conclusions (Kodlin et al. 1977).

Our approach to anatomic classification of epithelial lesions has been to separate qualitative and quantitative features rather than placing them in an ascending order with combined complexity. This has produced a stratification of benign breast biopsies into three broad categories: no proliferative disease, proliferative disease without atypia, and atypical hyperplasia. An almost identical approach was utilized by Prechtel (1972). We recognize, as did Foote and Stewart (1941) and Wellings et al. (1975), two series or patterns of hyperplasia based largely on cytologic features: a lobular series, and a series of usual hyperplasias termed "ductal", "papillomatosis", or type A of Wellings et al. (1975). In the lobular series, only atypical lobular hyperplasia (ALH) and lobular carcinoma in situ (LCIS) are recognized since the definition of lesser examples in this series has not been achievable with reliable reproducibility or linkage to subsequent increased risk of cancer (Dupont and Page 1985).

The usual hyperplasias are so termed because they are the most commonly found within the breast and despite the frequent appellation "ductal" they most often occur within lobular units. Mild examples of epithelial hyperplasia of the usual type are not associated with unusual risks, and for that reason were placed in a no risk category by a recent consensus conference of the College of American Pathologists and the American Cancer Society (Hutter et al. 1986). These mild hyperplasias may also be placed in the category of no epithelial proliferative disease with the word *disease* in the phrase "proliferative disease" (Rogers and Page 1979) taken to indicate an increased risk of cancer. As hyperplasia indicates an increased number of cells, these mild hyperplasias of the usual type must have an increased cell number greater than the two cells above the basement membrane normally found in the breast. They usually have three or four cells above the basement membrane. They have little tendency to cross over or distend spaces. The moderate and florid hyperplasias of the usual type, which constitute the most common form of proliferative disease without atypia in the breast, usually have five or more cells above the basement membrane and tend both to cross and distend involved spaces (Figs. 1, 2). These latter, slightly increased risk lesions, are often recognized as "papillomatosis" or "epitheliosis".

Intermediate in both histologic appearance and magnitude of cancer risk between the proliferative lesions and carcinoma in situ are the atypical hyperplasias (Page et al. 1985). The atypical hyperplasias are recognized by their demonstration of some but not all of the determinant histologic features of carcinoma in situ. These features are evaluated largely in a qualitative and not a quantitative fashion, i.e., the number of cells or size of the lesion is not a defining feature. Thus, the diagnosis of atypical hyperplasia must take into account criteria for the diagnosis of carcinoma in situ. Cribriform and micropapillary carcinoma in situ (ductal carcinoma in situ, DCIS) must have a uniform population of cells throughout an entire area bounded by basement membrane. The pattern is of neatly rounded, geometric spaces or bulbous, well-defined papillary fronds. Also important, but less so, is the random yet even placement of nuclei which are round, usually hyperchromatic, and monotonous. In other words, the characteristic finding of varied oblong and rounded nuclei with a tendency toward swirling which characterizes

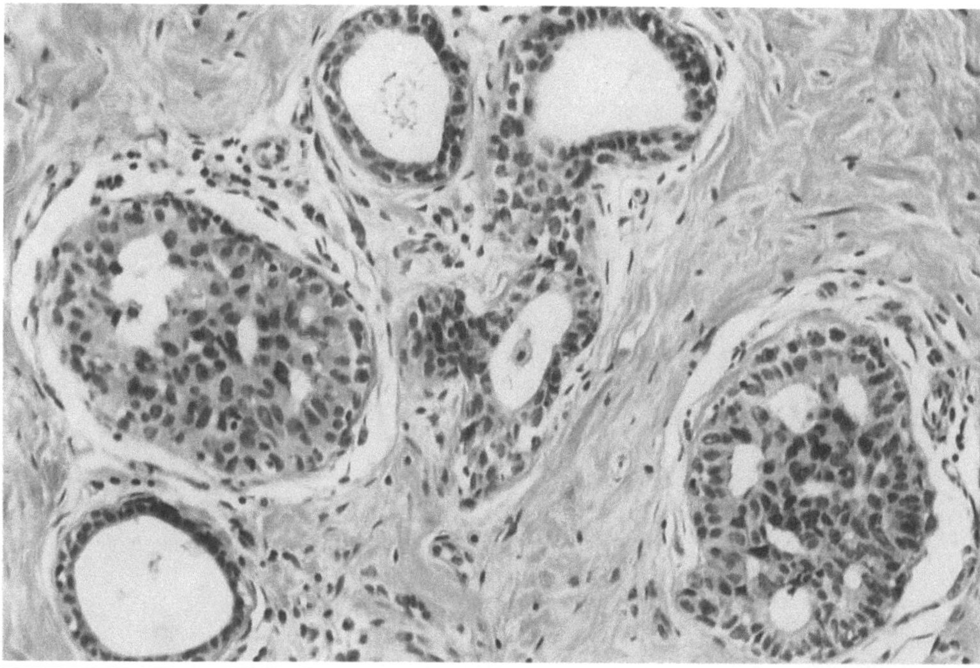

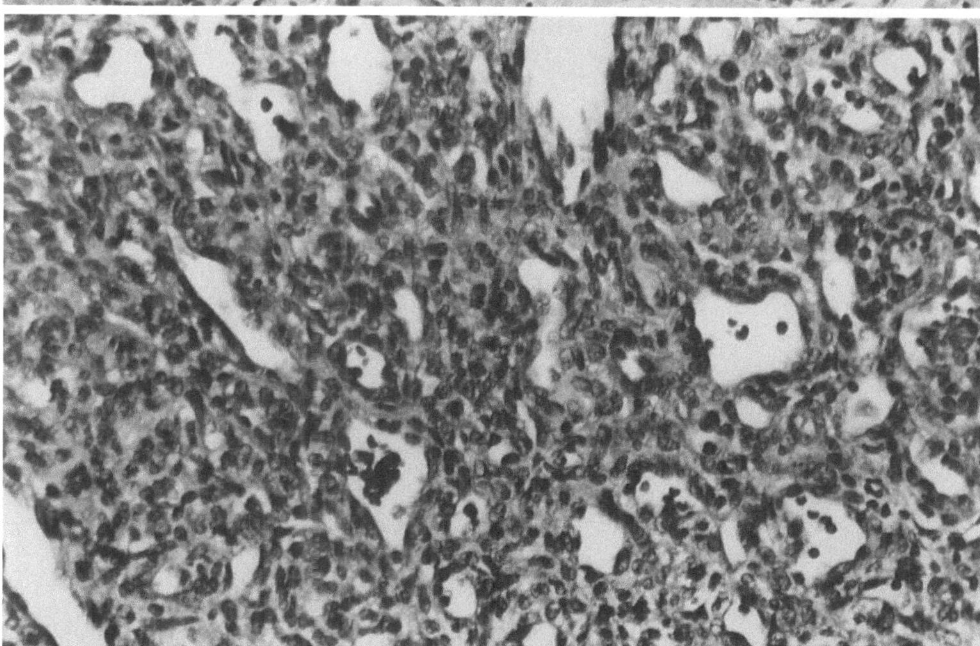

Fig. 1 *(above)*. An example of moderate hyperplasia of the usual type, the most common form of proliferative disease without atypia in benign breast biopsies. Note the two distended acinar spaces with hyperplastic cells crossing the spaces producing irregular secondary lumina, and having a heterogeneous cytology and cell placement. H & E, ×250

Fig. 2 *(below)*. This example of florid hyperplasia of the usual type has irregular intercellular spaces obviously present in a greatly distended acinar or ductal space. Nuclei vary from oblong to round and placement suggests a swirling pattern. No feature of atypia is present. H & E, ×250

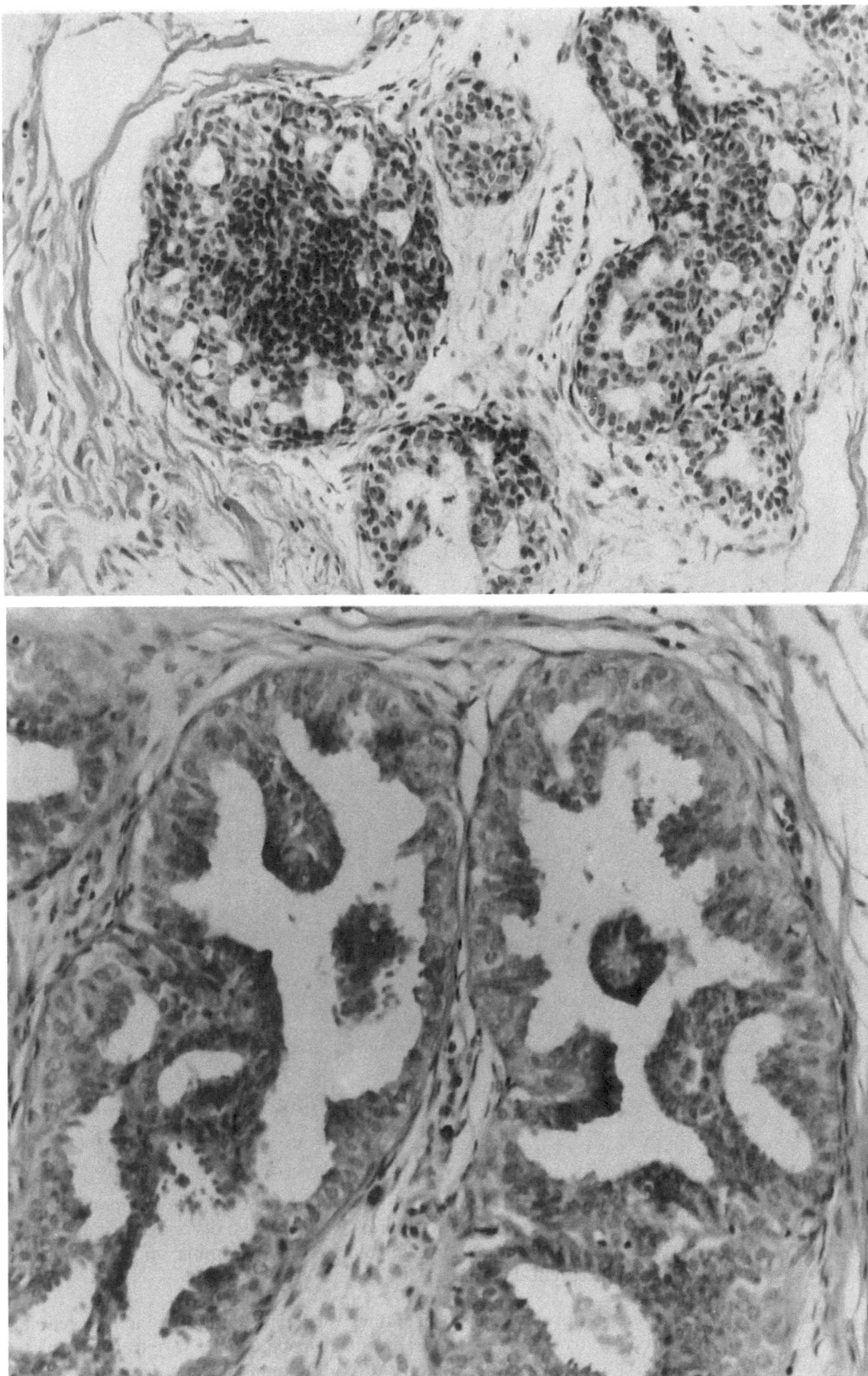

the usual hyperplasias is absent. The defining features of DCIS should be present in at least two spaces, a helpful criterion for the diagnosis of DCIS in difficult cases. Atypical hyperplasia of "ductal" type is diagnosed if these defining elements of DCIS are suggested, present in poorly developed form, or if one is present without the others (Figs. 3, 4). Many cases of atypical ductal hyperplasia as defined in our studies are characterized by the presence of a quite uniform population of hyperchromatic cells centrally within a space with a normal cell population at the basement membrane, at least focally. The histologic criteria for lobular carcinoma in situ (LCIS) involve the presence of characteristic and uniform cells comprising the entire population of a lobular unit (Foote and Stewart 1941). All of the acini must be filled, i.e., there must be no interspersed, intercellular spaces between the cells. Expansion and/or distortion of at least one-half of the acini of the lobular unit completes the definition of lobular carcinoma in situ. Cytologically identical lesions which do not have all of these criteria are recognized as atypical hyperplasia of the lobular type (Fig. 5). Atypical lobular hyperplasia (ALH) must have at its lower bound of histologic definition at least the certainty that an abnormally increased number of cells are present within acini having the characteristic cytologic features. If this is not present, changes long recognized as mimickers of lobular neoplasia may be ignored for diagnostic purposes as in follow-up they did not recognize an increased risk of subsequent cancer development (Dupont and Page 1985). In follow-up studies done in Nashville, Tennessee, over the last 10 years, these histologic categories were assigned to over 10000 biopsies originally diagnosed as benign and performed between 1950 and 1968. Follow-up of all women with atypical lesions, as well as those with proliferative disease without atypia and a control group of women without proliferative disease, has produced a stratification of these groups in terms of cancer risk predictability. The subsequent risk of invasive breast cancer development in these women was determined over a follow-up period averaging more than 17 years and representing successful contact of over 85% of the women. The risk of subsequent breast cancer in women in our study group was compared with women in the general population followed for the same number of years controlled for age. Women without proliferative changes had a risk slightly less than that of the general population. Women with proliferative disease without atypia, representing approximately one-fourth of the population, had a risk approaching twice that of the general population, being 1.6 if evaluated against the general population and 1.9 if evaluated against women from our own study without proliferative changes by the Cox Proportional Hazards Method (Dupont and Page 1985). Both types of atypical hyperplasia were associated with risk greater than four times that of the general population (Page et al. 1985). This magnitude of risk was the same for each type of atypia and the risk was evenly distributed between the breasts, not showing the tendency

◁ **Fig. 3** *(above).* This pattern may be accepted as a lesser or milder example of atypical ductal hyperplasia. This is largely supported by the hyperchromatic and quite homogeneous cell population in the larger rounded space as well in the somewhat elongated space at the right where the ridged and narrow bars found in cribriform ductal carcinoma in situ are suggested. Note that a completely uniform cell population is not present. H & E, ×175

Fig. 4 *(below).* This example of atypical ductal hyperplasia suggests both the bulbous projections of micropapillary carcinoma in situ as well as the rigid bars or arches of cribriform ductal carcinoma in situ. However, the cell population is not uniform throughout the spaces and atypical ductal hyperplasia is diagnosed. H & E, ×200

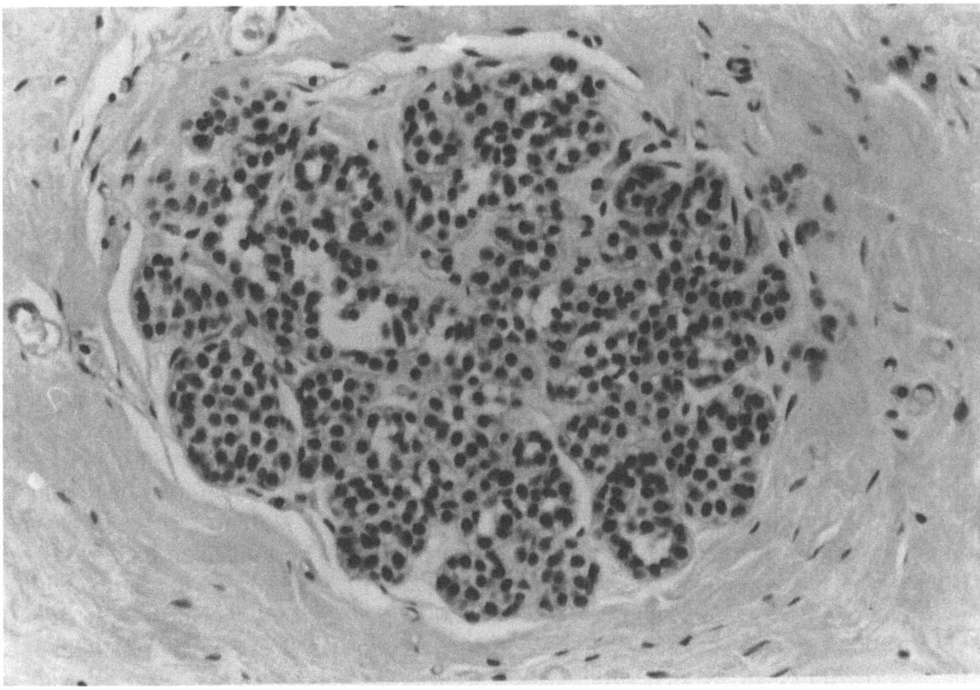

Fig. 5. This is an advanced example of atypical lobular hyperplasia. Note that some acinar spaces in this lobular unit are very evidently distorted, distended, and completely filled with a uniform population of cells characteristic of either atypical lobular hyperplasia or lobular carcinoma in situ. However, many of the spaces are not distended or filled. As fewer than 50% of the acinar units are filled and distended, this is an example of atypical lobular hyperplasia. H & E, ×250

toward homolateral breast cancer development demonstrated for the analogous carcinoma in situ lesions of ductal type (Betsill et al. 1978; Page et al. 1982).

These changes also have a strong interaction with family history of breast cancer (Dupont and Page 1985), long known to be an important indicator of increased risk (Ernster 1981; Kelsey 1979). Women with both the atypical hyperplastic (AH) lesions and positive family history (FH) in a mother, sister, or daughter (first-degree family history) have a doubling of risk over that recognized by AH alone. The interaction of histology and FH is also demonstrated at the opposite end of the histologic spectrum. When women with FH (associated with a risk of about twice the general population) had no proliferative disease, their risk was only 1.2.

Conclusions

Indeed, the wisdom of our predecessors extending back into the late portions of the last century has been borne out by our increase in knowledge of the past few decades. They diagnosed comedo carcinoma in situ as carcinoma and this approach carried into the early 1950s when comedo carcinoma was still diagnosed when invasion was inapparent or absent. Thus, larger and better developed in terms of nuclear atypia, these examples of comedo carcinoma in situ termed "ductal type" may certainly be accepted as incipient carcinomas despite the fact that the great majority may be cured at the time of diagnosis. We would suspect that in biological terms these cellular populations have attained the majority of those features necessary to kill the host and that if left untreated the majority of these lesions would progress to metastases. As we step down to lesser examples of epithelial proliferative changes which have been associated with subsequent elevated cancer risk, the appellation "incipient carcinoma" becomes less and less appropriate in both absolute and relative terms. Thus, examples of cribriform and micropapillary carcinoma in situ of the ductal type are less often as large as comedo carcinoma at the time of diagnosis, and are undoubtedly more satisfactorily treated by methods of breast conservation (Millis and Thynne 1975; Lagios et al. 1982; Lagios 1986, Zafrani et al. 1986). However, even microscopic examples of these changes are associated with increased risk of subsequent carcinoma development (10 × that of the general population) in the ipsilateral breast (Betsill et al. 1978; Page et al. 1982).

These lesser examples of DCIS are determinant premalignant changes because the later cancers develop at the same site, and are markers of elevated risk as well. The other conditions discussed here are better understood only as markers of increased breast cancer risk because subsequent invasive malignancies develop anywhere in the breasts. LCIS has the greatest associated risk in the range of 10 × the general population (Haagensen et al. 1978; Rosen et al. 1978), with atypical hyperplasias having about one-half the risk of CIS. Certainly lesions of proliferative disease without atypia which are associated with slightly increased risk (1.5-2) and are present in over one-fourth of benign biopsies should not be considered as part of the pathway to cancer. For clinical purposes at least, they are best considered as markers of slightly increased risk. What these markers are in biologic terms has yet to be established.

References

Betsill WL Jr, Rosen PP, Lieberman PH, Robbins GF (1978) Intraductal carcinoma. Long-term follow-up after treatment by biopsy alone. JAMA 239: 1863-1867

Black MM, Barclay TH, Cutler SJ, Hankey BF, Asire AJ (1972) Association of atypical characteristics of benign breast lesions with subsequent risk of breast cancer. Cancer 29: 338-343

Dupont WD, Page DL (1985) Risk factors for breast cancer in women with proliferative breast disease. N Engl J Med 312: 146-151

Ernster VL (1981) The epidemiology of human breast cancer. Epidemiol Rev 3: 184-202

Foote FW, Stewart FW (1941) Lobular carcinoma *in situ*. Am J Pathol 17: 491-495

Foote FW, Stewart FW (1945) Comparative studies of cancerous versus noncancerous breasts. Ann Surg 121: 6-53, 197-222

Haagensen CD, Lane N, Lattes R, Bodian C (1978) Lobular neoplasia (so-called lobular carcinoma in situ) of the breast. Cancer 42: 737-769

Hutter RVP et al. (1986) Consensus meeting: is "fibrocystic disease" of the breast precancerous? Arch Pathol Lab Med 110: 171-173

Jensen HM, Rice JR, Wellings SR (1976) Preneoplastic lesions in the human breast. Science 191: 295-297

Kelsey JL (1979) A review of the epidemiology of human breast cancer. Epidemiol Rev 1: 74-109

Kodlin D, Winger EE, Morgenstern NL, Chen U (1977) Chronic mastopathy and breast cancer, a follow-up study. Cancer 39: 2603-2607

Lagios M (1986) Biology of duct carcinoma *in situ* of limited extent. Prospective study of patients treated by tylectomy. Lab Invest 54: 34A

Lagios MD, Westdahl PR, Margolin FR, Roses MR (1982) Duct carcinoma in situ. Relationship of extent of non-invasive disease to the frequency of occult invasion, multicentricity, lymph node metastases, and short-term treatment failures. Cancer 50: 1309-1314

Millis RR, Thynne GSJ (1975) In situ intraduct carcinoma of the breast: a long term follow-up study. Br J Surg 62: 957-962
Page DL (1986) Cancer risk assessment in benign breast biopsies. Hum Pathol 17: 871-874
Page DL, Dupont WD, Rogers LW, Landenberger M (1982) Intraductal carcinoma of the breast: follow-up after biopsy only. Cancer 49: 751-758
Page DL, Dupont WD, Rogers LW, Rados MS (1985) Atypical hyperplastic lesions of the female breast. Cancer 55: 2698-2708
Prechtel VK (1972) Beziehungen der Mastopathie zum Mammakarzinom. Fortschr Med 90: 43-45
Rogers LW, Page DL (1979) Epithelial proliferative disease of the breast - a marker of increased cancer risk in certain age groups. Breast 5: 2-7
Rosen PP, Lieberman PH, Braun DW Jr, Kosloff C, Adair F (1978) Lobular carcinoma in situ of the breast: detailed analysis of 99 patients with average follow-up of 24 years. Am J Surg Pathol 2: 225-251
Wellings SR, Jensen HM, Marcum RG (1975) An atlas of subgross pathology of the human breast with special reference to possible precancerous lesions. JNCI 55: 231-273
Zafrani B, Fourquet A, Vilcoq JR, Legal M, Calle R (1986) Conservative management of intraductal breast carcinoma with tumorectomy and radiation therapy. Cancer 57: 1299-1301

Treatment Aspects of Minimal Breast Cancer

F. K. Beller, C. D. Nitsch, and H. Nienhaus

Zentrum für Frauenheilkunde, Westfälische Wilhelms-Universität, Albert-Schweitzer-Straße 33, 4400 Münster, FRG

The choice of treatment modalities for breast cancer relies primarily on histopathologic information, correlated with data from epidemiologic studies, including:

1. Multicentricity of a given lesion
   a) In the ipsilateral breast
   b) In the contralateral breast
2. General metastasis in relation to tumor size
3. Survival
   a) In relation to type of tumor
   b) In relation to size of tumor
4. Areola involvement

Although these areas have been discussed for the treatment of premalignant lesions, this is not the case for larger cancers T1 to T2. In the ipsi- and contralateral breast, multicentricity and survival in relation to histopathologic type are rarely discussed. Looking at the historical development of surgical treatment for breast cancer, it is apparent that radicality of surgical procedure has not increased in biological concept but in surgical skill. Sir James Paget began 1865 with lumpectomy, and the peak of radicality was reached nearly 100 years later, around 1965, with extended ultraradical mastectomy. During the past few years breast-preserving operative procedures like tumorectomy, quadrantectomy, and wedge resection have been proposed for breast cancer up to 4 cm. The terms lumpectomy, tumorectomy, and incisional biopsy are used synonymously. A more extensive surgical procedure is quadrantectomy, wedge resection, and extended excisional biopsy. The authors are aware of the controversy in terminology but this is not the topic of this paper. The difference between lumpectomy, performed by Sir James Paget, and lumpectomy as a breast-preserving procedure is that radiation is an integral part of the primary procedure. These operations should be performed in centers provided that surgeons, radiologists, and pathologists with special expertise work together, and follow-up is guaranteed by specialized personal (Fig. 1). The pros and cons have been discussed in numerous symposia on both sides of the Atlantic. There is no need to repeat this discussion in this context.

In contrast to various treatment modalities for the ipsilateral breast, the contralateral breast has been left out in the consideration of treatment a alternatives completely. Only a few surgeons have proposed a biopsy of the contralateral breast. But there is a lack of agreement as to whether the inner upper or lower or outer upper quadrant of the con-

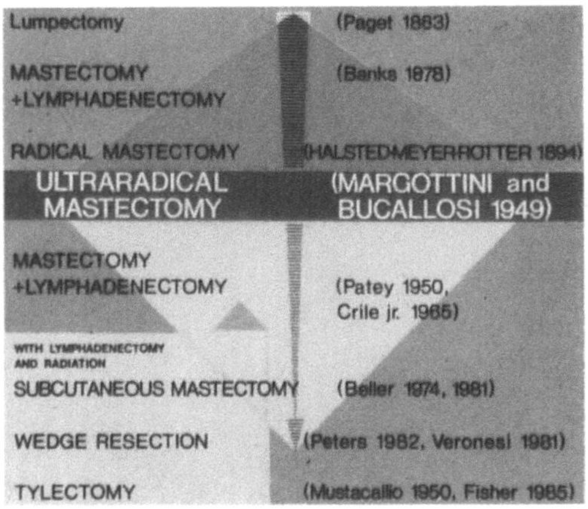

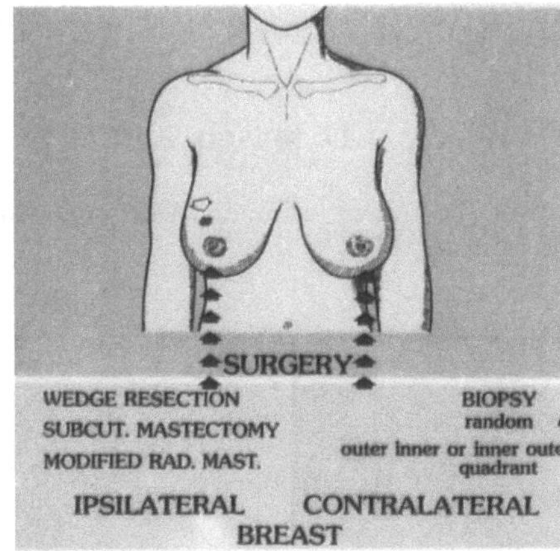

Fig. 1 *(left).* Historical development of surgery for breast cancer (schematically)

Fig. 2 *(right).* Surgical standard procedures for the ipsilateral breast for the treatment of breast cancer. For the contralateral breast only unstandardized biopsies are recommended

tralateral breast should be biopsied, as emphasized by Fracchia et al. (1985) and Urban (1977) (Fig. 2).

Why should the treatment of minimal breast cancer be different from more advanced stages? The answer requires a definition of minimal breast cancer. But this is difficult for the clinician to understand since the definitions of the pathologist vary. Also pathologists have been unable to agree on terms like multicentricity, multifocality, occult, synchronous to name only a few. For instance Gallager's definition of minimal cancer (Gallager and Martin 1971) emphasizes the tendency of the tissue to become neoplastic. This definition implies that at least some stages of in situ cancers may be included in this definition. Page et al. (1981) have introduced the term "proliferative lesion", which is believed to have some, but not all, of the characteristic of the in situ lesion and may preceded the in situ lesion.

The schematic MacDonald curve is generally accepted (Fig. 3). It demonstrates that a cancer has grown unnoticed for 6–8 years, until it has reached the tumor diameter of 1 cm or equivalent tumor mass or number of cells. But where is the beginning of the tumor growth if we plot the curve against premalignant lesions? This seems to indicate that there is no point 0 since carcinomata in situ, proliferate lesions, and even fibrocytic disease in one or the other form may preceded minimal cancer (Fig. 4). Therefore a rather large gray zone exists at least for the clinician. Whether an observed precancerous lesion progresses to invasive cancer and under what conditions a lesion metastasizes still remain unsettled questions. Generalized disease may be expected with a tumor size of 0.5 mm in a palpable range of 15% (Kindermann 1977) and lymph node involvement in 17.2% (Smart et al. 1978). At present a tumor which is identified by a lump, mammography, and/or ultrasonography is already cancerous. Although this is finally demonstrated after biopsy by histopathology (exceptionally by cytology), usually the lesion is cancerous and larger than 0.5 cm and requires cancer treatment with consequences, which the surgeon determines. To prevent this rather late development the idea of a prophylactic operation was considered. However, what is a prophylactic operation? The modified radical mastectomy as a bilateral operation seemed unacceptable for cosmetic reasons.

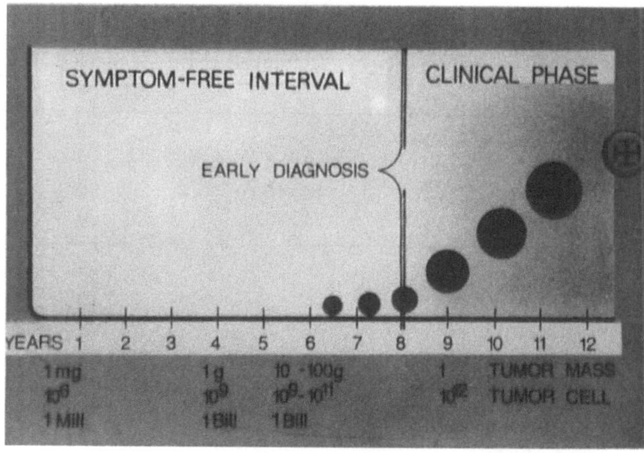

Fig. 3. Schematic representation of tumor growth up to 1 cm in diameter. The tumor has grown unnoticed for at least 6 years based on the multiplying rate of breast cancer. (Modified MacDonald curve)

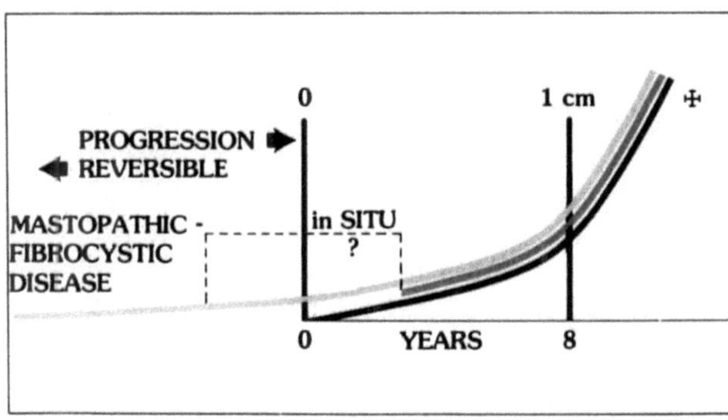

Fig. 4. Modified MacDonald curve as in Fig. 3. The various beginnings of the curve indicate the significance of minimal breast cancer

On the other hand, lumpectomy had the fallacy of incomplete resection lines. Therefore pathologists and surgeons attempted to identify risk groups for proliferate lesions and in situ cancers to minimize the candidates for such a prophylactic operation.

It is obviously taken for granted that tumors smaller than 0.5 mm rarely metastasize. Therefore the smaller the lesion, the less important are considerations about generalization of the disease. This means in turn that treatment aspects for premalignant lesions and minimal breast cancer rely entirely upon on operations which guarantee local control.

Foote and Stewart in 1941 noted the multicentricity of premalignant lesions, and some 10 years ago the different behavior of carcinoma lobulare in situ and ductal carcinoma in situ were identified. The risk factors which are given in the literature are shown in Table 1. These observations influenced treatment aspects of premalignant lesions and minimal cancer as well.

Table 1. Factors indicating increased risk of carcinoma

Risk factor	Increased risk	If mother affected
Fibrocystic breast disease		
Atypical proliferation	2- 4	4- 8
LCIS	10-40	20- 80
DCIS	25-75	50-100

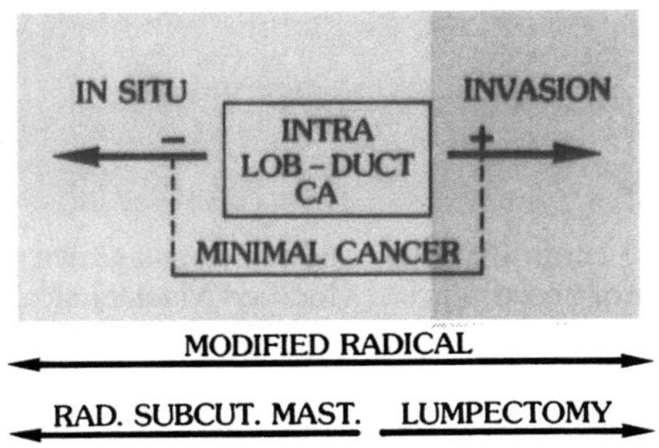

Fig. 5. Surgical procedures available for minimal cancer

What surgical procedures (Fig. 5) are available? Modified mastectomy was advised by Foote and Stewart (1941). However, the radicality seemed to be too extensive for the desired result. Subcutaneous mastectomy was advised for precancerous lesions and tumorectomy for larger cancers up to 4 cm. This differentiation does not seem logical. The reason that surgeons used tylectomy for larger cancers is that radiation is an integral part of treatment. It is quite apparent from B. Fisher's series that patients radiated had less recurrent tumors after tylectomy than wedge resection alone. I assume therefore that earlier or later radiation will be discussed for the treatment of precancerous lesions to stop progression.

The plastic surgeons Freeman in the United States in 1973 and Gynning in Australia in 1975 began to use subcutaneous mastectomies (SMs) for the treatment of cancer. They designed special surgical procedures but did not give follow-up results. However, SM was not used by plastic surgeons for the treatment of cancer, not even minimal cancer. They began to perform subcutaneous mastectomies as a prophylactic operation to eliminate precancerous lesions, whatever that may be. To perform "an exchange" mastectomy as it was called, using a silicone implant for the resected glandular part of the breast, became in vogue in the early 1970s. There was so much confidence among plastic surgeons that they performed this operation bilaterally. And indeed, provided that the pathologist in the group had rigid standards for premalignant lesions, a rather high recovery rate of 10% for occult cancers was achieved. Table 2 shows nearly identical results from two centers where such rigid standards were employed.

The plastic surgeon Strömbeck (1976) requested for subcutaneous mastectomy removal of at least 90% of the glandular part of the breast. This means that nearly all the fat had to be removed with only the skin left. A silicone implant was then placed under the skin and above the large pectoral muscle either in a one- or two-stage procedure. By the end of the decade it became appearent that the cosmetic results were not as good as expected. Capsule contracture was the main reason for failure. This in turn inaugurated a great debate among plastic surgeons. The value of a prophylactic operation was ques-

Table 2. Occult cancer after bilateral subcutaneous mastectomy for precancerous lesions

	Heidelberg Kubli et al.	Münster
n	106	100
Invasive carcinoma	8	12
LCIS/DCIS	31	34

Table 3. Residual cancer after wide excisional biopsy

When the original tumor was LCIS						
Author		*n*	Inv.	DCIS	LCIS	CIS
Shah et al.	(1973)	40	2	–	–	26
Wanebo et al.	(1974)	49	2	0	41	–
Carter and Smith	(1977)	49	3	–	–	31
Rosen et al.	(1979)	50	2	2	28	–

Table 4. Residual cancer after wide excisional biopsy

When the original tumor was DCIS						
Author		*n*	Inv.	DCIS	LCIS	CIS
Shah et al.	(1973)	45	8	–	–	21
Wanebo et al.	(1974)	37	5	16	3	–
Carter and Smith	(1977)	47	7	–	–	25
Rosen et al.	(1979)	50	3	26	1	–

tioned because appropriate indications had not been identified by the pathologists. However, somewhat ironically it was the time when general surgeons begun to treat larger lesions by tumorectomy and quadrant resection. Some surgeons felt that subcutaneous mastectomy was an incomplete operation. The opposite, however, is correct: SM was already too radical in comparison to the tylectomy approach.

One of the arguments for breast-preserving surgery was that the less extensive operations would be the result of earlier diagnosis. However, if the surgery for minimal cancer was more extensive than for earlier stages than this, the goal of earlier diagnosis could not be achieved. Therefore treatment modalities for premalignant lesions and minimal cancer were again evaluated.

Could tumorectomy for lobular carcinoma in situ (LCIS) or ductal carcinoma in situ (DCIS) be sufficient for treatment? Some data in the literature indicate a large number of residual cancers after excisional biopsy. The most significant papers in the literature show 5% invasive cancers and approximately 50%–60% LCIS if the lesion in the biopsy was LCIS. When the tumor was DCIS, around 30%–40% remaining DCISs were found (Tables 3, 4). It should be stressed that not all these lesions progress into invasive cancer. But yet it is unknown which will and which will not progress. Is it just the incision line or reduction of tumor mass which should be the inhibiting factor? Figure 6a, b demonstrates the incision lines of biopsy. The incision may cut through the tumor or leave in

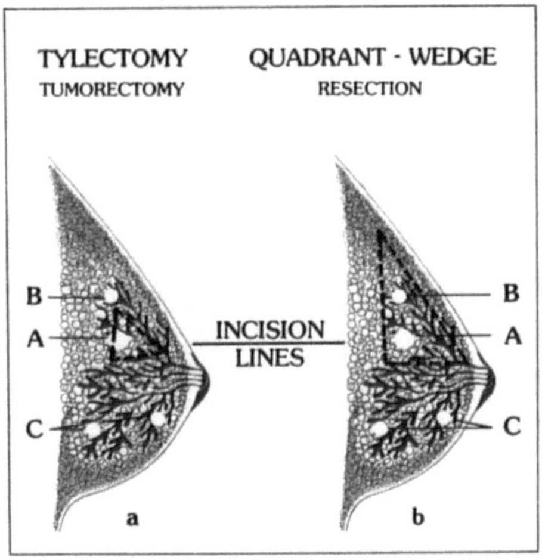

Fig. 6a, b. Incision lines for tumorectomy. **a** Note the cut through the tumor *(A)* and the untouched multicentric lesions *(B, C)*. In **b** the tumor *(A)* is excised with closed located satellite tumors *(B)* but not the more distant lesions *(C)*

situ lesions untouched (Fig. 6a). The tumor cut is avoided by larger - wedge resection - biopsies, but precancerous lesions may still be left (Fig. 6b). This seemed to exclude excisional biopsy as a breast-preserving operation. However, later data in regard to DCIS revealed long-term survival equal to that of modified mastectomy (Millis and Thynne 1975; Betsill et al. 1963; Peters et al. 1977). It was speculated that the explanation would be that ductal in situ foci would be close to the original lesion (Betsill et al. 1963) and therefore a wide excision would be sufficient for treatment.

If tumorectomy was sufficient for treatment this seemed to render subcutaneous mastectomy a historical reminiscence. However, it should be stressed that segmental biopsy of the ipsilateral breast again leaves the contralateral breast out of diagnostic evaluation. Not even a biopsy was requested of those who used segmental resection biopsy. Is this justified? There is a high incidence rate of LCIS and DCIS in both breasts. Fracchia et al. (1985) reported a 16% recurrence rate in the ipsilateral breast in stage I and 29% bilaterally. In the earlier paper of Robbins and Berg (1964) the expectation of a 1% incidence for the next 10 years is well known. According to Rosen et al. (1980), the incidence of LCIS in both breasts is similar. The increase for the other breast was nine times the expected rate of the control population and the mortality ten times. For understandable reasons data for both breasts are less available than for multicentricity of the ipsilateral breast. A review from the literature indicates the involvement rate (Tables 5, 6). The same is indicated in a summary curve of McDivitt et al. (1967). We have plotted both curves for cumulative risks in one graph in order to show the high incidence in both the ipsilateral and the contralateral breast (Fig. 7). For the evaluation of this question survival of cancer in the contralateral breast is of significance: Table 7 shows data from our material of 365 bilateral subcutaneous mastectomies. The high incidence of minimal cancer rate supports Andersen's et al. (1985) statements that a least if LCIS occurs the breasts should be regarded as one organ.

When modified radical mastectomy seemed too radical for a *bilateral* operation, subcutaneous mastectomy was perhaps the more acceptable procedure. One argument against was areolar involvement. Data in the literature indicate a high proportion of involvement (Table 8). Similar high incidence rates can be found for invasive cancers (see Beller 1985). However, these data are not comparable in regard to stage, distance from tumor, age, and other parameters. We have searched the literature and among

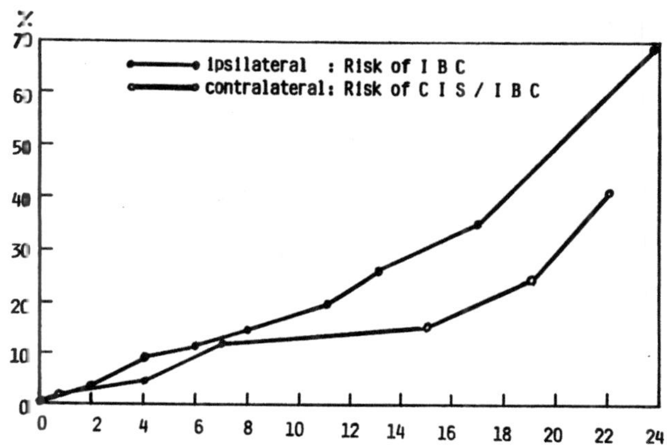

Fig. 7. Subsequent cumulative risks of carcinoma after local excision of LCIS. (Based on McDivitt et al. 1967)

Table 5. Data from the literature for in situ cancers in the ipsi- and contralateral breast

		LCIS		
Author		*n*	Ipsilateral	Contralateral
Rosen et al.	(1980)	10	6	4
Carter and Smith	(1977)	39	25	14
Farrow	(1970)	200	151	49
Hutter and Foote	(1969)	4	3	1

Table 6. Data from the literature for in situ cancers in the ipsi- and contralateral breast

		DCIS		
Author		*n*	Ipsilateral	Contralateral
Webber et al.	(1981)	123	–	6
Rosen et al.	(1980)	4	3	1
Farrow	(1970)	51	47	4

Table 7. Incidence of cancers in ipsilateral and contralateral breast at the time of primary treatment (radical and modified subcutaneous mastectomy). (Beller et al. 1986)

	Ipsilateral breast	Contralateral breast				
		Secondary cancer (T1)	Primary cancer (TIS)	Metastasis	Σ	Precancerous lesions
n	365	15	28	4	47	111
%	100	4	8	1	13	30

Table 8. Nipple involvement related to DCIS

Author		%
Brown	(1976)	15
Wertheim	(1980)	38.5
Lagios et al.	(1982)	7.5
LCIS		
Wertheim	(1980)	0
LCIS + DCIS		
Kochem	(1980)	1

5000 patients treated by an operative procedure for cancer, where the areola was preserved (tylectomy, quadrantectomy, or subcutaneous mastectomy), we have found not a single report of a recurrence in the areola. Areolar involvement can therefore not be a consideration in rejecting this technique.

In 1974, when data about the frequency of multicentric lesions became available, but data on tylectomy and quadrantectomy were lacking, we had begun to perform extended subcutaneous mastectomies with subsequent radiation for cancers up to stage T2, N0, or 1. In more than 100 patients the procedure was performed bilaterally. This is an unusual series since it is the only data in the literature where extended subcutaneous mastectomy was used for primary treatment of cancer. The 10-year survival rates are 90% for stage T1 and 85% for stage T2 (Beller and Schnepper 1981; Beller and Schmidt 1985):

1. Resection of glandular tissue by approximately 95%
2. Frozen section of both areola and mammilla
3. Lymphadenectomy
4. Irradiation
   + adjuvant chemotherapy by N1

The recurrence rate of 3% was extremely low. There was not a single recurrence in the areolar region and there was no recurrence in the contralateral breast. Our data indicated to us that SM is a procedure sufficient to remove cancer and multicentric lesions. But again for cosmetic reasons the operation seemed to be acceptable as a bilateral operation only in very selected patients who were considered high risks, although recent surgical developments have improved cosmetic results (submuscular extension prothesis, Beller 1985).

When data became available indicating that wedge resection may be sufficient for treatment of LCIS and DCIS, we developed a new operation technique based on a operation for reduction mammaplasty (Beller and Wagner 1980). Instead of resection of 90%–95% of the glandular part, only 70%–80% was removed. This allowed in turn preservation of tissue from which fat flaps could be used to form a new breast. The incision line of extended or radical versus reduced or modified subcutaneous mastectomy is indicated in Fig. 8 a, b.

Since January 1981 we have performed the new surgical procedure. Instead of extended subcutaneous mastectomy the modified operation was used for all stages of cancer and precancerous lesions as well. Glandular tissues with connective tissue septa (Cooper's ligaments), which are close to and run into the panniculus adiposus and overlying breast skin, remain in situ. Thus the glandular, connective, and adipose tissue left

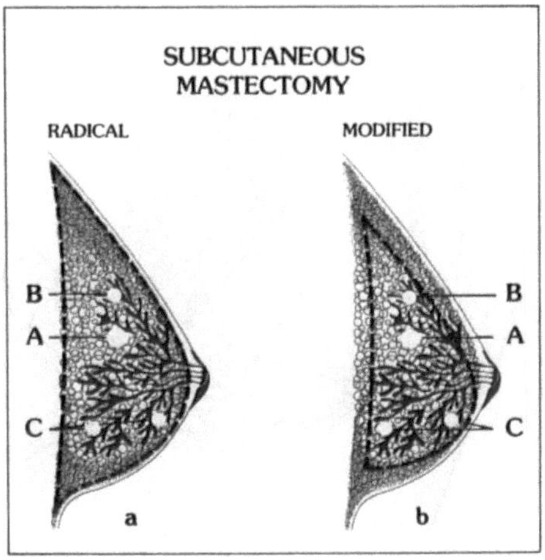

Fig. 8. **a** Incision lines after extended radical subcutaneous mastectomy. **b** After modified subcutaneous mastectomy. Note: Multicentric areas *A, B, C* are removed in both instances

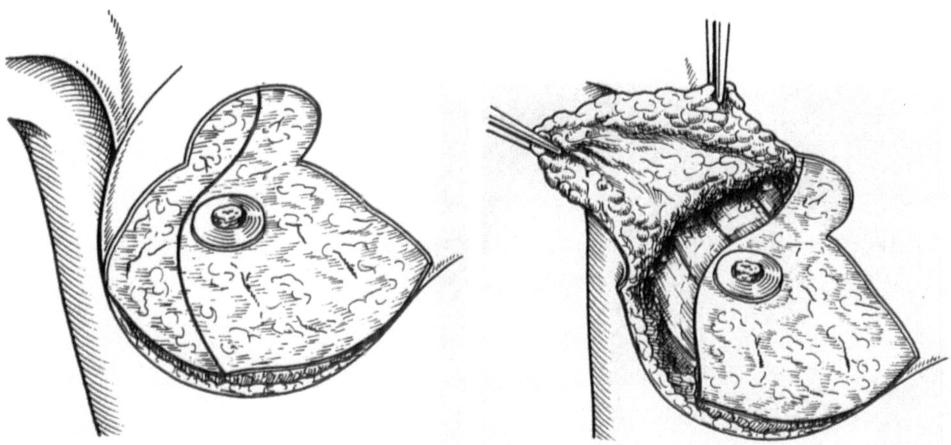

Fig. 9. The right breast is deepithelialized and the base incised. The *black, shaped line* is the incision line which enables the breast to be opened up and the glandular part with or without the cancer under sight to be excised

behind is used to construct a smaller breast by a technique slightly modified from the reduction mammaplasty we described earlier. The preoperative marking of the breast skin is accomplished by a modified Strömbeck pattern and the entire figure is deepithelialized. Subsequently, the glandular body is separated from the underlying pectoral fascia in the caudocranial direction, and the pectoral fascia is removed (Fig. 9 a). An incision described by Biesenberger in 1930 is used which allows both flaps to be turned up, enabling resection of the tumor or glandular tissue to be carried out (Fig. 9 b). Fat flaps are prepared for reconstruction of the new breast (Fig. 10 a, b). The cosmetic results were found satisfactory enough in the patients to propose this procedure bilaterally (Fig. 11). It was accepted by 95% in more than 250 patients. In 365 bilateral operations 13% occult cancers were observed in the contralateral breast and more than 30% precancerous lesions (Table 7).

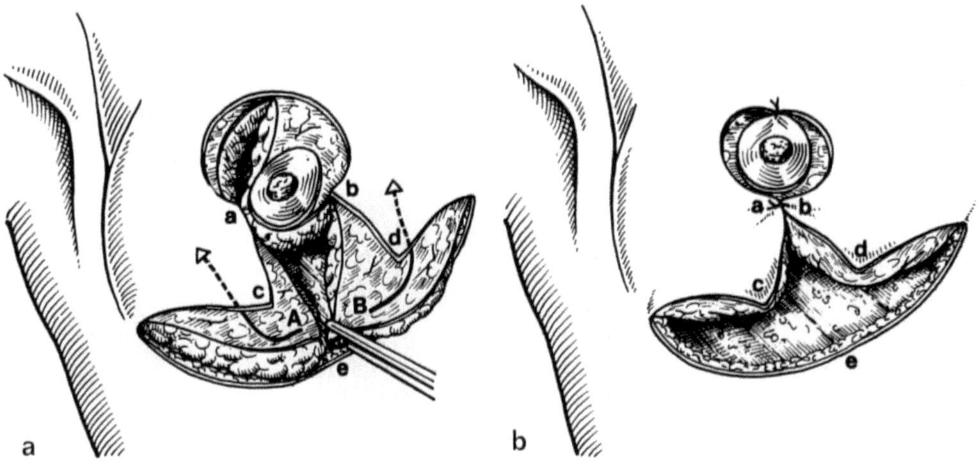

Fig. 10. **a** The flaps *A* and *B* will be used to form the new breast together with the fat left on the base. **b** The areola is placed in the new bed. After suturing point *c* to *d* to *e* the final suture lines are prepared for closure

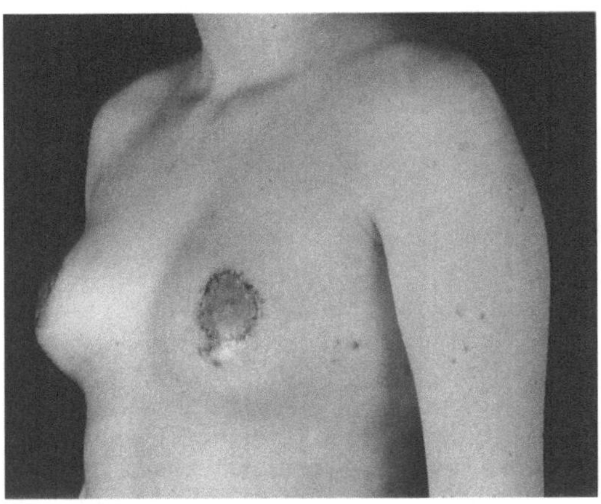

Fig. 11. Patient after modified subcutaneous mastectomy

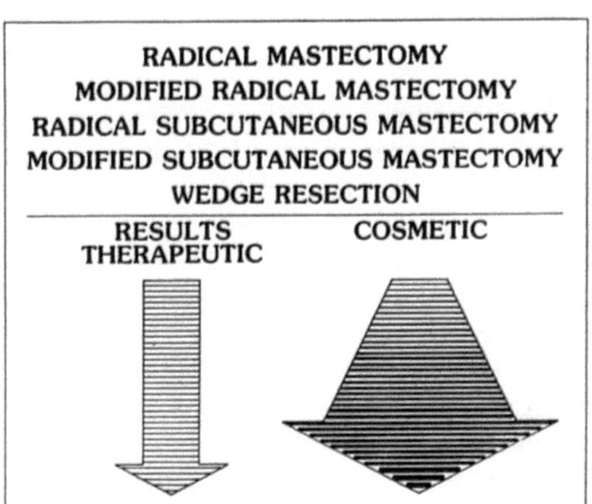

Fig. 12. Surgical treatment modalities and therapeutic versus cosmetic results

Since women obviously accept the cosmetic results of modified subcutaneous mastectomy it can be performed as a prophylactic operation. It is a better surgical procedure, regarding minimal cancer as a multicentric lesion. This type of surgery may prevent fear of screening procedures. When surgical procedures have identical treatment values at least the unilateral ones should be used (Fig. 12). This is not necessarily tylectomy but may be modified subcutaneous mastectomy because the breast is also lifted and therefore cosmetically improved.

References

Adami HO, Bergström R, Hansen J (1985) Age at first primary as a determinant of the incidence of bilateral breast cancer. Cancer 55: 643

Andersen JM, Nielsen, Christensen L (1985) New aspects of the natural history of in situ and invasive carcinoma in the female breast. Verh Dtsch Ges Pathol 69: 88

Beller FK (1985) Atlas der Mammachirurgie. Schattauer, Stuttgart

Beller FK, Schmidt EH (1985) Subcutaneous mastectomy with lymphadenectomy and irradiation for primary treatment of breast cancer. In: Zander J, Baltzer J (eds) Early breast cancer. Springer, Berlin Heidelberg New York, p 296

Beller FK, Schnepper E (1978) Die mammillenerhaltende Operation zur Behandlung kleiner Mammakarzinome. Senologia 3: 27

Beller FK, Schnepper E (1981) Konservative Primärbehandlung des Mammakarzinoms; subkutane Mastektomie, Lymphadenektomie und Bestrahlung. Dtsch Med Wochenschr 106: 329

Beller FK, Wagner H (1980) Klinische Ergebnisse nach Reduktionsplastiken der weiblichen Brust. Geburtshilfe Frauenheilkd 40: 412

Beller FK, Nienhaus H, Niedner W, Holzgreve W (1986) Bilateral breast cancer: the frequency of undiagnosed cancers. Am J Obstet Gynecol 155 (2): 247

Betsill WL, Rosen PP, Lieberman PH, Robbins GF (1963) Intraductal carcinoma. Long term follow up after treatment by biopsy alone. JAMA 239: 63

Biesenberger H (1930) Eine neue Methode der Mammaplastik. Ergänzungen zum gleichnamigen Aufsatz im Zentralbl Chir 33 (1928). Zentralbl Chir 48: 2971

Brown PW, Silverman J, Owens E, Tabor DC, Tertz JJ, Lawrence W (1976) Intraductal "not infiltrating" carcinoma of the breast. Arch Surg 111: 1063

Carter D, Smith RL (1977) Carcinoma in situ of the breast. Cancer 40: 1189

Dupont WD, Page DL (1985) Risk factors for breast cancer in women with proliferative breast disease. N Engl J Med 312: 146

Farrow JH (1970) Current concepts in the detection and treatment of early breast cancers. Cancer 102: 468

Fisher ER, Gregorio R, Redmond C et al (1975) Pathologic findings from the National Surgical Adjuvant Breast Project (protocol no 4). Observations concerning the multicentricity of mammary cancer. Cancer 35: 247

Fisher ER, Fisher B, Sass R, Wickerham L (1984) Pathologic findings from the National Surgical Adjuvant Breast Project (protocol no 4). Bilateral breast cancer. Cancer 54: 3002

Fisher B, Bauer M, Margolese R et al (1985) Five year result of a randomized clinical trial comparing total mastectomy and segmental mastectomy with or without radiation in the treatment of breast cancer. N Engl J Med 312: 665

Foote FW, Stewart FW (1941) Lobular carcinoma in situ. A rare form of mammary cancer. Am J Pathol 17: 491

Fracchia AA, Robinson D, Legaspi A, Greenall MJ, Kinne DW, Groshen S (1985) Survival in bilateral breast cancer. Cancer 55: 1414

Freeman BS (1973) Subcutaneous mastectomy in the treatment of minimal breast cancer. In: Snyderman RK (ed) Symposium on neoplastic and reconstructive problems of the breast. Mosby, St Louis, p 24

Gallager HS, Martin J (1971) An orientation on the concept of minimal breast cancer. Cancer 28: 1505

Gynning J, Jacobsen S, Linell F, Rothman V, Ostberg OG (1975) Subcutaneous mastectomy in 80 patients with breast tumors. Acta Chir Scand 141: 480
Hutter RVP, Foote FW Jr (1969) Lobular carcinoma in situ. Cancer 24: 1081
Kindermann G (1977) Über Definition, Diagnostik und Frühfälle des Mammakarzinoms. Geburtshilfe Frauenheilkd 37: 829
Kochem HG, Schremmer H, Hircher H (1980) Zur Bedeutung der Mamille beim Brustkrebs der Frau, Geburtshilfe Frauenheilkd 40: 32
Kubli F, Lorenz V, Müller A, Weiger H (1984) Die subcutane Mastektomie. Komplikationen und Indikationen. In: Kubli F, von Fournier D (eds) Neue Konzepte der Diagnostik und Therapie des Mammakarzinoms. Springer, Berlin Heidelberg New York
Lagios MD, Gates EA, Westdahl PR et al (1979) A guide to the frequency of nipple involvement in breast cancer. Am J Surg 138: 135
Lagios MD, Westdahl PR, Margolin FR, Rose MR (1982) Duct carcinoma in situ. Cancer 50: 1309
McDivitt RW, Hutter RVP, Foote FW, Stewart FW (1967) In situ lobular carcinoma: a prospective follow up study indicating cumulative patient risk. JAMA 201: 82
Millis RR, Thynne GSJ (1975) In situ intraduct carcinoma of the breast. A long term follow up study. Br J Surg 62: 95
Page DL, Dupont WD, Rogers LW et al (1981) Intraductal carcinoma of the breast: follow up after biopsy only. Lab Invest 44: 49
Peters TG, Donegan WL, Burg EA (1977) Minimal breast cancer: a clinical appraisal. Ann Surg 186: 704
Ringberg A, Palmer B, Linell F (1982) The contralateral breast at reconstructive surgery after breast cancer operation: a histopathological study. Breast Cancer Res Treatm 2: 151
Robbins GF, Berg SW (1964) Bilateral primary breast cancers. Cancer 17: 1501
Rosen PP, Senie R, Schottenfeld D, Ashikari R (1979) Non invasive breast carcinoma. Ann Surg 189: 377
Rosen PP, Braun DW, Kinne DE (1980) Clinical significance of pre-invasive breast carcinoma. Cancer 46: 919
Rosner D, Bedwaniy RN, Baker VJ (1980) Non invasive breast carcinoma. Results of a national survey of the American College of Surgeons. National Survey ACS. Ann Surg 192: 139
Ryan AJ, Griswold MH, Allen EP et al (1958) Breast cancer in Connecticut 1935–1953. JAMA 167: 298
Shah JP, Rosen PP, Robbins GF (1973) Pitfalls of local excision in the treatment of carcinoma of the breast. Surg Gynecol Obstet 136: 721
Smart CR, Myers MH, Gloechler LA (1978) Implications from SEER data on breast cancer management. Cancer 41: 787
Strömbeck JO (1976) Technik und Ergebnisse der subcutanen Mastektomie. 41 Tagung Dtsch Ges Gyn Geb, Hamburg, 28 Sept–2 Oct
Urban JA (1977) Bilateral breast cancer. Biopsy of the centralateral breast. Prog Clin Biol Res 12: 517
Wanebo HJ, Hucos AG, Urban JA (1974) Treatment of minimal breast cancer. Cancer 33: 349
Webber BL, Heise H, Neifeld JP, Cost J (1981) Rise of subsequenz breast carcinoma in a population of patients with in situ. Cancer 47: 2928
Wertheim V, Ozzello L (1980) Neoplastic involvement of the nipple and skinflap carcinoma of the breast. Amer J Surg Path 4: 543

Incipient Prostate Cancer: Definition, Histology, and Clinical Consequences

G. Dhom

Institut für Pathologie, Universität des Saarlandes, 6650 Homburg/Saar, FRG

Initiation, latency, and promotion are the critical phases of malignant growth. Initiation of cancerous growth in the prostate of the aging man is the rule rather than the exception. Examining by step-section prostates taken from autopsies we find latent carcinomas in over 30% of patients over 45 years old (Table 1) (Dhom 1983). Evidence of tumors rises to more than 50% in males over 75 years. With age, tumor volume and the number of tumorous foci in the organ increase. About one-half of tumorous foci reach a diameter of more than 1 cm after the age of 70 years (Fig. 1). Histologically, one can see predominantly well-differentiated carcinomas with increasing tumor volume. However, we also find less-differentiated tumors. Certainly, we deal with a very slow, but constant, cancer growth in the prostate. Unequivocally, this slow growth prevents the majority of tumorous foci from becoming manifest during the patients' lifetime. On the other hand, the malignant process is overtaken by other age-related disorders, for example, by diseases of the cardiovascular system or by secondary tumors, which consequently determine morbidity and mortality.

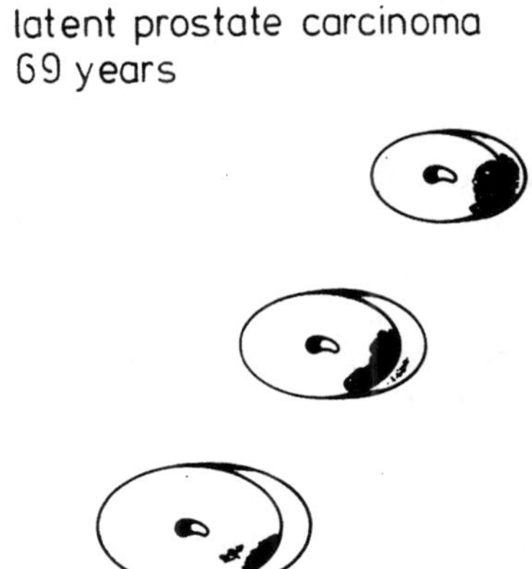

autopsy: 65 to 75 years	n	50
latent carcinomas	n	19
affected slices of the organ	$\bar{x}$	2.5

Fig. 1. Latent cancer at autopsy: tumor focus in three slices: 69-year-old man. Frequency of latent carcinoma in age group 65–75 years

Recent Results in Cancer Research, Vol. 106

Table 1. Frequency of latent prostate carcinoma in autopsy material

Age (years)	*n*	Latent carcinoma	Tumors Ø > 1 cm
45–54	43	8	1
55–64	49	20	6
65–74	50	19	6
> 75	31	16	8
Total	173	63 (36.4%)	21 (12.1%)

Table 2. Prevalence of latent prostate carcinoma

Male population of the Saarland over 45 years of age	168386
Rate of latent carcinomas	36% 60588
First detected clinical carcinomas 1978	245 0.4% of all latent carcinomas

From autopsy findings one can calculate the prevalence of latent prostate carcinomas in a population (Table 2). There is a male population of about 168000 over 45 years of age in the Saarland and a latent carcinoma rate of 36% with a prevalence of 60588 cases. In 1978 – the year concerned – 245 prostate carcinomas were clinically detected, amounting to 0.4% of the rate of prevalence. This low rate is sufficient, however, to put prostate carcinoma in third place of incidence of male cancer diseases.

As worldwide incidence and mortality for prostate cancer differ greatly, some studies have reported on investigations on whether the incidence of latent prostate carcinoma correlates with the incidence of the clinically manifest prostate carcinoma and its mortality. First Akazaki (1973) and Akazaki and Stemmermann (1973) were able to show that the prevalence of latent prostate carcinoma in Japanese in Japan and in Japanese in Hawaii does not differ significantly. There is only a difference when distinguishing histologically between a nonproliferative and a proliferative type. In this case, Japanese migrants to Hawaii show a significantly higher proportion of proliferating but latent carcinomas. Similar conditions were observed by Akazaki (1973) comparing the prevalence of latent carcinomas among Japanese inhabitants from Texas and Louisiana, Hawaii, and Colombia.

The study on latent prostate carcinoma in seven different geographic regions conducted by IARC, Lyon, and published by Breslow et al. (1977) is well known. The Federal Republic of Germany, Sweden, and Jamaica show a relatively high mortality, and Singapore, Hong Kong, Uganda, and Israel a low mortality for prostate carcinoma among the populations involved (Table 3). Analysis of latent carcinoma by a regression model (Fig. 2) shows statistically significant differences between the populations of Singapore and Hong Kong on the one hand, and of Jamaica, the Federal Republic of Germany, and Sweden on the other hand. The differences disappear if only small tumorous foci are considered but appear again if only large tumorous foci are counted. Countries

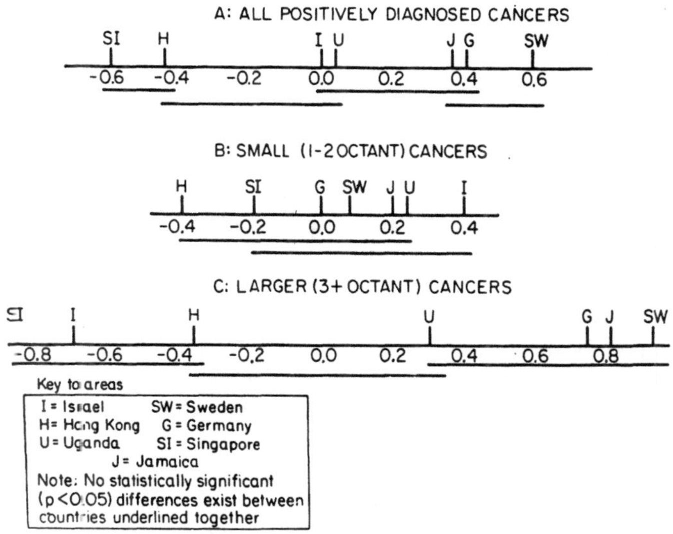

Fig. 2. Latent cancer of the prostate in seven areas. Regression coefficients for area effects. (Breslow et al. 1977)

Table 3. Clinical and latent prostate cancer rates in the seven areas. (Breslow et al. 1977)

Area	Mortality	Incidence	Prevalence
	(per 100000 per year)		(Latent cancer, %)
Singapore	–	3.6	13.2
Hong Kong	2.2	–	15.8
Uganda	–	4.4	19.5
Israel	7.9	14.3	22.0
Jamaica	13.9	20.7	29.8
German Federal Republic	13.9	21.1	28.4
Sweden	18.4	38.8	31.6

with a low mortality have low rates: Singapore, Israel, and Hong Kong, whereas the Federal Republic of Germany, Jamaica, and Sweden have higher rates.

The study proves clearly that not the initiation of cancer growth is responsible for the different mortality rates in the populations examined, but that definite promoting factors must be responsible for tumor progression in populations with high mortality. It is well known that the absolute top position is occupied by the black population of the United States, who have a considerably higher rate of prostate cancer than the white population of the United States.

To date, analytical epidemiology has given only greatly insufficient answers to the question of why prostate carcinoma shows such a worldwide difference in frequency. The remarkably high number of latent prostate carcinomas and its growth tendency with age – a fact that has been known for a long time – have two practical important consequences for all of us, for the patient, for the attending physician, and for the pathologist:

1. So-called precancerous lesions have to be of less importance in the prostate than in other organs.

2. Cancerous foci detected during a patient's lifetime will represent greatly different phases of promotion.

With that we have now come to the topic "minimal neoplasias".

Inevitably, every epithelial neoplasia passes through an in situ stage. We also see intraglandular epithelial atypias in the prostate - mostly in the direct neighborhood of invasively growing carcinomas, which may show the characteristics of cancer cells. A number of studies have dealt with these changes. They use common terms such as atypia or atypical hyperplasia, dysplasia, and carcinoma in situ (Dhom 1985; Helpap 1980, 1983; Kastendieck 1980; McNeal and Bostwick 1986; Tannenbaum 1975). In contrast to respective changes in epithelial surfaces, however, there is no opportunity to follow up concretely the fate of such epithelial variants in solid glandular organs. The structure considered atypical is surgically removed. Thus, we are content with determining whether this change coincides with a carcinoma or not, and we are looking for "transitions".

There is a great margin of interpretation, especially if alterations of the glandular architecture are associated with the definition of atypia and dysplasia. Taking into consideration the variety of age-dependent alterations in the human prostate - hyperplasia and atrophy are parallel processes - we think the terms "atypia" or "dysplasia" for such structural alterations are misinterpreted. Here, cribriform hyperplasia as a special form of benign nodular hyperplasia may be taken as example (Wernert and Dhom 1984).

As we know from epithelial surfaces, the terms "atypia" or "dysplasia" should exclusively be used for cytological or karyological alterations that occur intraglandularly. Such alterations can actually be seen frequently in the neighborhood of manifest carcinomas. There is still the unanswered question of whether a manifest carcinoma secondarily invades still intact glands or whether these epithelial alterations are a true precursor. Hamperl (1974) has reported on the problems of such tissue alterations in the marginal region of a carcinoma. These phenomena only gain practical importance if they occur isolated in biopsy material - without simultaneous proof of an invasively growing carcinoma. In this case, the biopsy has to be repeated. In our biopsy material, lesions solely diagnosed as atypia or suspected tumor are very rare. The reason for that is probably that we prefer to make a definite diagnosis: benign or malignant. Out of 1191 punch biopsies, only 7 cases (or 0.6%) are concerned, i.e., they are suspected cases (Table 4).

According to Mostofi and Price (1973), we do not use the term "carcinoma in situ" in our histologic reports. There is no conformity in its definition and it is without clinical relevance. Of course, it is not at all the right term for the so-called incidental carcinoma found occasionally in nodular hyperplasia. This incidental carcinoma has now been

Table 4. Morphologic findings in punch biopsies of the prostate on clinical suspicion of carcinoma ($n = 1191$)

	n	%
Not representative	103	8.6
Tumor free	674	56.6
Suspicion of carcinoma	7	0.6
Carcinoma	407	34.2

designated as T1 carcinoma in the nomenclature of the UICC, in alteration of the prevailing stage classification (Hermanek 1986). Its practical relevance increases gradually, especially when discussing early detection of prostate cancer. On the long way from latent phase to clinical manifestation, the incidental carcinoma can indicate very different stages of cancerous development. Therefore the differentiation into state T1a and T1b - as already proposed by Jewett in 1975 - is reasonable. These tumors have been classified into A1 and A2 carcinomas in the hitherto existing nomenclature.

The T0 carcinoma is still mentioned in the UICC classification, but unequivocally this term has now become insignificant: It signifies a phantom, a tumor that cannot be seen microscopically. With regard to its definition, the incidental carcinoma cannot be detected by clinical methods. The rectal palpation finding is unsuspected and is mostly determined by simultaneously present benign nodular hyperplasia. So far, the modern imaging techniques have not helped to detect such nonpalpable tumorous foci. These are still dreams of the future to find carcinomatous foci of stage T1 by transrectal sonography (Peeling et al. 1986). Of course, the definition of T1 carcinoma requires normal skeletal findings and normal serum values.

Thus, the detection is reserved for the pathologist who receives biopsy material on the occasion of transurethral resection for benign nodular hyperplasia. The task of finding an incidental carcinoma in such resection material resembles the well-known game at the festival of the bean king. The cake is divided into many slices, but the bean can only be in one slice. The resection material (Table 5) taken by the urologist varies widely, and it stands to reason that our chance of detecting a carcinoma depends on the expansion of our examination. A weight table shows that about 75% of the material we received had a weight up to 30 g. This tissue of 30 g is put into ten paraffin blocks of normal size. In the case of voluminous resection material, most of the histopathologic laboratories make a compromise that should be between the intensity of search for the "bean" and reasonable labor effort (Kastendieck 1984). Our compromise is as follows: The tissue up to 30 g is embedded and examined by step section. If a carcinomatous focus is found in this material, the whole residual material will be embedded and examined.

Proceeding in this way we have detected an incidental T1 carcinoma in 12.1% of all resection material received (Table 6). Formerly, we used to take random samples, obtain-

Table 5. Resected quantity of prostate TUR material

Weight	*n*		Percentage	
Up to 5 g	81		15.1	
Up to 10 g	73		13.6	
Up to 15 g	93		17.4	
Up to 20 g	58		10.8	
Up to 25 g	46		8.6	
Up to 30 g	55	406	10.3	75.8%
Up to 40 g	62		11.6	
Up to 50 g	28		5.2	
Up to 60 g	12		2.2	
Up to 70 g	7		1.3	
Over 70 g	21		3.9	
Total	536		100.0%	

Table 6. Frequency of incidental carcinoma in TUR material

	n	Carcinomas	%
Random sample	523	54	10.3
Complete examination by step section up to 30 g (10 blocks)	653	79	12.1

Table 7. Prostate carcinoma in punch biopsies (1981-1986) and in transurethral resections (1983-1986)

	n	Carcinoma positive	%
Punch biopsies	1191	407	34.2
TUR in BNH	1176	133	11.3

Table 8. Age-dependent frequency of incidental prostate carcinoma in TUR material ($n = 131$ of 1176)

Age	Total number of cases	Incidental prostate carcinomas	
		n	%
30-39	3	0	0
40-49	16	0	0
50-59	165	6	3.6
60-69	391	37	9.5
70-79	493	68	13.8
80-89	105	19	18.1
90-99	2	1	50.0
100-109	1	0	0
Total	1176	131	11.1

ing a result of 10.3%. Let us compare our findings in punch biopsies with those in transurethral resection material: The clinically suspected palpation finding - according to stages T2-T4 - gives rise to a punch biopsy. On the other hand, the indication for transurethral resection is predominantly the obstruction of the urinary tract caused by benign nodular hyperplasia. One can see that there are three histologically confirmed carcinomas of all stages to each incidental carcinoma T1 in examination material of the same volume (Table 7). This is the pathologist's contribution to the subject "early detection of prostate carcinoma".

Looking at the age distribution there is evidence that the rate of incidental carcinoma increases with age (Table 8).

Now, these "early" detected carcinomas have to be classified into T1a and T1b or - as it has been common in the United States-American nomenclature - into A1 and A2 carcinomas (Table 9). With regard to the proposal by the UICC there is primarily only a quantitative classification: up to a maximum of three foci or tumor-positive resection chips we call it a focal T1a carcinoma. If there is an expansion beyond that, it is classified T1b and is considered as a diffusely growing tumor or a multicentric carcinoma.

Table 9. UICC classification of incidental carcinoma of the prostate. (Hermanek 1986)

T1	Incidental histologic finding
T1a	Not more than three microscopic carcinomatous foci
T1b	More than three microscopic carcinomatous foci

Table 10. Histological grading score of prostate carcinoma

	Score	
Highly differentiated adenocarcinoma	0	
		0 poor nuclear anaplasia
Poorly differentiated adenocarcinom	1	
		1 moderate nuclear anaplasia
Cribriform carcinoma	2	
		2 pronounced nuclear anaplasia
Solid carcinoma	3	
Score in total	Grade of malignancy of carcinoma	
0-1	I	
2-3	II	
4-5	III	

Table 11. T1a and T1b carcinomas and histologic grade of malignancy

	n T1a	%	*n* T1b	%
GI	45	70.3	25	41.0
GII	17	26.5	20	32.8
GIII	2	3.2	16	26.2
Total	64	100	61	100

The histologic grading is added to this purely quantitative, but fully schematic, demarcation. I cannot go into further details of the different grading systems here. A pathologic-urologic workshop in the Federal Republic of Germany has agreed on a system based on the proposal by Mostofi (1976) and formulated as a score by Böcking et al. (1982) in which the histologic architecture and degree of nuclear anaplasia are evaluated. The total values are summarized as three degrees of malignancy (Table 10) (Helpap et al. 1985).

Among the T1a carcinomas, about 70% are GI carcinomas. This proportion is about seven times higher than is seen in clinically manifest carcinomas in our biopsy material. In the Tb1 carcinoma the proportion decreases to 41%. On the other hand, here we have 26.8% of GIII carcinomas (Table 11).

Two cases of GIII carcinomas remained in the group of T1a cases, as we want to show that there are individual cases of still small carcinomas which may be malignant.

The subdivision of degrees of malignancy makes it obvious that incidental carcinomas detected by the pathologist represent a very heterogeneous group. Small uniformly well differentiated carcinomas of stage T1a are probably detected in a phase of latency that no longer has any consequences for the patient. Of course, age and life expectancy of the patient are of importance. No major tumor progression occurs. On the other hand, T1b carcinomas represent different phases of promotion. In some cases, the rectal palpation finding has been misdiagnosed by the attending physician. In future, the transrectal sonography should above all enable us to obtain the right diagnosis and a better stage assessment presurgically. This refers mainly to tumors having already exceeded the capsule of the organ. The life expectancy of patients suffering from T1a carcinomas with classification nOMO does not deviate from that of a healthy comparative population. Cantrell et al. (1981) followed up 117 patients with untreated T1 carcinomas for a period of 15 years. None of the patients with A1 or T1a carcinomas showed a tumor progression during the observation period. The extension of the carcinoma and histologic degree of malignancy turned out to be prognostically relevant.

The widely accepted conclusion is now that a prostate carcinoma of stage T1a simultaneously showing a high degree of differentiation requires no therapy. This patient should only be kept under control.

The pathologist's task is to help clinical colleagues arrive at the right diagnostic decision by submitting a reliable diagnosis.

References

Akazaki K (1973) Comparative studies on the prevalence of latent prostate cancer among Japanese, American, and Colombian males. Director's report 1968/69. Aichi Cancer Center Research Institute, Nagoya

Akazaki K, Stemmermann GN (1973) Comparative study of latent carcinoma of the prostate among Japanese in Japan and Hawaii. JNCI 50: 1137-1144

Böcking A, Kiehn K, Heinzel-Wach M (1982) Combined histologic grading of prostatic carcinoma. Cancer 50: 288-294

Breslow N, Chan CW, Dhom G, Drury AB, Franks LM, Gellei B, Lee YS, Lundberg S, Sparke B, Sternby NH, Tulinius HJ (1977) Latent carcinoma of prostate at autopsy in seven areas. Int J Cancer 20: 680-688

Cantrell BB, Deklerk DP, Eggleston JC, Boihott JK, Walsh PC (1981) Pathologic factors that influence prognosis in stage A prostatic cancer. The influence of extent versus grade. J Urol 125: 516-520

Dhom G (1983) Epidemiologic aspects of latent and clinically manifest carcinoma of the prostate. J Cancer Res Clin Oncol 106: 210-218

Dhom G (1985) Histopathology of prostate carcinoma. Diagnosis and differential diagnosis. Pathol Res Pract 179: 277-303

Hamperl H (1974) Präcancerose und Carcinoma in situ. In: Grundmann E (ed) Geschwülste/Tumors I. Springer, Berlin Heidelberg New York, pp 351-416 (Handbuch der allgemeinen Pathologie, vol 6/5)

Helpap B (1980) The biological significance of atypical hyperplasia of the prostate. Virchows Arch [Pathol Anat] 387: 307-317

Helpap B (1983) Praeneoplasien der Prostata. Extr Urol 6: 287-317

Helpap B, Böcking A, Dhom G, Faul P, Kastendieck H, Leistenschneider W, Müller HA (1985) Klassifikation, histologisches und cytologisches Grading sowie Regressionsgrading des Prostatakarzinoms. Pathologe 6: 3-7

Hermanek P (1986) Neue TNM/pTNM-Klassifikation und Stadieneinteilung urologischer Tumoren ab 1987. Urologe [Ausg B] 26: 193-197

Jewett HJ (1975) The present status of radical prostatectomy for stages A and B prostatic cancers. Urol Chir N Am 2: 105

Kastendieck H (1980) Correlations between atypical primary hyperplasia and carcinoma of the prostate. Pathol Res Pract 169: 366-387

Kastendieck H (1984) Klassifikation, Morphologie und Pathogenese des incidenten Prostatakarzinoms. In: Helpap B, Senge T, Vahlensieck W (eds) Prostatacarcinom 2. Prostata-Workshop. pmi, Frankfurt, pp 133-152
McNeal JE, Bostwick DG (1986) Intraductal dysplasia: a premalignant lesion of the prostate. Hum Pathol 17: 64-71
Mostofi FK (1976) Problems of grading carcinoma of prostate. Semin Oncol 3: 161-169
Mostofi FK, Price EB (1973) Tumors of the male genital system. AFIP, Washington (Atlas of tumor pathology, 2nd ser, fasc 8)
Peeling WB, Griffiths GJ, Evans KT (1986) Clinical staging of prostatic cancer. In: Blandy JP, Lytton B (eds) The prostate. Butterworth, London, pp 121-146
Tannenbaum M (1975) Differential diagnosis in uropathology: carcinoma in situ of prostate gland. Urology 5: 143-146
Wernert N, Dhom G (1984) Morphologie und Differentialdiagnose der cribriformen Prostatahyperplasie. Pathologe 5: 27-32

Incipient Cancer of the Colon: Definition and Histology

B. Wiebecke

Institut für Pathologie, Universität München, Thalkirchner Straße 36, 8000 München 2, FRG

In spite of the fact that we know some pathogenetically significant factors, the etiology of colon carcinoma is basically unknown and this has so far prevented a well-founded concept of prevention. For that reason, all activity in clinical medicine has been directed at the recognition and adequate treatment of the very earliest forms of and preliminary changes in this frequent tumor. The resulting interest, which has now been sustained for decades in formal tumor pathogenesis and its individual steps, is an expression of the fact that in this field all problems are by no means solved. Without doubt, however, in the past decades some progress has been made, not least in the conceptual definition of the carcinoma and its early and preliminary stages.

Carcinoma of the colon was defined in 1976 by WHO (Morson and Sobin 1976) as a neoplastic process that crosses the line of the muscularis mucosae. This definition followed indirectly from removing the "focal carcinoma" or "mucosal carcinoma" within adenomas from the concept of carcinoma, which until then was based on purely morphological considerations. On the other hand, the new definition has a pragmatic basis, since statistically lymphogenous metastasis occurs only after infiltration into the submucosa has taken place.

The theoretical background of this definition, which is also adopted for tumors of the colon in animal experiments, is the finding by Fenoglio et al. (1973) that the mucosa of the colon contains practically no proper lymph vessels which a tumor could invade; some lymph vessels are found only directly above the muscularis mucosae (Fig. 1).

In the new version of the TNM classification for 1987 (UICC 1987), the UICC also takes this finding into account and deletes the "mucosal carcinoma" from the T1 category. Whether a signet ring cell carcinoma limited to the mucosa should consequently be termed a "severe signet ring cell dysplasia" is, however, because of the rare occurrence of this observation, rather an academic question.

The category of precancerous neoplasms applies to the adenomas and dysplasias. While it is not difficult to conceive of adenomas in their tubular, tubulovillous, and villous manifestations as of benign neoplasms, especially since histologically they stand out against the surrounding mucous membrane, dysplasias have largely been understood so far as a spectrum of epithelial changes ranging from reactive and reversible to premalignant and irreversible and denoting an indistinct transitional scope between neoplastic and nonneoplastic lesions.

The study of the development of carcinomas in chronic ulcerative colitis by a group of experts under the direction of Riddell (1984; Riddell et al. 1983) has led recently to

Recent Results in Cancer Research, Vol. 106

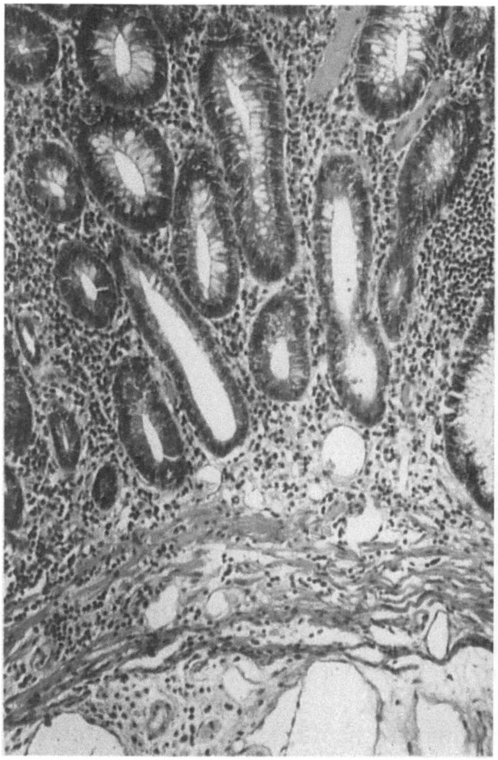
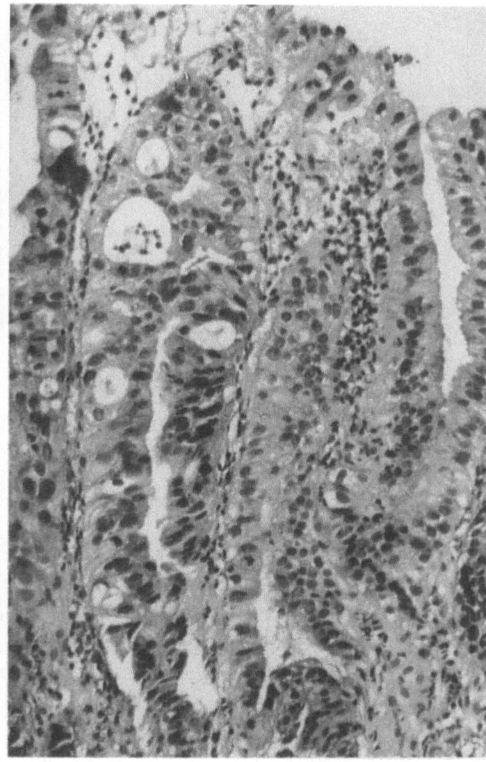

Fig. 1 *(left).* Dilated lymph vessels in submucosa, muscularis mucosae, and just above the muscularis mucosae

Fig. 2 *(right).* Severe epithelial dysplasia in chronic ulcerative colitis, with loss of nuclear polarity and polymorphy of nuclei also present in the upper half of the mucosa

the strong recommendation that only definitively neoplastic epithelial changes in the flat or more or less polypous mucosa should be described as dysplasias and that they should be graded as mild or severe. Essential characteristics of mild dysplasia are a maintained nuclear polarity, nuclear organization only in the basal half of the epithelium, hyperchromasia, and moderate polymorphism. The cytoplasmic differentiation can be very well maintained. This is not the case with severe dysplasia (Fig. 2). Here the nuclear polarity is mostly lost and the pseudostratification of the nuclei is pronounced, extending into the upper half of the epithelial layer.

The definition of dysplasia as a definitive neoplastic change gives rise to a necessary clarification. It is based on the observation, also made occasionally in the past, that in ulcerative colitis even low-grade dysplasia can change directly into infiltrating carcinoma. Consequently, all questionable epithelial changes are no longer covered by the new concept of dysplasia and must therefore be characterized separately.

The mucosal changes preceding adenomas and dysplasias are referred to as preneoplastic. Morphologically they are frequently hyperplasias or deviations of proliferative behavior from the norm. As such, these changes are mostly unspecific. However, in the course of carcinogenesis in animal experiments or in the follow-up of patients with a high risk of colon carcinoma, they are part of a definite pathogenetic sequence.

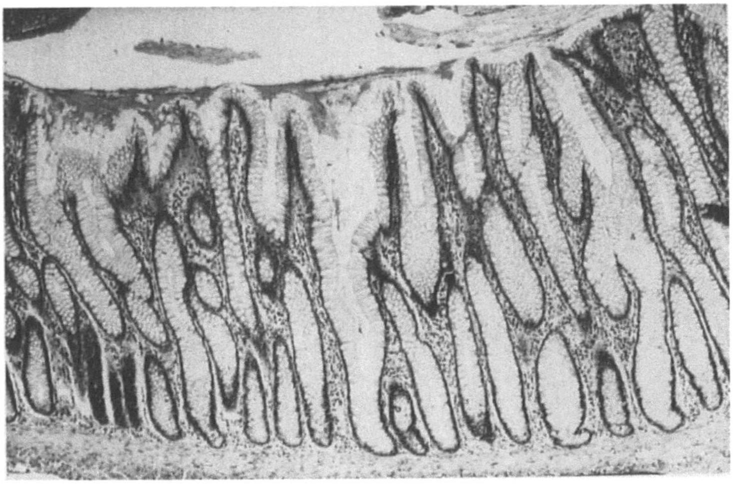

Fig. 3. So-called transitional mucosa from the vicinity of a colon carcinoma: well-differentiated mucosa with crypt divisions

If we now turn to formal pathogenesis, animal experiments show frequent early hyperplastic changes, though these are not regularly confirmed microscopically. They are caused by a permanently increased cell proliferation in a widened proliferative zone (Wiebecke et al. 1973).

Hyperplastic mucosal areas have also been found in high-risk patients, in particular also in asymptomatic relatives of polyposis coli patients, moreover regularly in the vicinity of carcinomas and adenomas (Filipe and Branfoot 1974; Schmidbauer and Heilmann 1985). In addition to crypt divisions (Fig. 3), these areas are characterized by an altered mucus production, with an increase in sialomucins and a reduction in sulfomucins. This type of mucus production is found in neoplasms. The assumption of a frequent transition of these hyperplastic mucosal areas into neoplasms has led to the, in my opinion unfortunate, designation of "transitional mucosa" (Filipe 1969), and by now even so-called transitional polyps (Franzin et al. 1982) are being mentioned. For, the certainty of a progression to neoplasia suggested by this term is, in the majority of such changes, in particular in nonrisk patients, very improbable. The so-called transitional mucosa was found by us and others (Isaacson and Attwood 1979; Lev et al. 1985) also in nonspecific inflammatory intestinal deseases and moreover in the vicinity of metastases, e.g., of a malignant melanoma. Besides, it is remarkable that small and large carcinomas of the colon are invariably surrounded by an approximately 1- to 3-cm-wide ring of transitional mucosa. While, however, for instance an adenoma remnant at the margin of a carcinoma is destroyed by the increasing malignant growth, this border of transitional mucosa around the tumor is always maintained, i.e., it grows with the tumor. This contradicts the preneoplastic precursor status of this change. It seems more likely that this ring of transitional mucosa that becomes shallower according to the distance from the tumor must be attributed to the paracrine influence of growth factors (Coffey et al. 1986) produced by the tumor. Hence the so-called transitional mucosa is an ambiguous alteration and only in high-risk patients is it a possible indicator of a developing neoplasm; frequently, however, it is a reactive and presumably also a reversible phenomenon.

The earliest kinetic proliferation abnormality in the course of cancerogenesis that can be observed in a histologically completely normal mucosa consists of the displacement

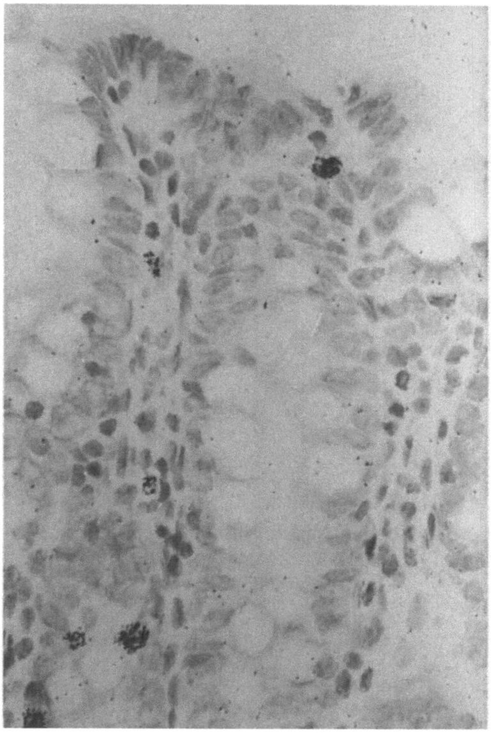

Fig. 4. Autoradiographically labeled DNA-synthesizing cells near the surface in the normal mucosa of a patient with colon carcinoma

of single DNA-synthesizing cells from the proliferative zone in the lower two-thirds of the crypts, up to the mucosal surface. This phenomenon, designated by Deschner (1980) as "stage I abnormality", is observed both experimentally in the rat and in incubated colonic mucosa of high-risk patients (Fig. 4). It is, however, still relatively noncharacteristic and occurs also, as we and others have shown (Wiebecke et al. 1980), as a reversible change in the course of increased regeneration, e.g., in nonspecific inflammations. According to more recent investigations by Deschner (1982), the phenomenon was found in fact in three-fourths, of normal control persons.

Of a different quality and importance is, on the other hand, the transformation designated as stage II (Deschner 1980), in which the proliferative zone has spread to the mouth of the crypts, and at the same time the main proliferative activity is shifted to the upper half of the mucosa.

This phenomenon was observed in 1963 by Cole and McKalen as well as by Deschner et al. (1963), independently of each other, in normal-appearing mucosa of patients with familial adenomatosis and is considered to be an essential cause of adenoma development. However, actual tumor formation ensues, according to Deschner (1980, 1982), only when the index of DNA-synthesizing cells in man exceeds 15% of the crypt population, apparently because cell regeneration is then greater than cell loss.

We have been able to confirm the basic proliferation kinetic transformations in cancerogenesis with an experimental model in rats and mice (Wiebecke et al. 1973). Even in the smallest sessile polyps, [^{3}H] thymidine autoradiography shows a shift in the main activity of DNA synthesis to the surface (Fig. 5). The quantitative evaluation of the index distribution in tubular adenomas (Fig. 6) confirms the optical impression gained histologically and shows the contrast to the conditions in normal and hyperplastic mucosa.

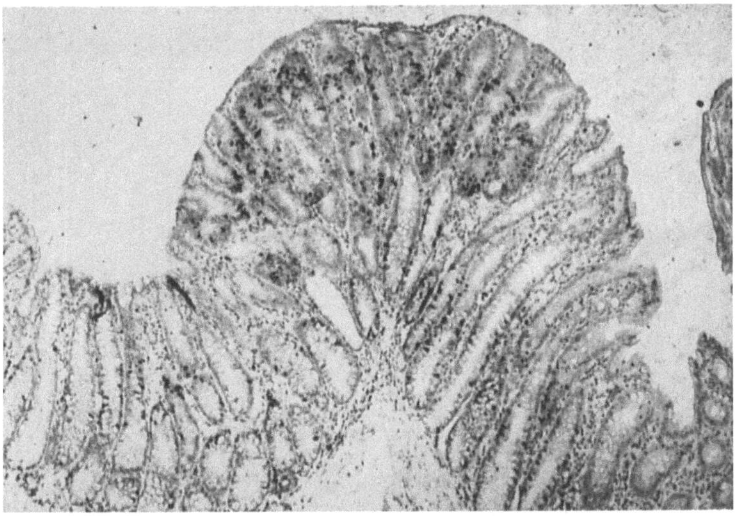

Fig. 5. Incipient sessile tubular adenoma, rat. ^{3}H-labeling pronounced near the surface. (Wiebecke et al. 1973)

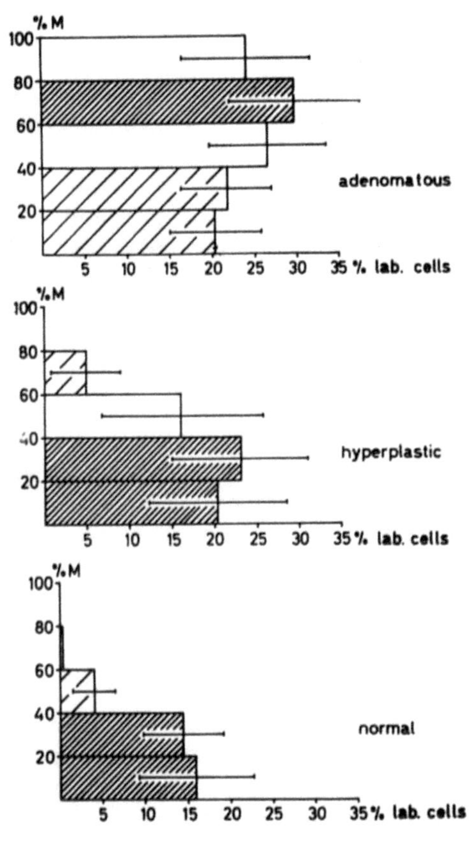

Fig. 6. Distribution of the ^{3}H-index in normal, hyperplastic, and adenomatous colon mucosa of rats. Shift of main activity toward the surface in adenomas. Differences between *loosely* and *closely hatched zones* are significant. (Wiebecke et al. 1973)

The same basic phenomenon is operative also in the development of the very rare villous adenomas in rats (Wiebecke et al. 1973).

The analysis of cellular proliferative activity in human tubular and villous adenomas could only be made with the aid of the mitotic index, which is of course considerably lower than the ^{3}H-labeling index (Wiebecke et al. 1974). Nevertheless, in contrast to normal mucosa and hyperplastic polyps, tubular and villous adenomas showed the same phenomenon of extension of the proliferative zone up to the mucosal surface and a simultaneous upward shift in the main proliferative activity. As substantiated by partial reconstructions, the formal pathogenetic development of tubular adenomas follows a principle well known since at least the 1930s (Patzelt 1936) for the growing intestine. At the site of the most intensive epithelial proliferation in the bottom of the crypts, induction of a connective tissue septa formation takes place which results in a progressive longitudinal subdivision of the crypts from below upward. This phenomenon is also induced in tubular adenomas, though not basally but rather in the particularly strongly proliferating upper mucosal zone, so that here in addition to windings and dilatations, a predominantly glandular division occurs (Fig. 7). The horizontal growth pressure resulting from this mass increase in the upper mucosal layers leads to a fan-shaped expansion of the adenomatous focus in all directions and so to the typical mushroom form of tubular adenomas (Fig. 8). From the above description it follows that tubular adenomas can theoretically arise from a single crypt and hence they may possess a relatively homogeneous cell population.

This does not apply, as we shall see, to the villous adenoma. In the same basic kinetic phenomenon of proliferation, namely a shift of the main proliferative activity to the surface, here the connective tissue induction leads not so much to crypt divisions as to an outsprouting of the intercryptal ridges and so to the formation of villi (Fig. 9). Villous adenomas arise from several to many crypts and, therefore, consist of an inhomogeneous cell population, which is a possible reason for their greater frequency of degeneration.

The key phrase "malignant degeneration" touches upon the theme of the adenoma-carcinoma sequence and so upon a controversy that has been going on for decades and

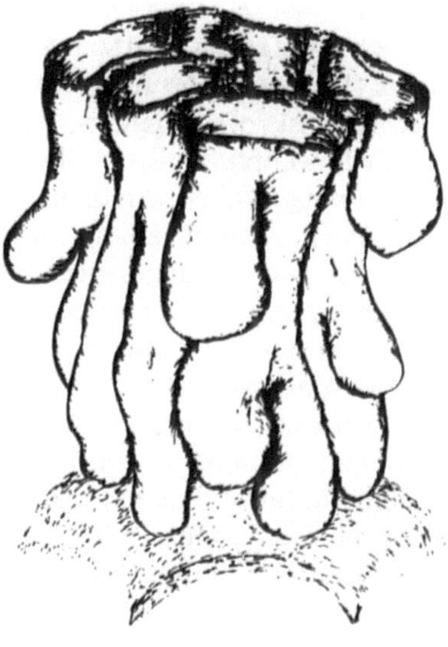

Fig. 7. Graphic reconstruction of a glandular complex with numerous divisions especially *in the upper part.* (Wiebecke et al. 1974)

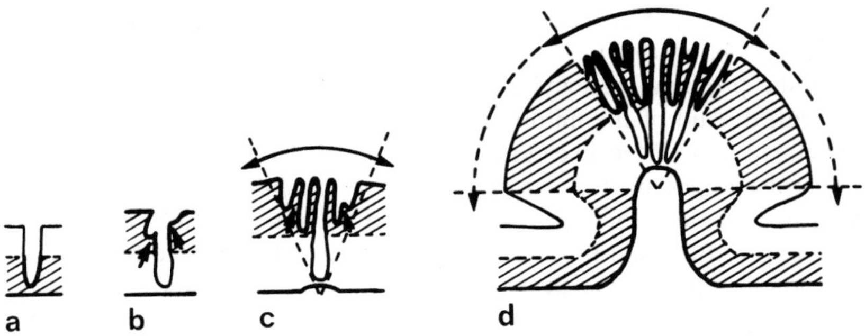

Fig. 8 a–d. Morphogenesis of tubular adenomas (for explanations see text). Zones of main proliferative activity are *hatched;* **a** normal crypt. (Wiebecke et al. 1974)

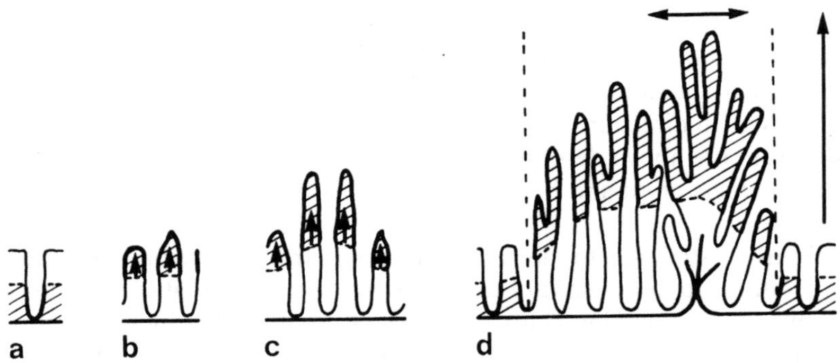

Fig. 9 a–d. Morphogenesis of villous adenomas (for explanations see text). Zones of main proliferative activity are *hatched;* **a** normal crypt. (Wiebecke et al. 1974)

will not come to an end in the near future, because the second step of carcinoma development discussed here can only be proved indirectly. Some of the evidence, however, is very significant and justifies the concept of carcinoma prophylaxis by removing the adenomas, the so-called polypectomy.

High-risk factors for the malignant degeneration of adenomas are by now generally known (Day and Morson; Hermanek et al. 1983). Significant is first of all the histologic type. The risk of malignant degeneration increases considerably from tubular to the tubulovillous and finally to villous adenomas. An equally important factor is the size of the adenoma. While the risk of malignant degeneration of tubular adenomas up to 1 cm in diameter is 1%, it rapidly increases with increasing size of the adenomas. A fundamental support for the assumption of an adenoma-carcinoma sequence is the observation that in large-scale endoscopic statistical surveys no carcinoma foci could be found in adenomas under 4 mm in diameter (Matek 1985).

The form of growth is also important (Hermanek et al. 1983). Broad-based and sessile adenomas degenerate more frequently than pedunculated ones, though here an important additional factor is time, since the early forms of adenomas are always broad based or sessile at first and pediculation ensues as a secondary event. Finally, the degree of atypia is important. In adenomas with a high degree of atypia, carcinomas are found more often than in those with mild atypia. The correlation, however, is not absolute. It is by no means necessary that a severe dysplasia be present, before a carcinoma develops.

At least the Morson group (Day and Morson 1978) has found in one-third of cases of villous adenoma with carcinoma only a slight atypia in the adenoma portion. Frequently, in such cases the carcinomas are also well differentiated.

The infiltration into the submucosa as the decisive histologic criterion of malignancy is not always possible to assess on biopsy material with the desired certainty. In particular, differentiation from a pseudocarcinomatous invasion (Morson and Sobin 1976) should be made. This latter is conceived of as a more or less passive displacement of adenomatous mucosa into the submucosa through the split muscularis mucosae. Aids for the decision are the greater degree of atypia and the desmoplastic stromal reaction in the case of the carcinoma focus, as against the "endometriosis-like" picture with siderin deposition in the case of the pseudoinvasion.

The results of animal experiments concerning the question of an adenoma-carcinoma sequence vary with the species. Mice tend to form exophytic tumors; we have found in the early stages of these tumors predominantly adenomas and later invasive carcinomas with and without surrounding adenomatous parts (Weitz et al. 1984).

In the rat, the detection of purely pedunculated adenomas is very much less common. Generally broad-based polypous and infiltrating tumors develop. We did, however, clearly substantiate that in the rat early infiltrating carcinomas develop in the mucosa of the colon which do not project beyond the level of the mucosa (Wiebecke et al. 1973). These carcinomas fulfill the criteria of a de novo carcinoma, i.e., they do not arise from a polypous adenomatous precursor, but from a flat dysplasia. It is interesting, moreover, that in the autoradiogram of such carcinomas the main proliferative activity is not shifted upward, but remains more or less in the lower half of the mucosa and correlates with the downward direction of the infiltrating growth (Wiebecke 1975). Similar observations have been made in rats by Deschner and Maskens (1982) as well as by Shamsuddin and Trump (1981).

The so-called de novo carcinomas in man have been observed especially following ulcerative colitis, where they may even develop from low-grade dysplasias (Riddell 1984). Apart from this situation in ulcerative colitis, however, de novo carcinoma devel-

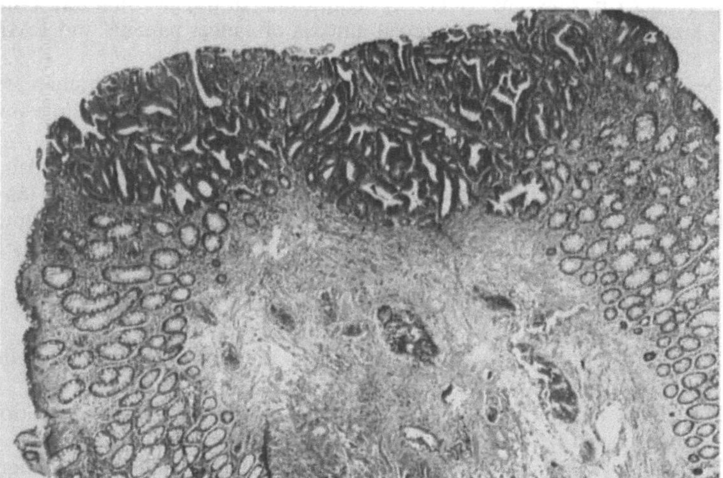

Fig. 10. Small so-called de novo carcinoma in human colon mucosa. Submucosal invasion without exophytic growth or adenoma formation

opment in man is widely considered to be practically nonexistent. This, however, is probably a mistake because, on the one hand, in the biopsy material one still sees occasionally small invasive carcinomas in which no adenoma remnants can be detected (Fig. 10). On the other hand, there are families with a high risk of colon carcinoma which do not develop any associated adenomas (Lipkin 1977).

The fact that during endoscopy the clinician practically does not see any de novo microcarcinomas can be, in addition to the difficulty of detecting small foci and their relatively rare occurrence, also a problem of selection: A tumor that is without early symptoms and grows and infiltrates relatively quickly is at its detection already a surgical case. Thus the question is in fact whether a larger proportion of carcinomas in which no adenoma remnant can be found in the marginal area and where are no associated adenomas in the rest of the colon do not represent the so-called de novo carcinomas after all. And if frequency estimations of 10%-20% for this tumor group (Fenoglio et al. 1973) should prove to be valid, then surely this would no longer be a *quantité negligeable*. The frequently voiced opinion that in man practically all carcinomas of the colon develop from adenomas in any case seems by no means established.

References

Coffey RJ, Shipley GD, Mores HL (1986) Production of transforming growth factors by human colon cancer lines. Cancer Res 46: 1164-1169

Cole JW, McKalen A (1963) Studies on the morphogenesis of adenomatous polyps in the human colon. Cancer 16: 998-1002

Day DW, Morson BC (1978) The adenoma-carcinoma sequence. In: Bennington JL (ed) The pathogenesis of colorectal cancer. WB Saunders, Philadelphia, pp 58-71 (Major problems in pathology, vol 10)

Deschner EE (1980) Cell proliferation as a biological marker in human colorectal neoplasia. In: Winawer SJ, Schottenfeld D, Sherlock P (eds) Colorectal cancer: prevention, epidemiology and screening. Raven, New York, pp 133-142

Deschner EE (1982) Early proliferative changes in gastrointestinal neoplasia. Am J Gastroenterol 77: 207-211

Deschner EE, Maskens AP (1982) Significance of the labelling index and labelling distribution as kinetic parameters in colo-rectal mucosa of cancer patients and DMH-treated animals. Cancer 50: 1136-1141

Deschner EE, Lewis CHM, Lipkin M (1963) In vitro study of human rectal epithelial cells. I. Atypical zone of H^3-thymidine incorporation in mucosa of multiple polyposis. J Clin Invest 42: 1922-1928

De Schryer-Keckemeti K (1986) Large intestine. In: Henson DE, Albores-Saavedra J (eds) The pathology of incipient neoplasia. Saunders, Philadelphia, pp 147-166

Fenoglio CM, Kaye IG, Lane N (1973) Distribution of human colonic lymphatics in normal, hyperplastic and adenomatous tissue. Its relationship to metastasis from small carcinomas in pedunculated adenomas, with two case reports. Gastroenterology 64: 51-66

Filipe MI (1969) Value of histochemical reactions for mucosubstances in the diagnosis of certain pathological conditions in the colon and rectum. Gut 10: 577-586

Filipe MI, Branfoot AC (1974) Abnormal pattern of mucous secretion in apparently normal mucosa of large intestine with carcinoma. Cancer 34: 282-290

Franzin G, Scarpa A, Dina R, Zamboni G, Fratton A (1982) "Transitional polyps" of the colon. Endoscopy 14: 174-175

Hermanek P, Frühmorgen P, Guggemoos-Holzmann J (1983) The malignant potential of colorectal polyps - a new statistical approach. Endoscopy 15: 16-20

Isaacson P, Attwood PRA (1979) Failure to demonstrate the specifity of the morphological and histochemical changes in mucosa adjacent to colonic carcinoma. J Clin Pathol 32: 214-218

Lev R, Lane P, Camora P (1985) Mucosa bordering rectosigmoid carcinomas. Hum Pathol 16: 151-161

Lipkin M (1977) The identification of individuals at high risk for large bowel cancer. An overview. Cancer 40: 2523-2530

Matek W (1985) Die Entwicklung kolorektaler Adenome. In: Bartelheimer H, et al. (eds) Gastroenterologie und Stoffwechsel, Bd 22. Thieme, Stuttgart, p 19

Morson BC, Sobin LH (1976) Histological typing of intestinal tumours. In: WHO (ed) International histological classification of tumours, no 15. World Health Organization, Geneva, p 56

Patzelt V (1936) Der Darm. In: Möllendorf W (ed) Handbuch der mikroskopischen Anatomie des Menschen, vol 5/3. Springer, Berlin

Riddell RH (1984) Dysplasia and cancer in ulcerative colitis: a soluble problem? Scand J Gastroenterol [Suppl 104] 19: 137-149

Riddell RH, Goldman H, Ransohoff DF, Appelman HD, Fenoglio CM, Haggitt RC, Ahren C, et al. (1983) Dysplasia in inflammatory bowel disease: standardized classification with provisional clinical applications. Hum Pathol 14: 931-968

Schmidbauer G, Heilmann KL (1985) Morphology and histochemistry of the mucosa surrounding small oligotubular adenomas of the large bowel. Pathol Res Pract 180: 45-48

Shamsuddin AKM, Trump BF (1981) Colon epithelium. II. In vivo studies of colon carcinogenesis. Light microscopic, histochemical, and ultrastructural studies of histogenesis of azoxymethane-induced colon carcinomas in Fischer 344 rats. INCI 66: 389-401

UICC (1987) TNM Klassifikation der malignen Tumoren 4. Aufl. Hermanek P, Scheibe O, Spiessl B, Wagner G (Hrsg). Springer, Berlin Heidelberg New York London Paris Tokyo

Weitz H, Kirscheneder C, Wiebecke B, Eder M (1984) The effect of cholecystectomy on the induction of colorectal tumors in mice by 1,2-dimethylhydrazine. Res Exp Med 184: 59-65

Wiebecke B (1975) Experimentelle Cancerogenese des Magen-Darm-Kanals. B. Darm. In: Grundmann E (ed) Geschwülste/Tumors III. Springer, Berlin Heidelberg New York, pp 731-767 (Handbuch der allgemeinen Pathologie, vol 6/7)

Wiebecke B, Krey U, Löhrs U, Eder M (1973) Morphological and autoradiographic investigations on experimental carcinogenesis and polyp development in the intestinal tract of rats and mice. Virchows Arch [A] 360: 179-183

Wiebecke B, Brandts A, Eder M (1974) Epithelial proliferation and morphogenesis of hyperplastic adenomatous and villous polyps of the human colon. Virchows Arch [A] 364: 35-49

Wiebecke B, Brandts A, Eder M (1980) Morphogenesis of hyperplastic polyps and tubular and villous adenomas of the colon with regard of underlying proliferative changes. 17th International Congress of SMIER (Société Internationale d'Endoscopie et de Ratiocinéma), Bruxelles 1980

*Immunological Approaches for Early Cancer Detection**

D. M. Goldenberg

Center for Molecular Medicine and Immunology, One Bruce Street, Newark, NJ 07103, USA

Immunological Markers and Early Cancer

Much discussion at this meeting has been devoted to the terms and definitions of "incipient" and "minimal" cancer. Since there is confusion in the literature on these issues, it is not surprising that we are also encountering difficulties. Defined as the initial stage of cancer, "incipient" is not recognized by biochemical or immunological means. If minimal refers to a clinical stage indicating localized disease, then the potential of a biochemical or immunological marker being recognized at this time is more likely than for a molecular or cellular alteration associated with incipient cancer. The diagnostic use of biochemical or immunological markers of cancer in body fluids, particularly blood, has been disappointing for diagnosing cancer since this appears to depend very much on tumor burden, or cell number. Thus, minimal cancer has generally escaped detection by biochemical or immunological means, but the likelihood is greater that a marker is determined at the site of neoplasia than peripherally, such as in body fluids. In summary, the current status of the use of cancer markers in the blood and most other body fluids does not allow early detection or even a definitive diagnosis of cancer to be made. The general application seems to be for the use of such markers in the blood for *monitoring* tumor growth, recurrence, or regression. A prototype marker has been the carcinoembryonic antigen (CEA) originally described by Gold and Freedman (1965). The severe limitation of most serum markers for cancer has been a poor specificity as compared with a relatively high sensitivity, thus precluding their diagnostic use, especially in early cancer. Nevertheless, markers which are quantitatively increased with neoplasia may be useful for locating sites of cancer which are missed by conventional, nonimmunological detection measures, particularly the visual approaches of radiology. This chapter will review the use of specific anticancer antibodies as targeting agents for radionuclides used in the external scintigraphic detection of cancer, a method termed "cancer radioimmunodetection" at an earlier meeting organized by the conveners of this meeting and its chairman, Professor Grundmann (Goldenberg 1979).

---

* The author's studies are supported in part by an Outstanding Investigator Grant Award (CA-39841) from the National Cancer Institute, NIH.

Recent Results in Cancer Research, Vol. 106

Animal Studies of Cancer Targeting with Radiolabeled Antibodies

When we began our studies of cancer radioimmunodetection in 1972, a body of literature already existed on the use of radiolabeled antibodies for cancer detection and therapy (reviewed by Goldenberg et al. 1979). Although some localization of tumors could be found in animal tumor models, it was not clear that this could be achieved in humans, particularly since specific antibodies against human cancers were not available. At the time of our initial interest, the two most prominent human tumor antigens were CEA and alpha-fetoprotein (AFP). Since both were released by tumors into the patient's circulation, it was commonly believed that antigen in the blood would bind any injected radiolabeled antibody, thus preventing tumor localization. Thus, even if animal models of human cancer were available, and showed that antibodies against human tumor antigens could localize in the antigen-bearing tumors selectively, the contribution or problem of the presence of the antigen in a patient's blood and possibly in small quantities in other organs was not predictable in such systems. On the other hand, clinical studies could not be justified if good tumor localization in these animal models was not demonstrated. Therefore, we needed to develop a suitable human tumor/antigen model, and evaluate the conditions for specific antibody localization.

Development of a Human Tumor/Antigen Model

Human tumors were xenografted to immunosuppressed rodents in the late 1950s and early 1960s for use in chemotherapy testing (Goldenberg 1967). Unfortunately, the low rate of establishment of human tumors in these models, and their general resistance to anticancer drugs, made them relatively unpopular. In 1964, Professor Grundmann, then associated with Farbenfabriken Bayer of Leverkusen, helped initiate my efforts to establish new human tumor transplant models, resulting in a number of human tumor xenografts, particularly the GW-39 and GW-77 human colonic carcinomas propagated in unconditioned, adult hamsters (Goldenberg et al. 1966; Goldenberg 1967). These were shown to have retained properties of their human and colon tumor origins, based upon karyotypic, isoenzymic, and immunologic evidence (Lampert et al. 1968; Goldenberg et al. 1970, 1976; Munjal and Goldenberg 1976). However, what proved to be an even more fascinating observation was the production of highly metastatic tumors in hamsters after grafting human tumors to their cheek pouches (Goldenberg 1968; Goldenberg and Gotz 1968). Karyological and biochemical evidence suggested to us that these highly malignant tumors in hamsters were of human/hamster hybrid origin, with a rapid loss of most of the human chromosomes of the tumor graft (Goldenberg 1971; Goldenberg et al. 1971, 1974a; Goldenberg and Pavia 1974). However, in situ hybridization methods were not available to us, so that the molecular demonstration of human genome in the resulting tumors was not achieved. Thus, it was not possible to secure definitive proof that the first examples of in vivo transfection were being observed. In later years, we were able to reproduce this or a similar phenomenon in nude mice receiving human tumor xenografts; we observed the production of highly malignant mesenchymal tumors in the murine stroma of human tumor xenografts (Goldenberg and Pavia 1981a, b; 1982).

The human colonic carcinoma xenografts in hamsters that retained their human properties and morphology provided the first evidence that an antigen such as CEA was in fact produced by the cancer cells themselves (Goldenberg and Hansen 1972; Goldenberg et al. 1972). Accordingly, these tumor systems could be used for antibody localization studies and for imaging these tumors by external photoscanning methods (Goldenberg et al. 1974b). Human choriocarcinoma xenografts producing chorionic gonadotropin (HCG) were also used for radioimmunodetection studies (Quinones et al. 1971).

Assessment of Tumor Xenograft Models for Antibody Targeting

Since human tumor xenograft models have negligible quantities of human tumor-associated antigens in the animal's normal tissues and blood, they are idealized methods for demonstrating tumor localization or therapy with anticancer antibody isotope- or drug-conjugates. Another very significant limitation is the discrepancy between antibody uptake in tumor xenografts and patients. Whereas tumor transplants in animals show values of 3%–40% of the injected dose per gram 2 or more days after antibody injection, patient tumors have only 0.001%/g, or less, uptake. Still another problem with animal models is the usual site of tumor growth. Human tumors are frequently transplanted in subcutaneous sites of the animal irrespective of the tumor's organ of origin in man, thus being highly artificial in growth pattern and vascularization to the autochthonous situation. Finally, neoplasms in man are more heterogeneous than their counterparts in cell culture or in serial xenografts, where population selection occurs with the processes of explantation or transplantation. Indeed, this may contribute to the higher antibody uptake seen in xenografts than in patient tumors. Accordingly, the animal systems of human xenografts are not to be considered as predictors of antibody localization or therapy of tumors in patients, where many more factors play a role. They merely provide comparative information on the localization and binding characteristics of different antibodies. Here again, the character of the tumor transplant is very important, since xenografts vary in antigen content and presentation, morphology, cell viability, vascularization, and vascular permeability, etc.

Despite these limitations, many interesting experimental studies related to tumor localization with anticancer antibodies have appeared, some of which have led to successful clinical findings. Of course, it is more difficult to assess which experimental results could not be corroborated clinically, since these findings usually are not reported.

Prior to venturing to clinical studies of radioimmunodetection, we decided to study this problem in a subhuman primate. Having successfully grafted human colonic carcinomas to the hamster cheek pouch, I sought to grow these same tumor systems in monkeys. Stumptail monkeys *(Macaca speciosa)* were available to us from a Tobacco and Health Research Institute study at the University of Kentucky, and since their smoking did not result in bronchial neoplasms, we were provided with an opportunity to utilize them in tumor transplantation studies. (It should be mentioned that the failure of bronchogenic tumors to develop is not surprising since the experimental subjects were taught merely to draw smoke into their mouths without inhaling. This was fortunate for the animals, for the tobacco supporters, and those of us in need of a gift of healthy monkeys for other research.) Transplantation of the GW-39 human colonic carcinoma from hamsters to the cheek pouch of these monkeys who received antilymphocyte serum for immunosuppression resulted in viable tumors for the 3 or more weeks required for radioimmunodetection studies. We found that goat anti-CEA IgG labeled with I-125, as compared with a radiolabeled, control goat antiperoxidase IgG, gave specific tumor localization and external imaging, with very high tumor/nontarget ratios (Goldenberg et al. 1979). Again, however, the monkeys did not have detectable CEA in other tissues or fluids, thus presenting an idealized situation as compared with humans. The ultimate results in patients could not be predicted, especially in the presence of high blood titers of CEA.

In our clinical experience, CEA has been a useful target for localizing radiolabeled antibodies (Goldenberg et al. 1978). However, the experimental and clinical results indicate some of the problems that are encountered with many human tumor antigen and antibody systems. Although we have been studying antibody localization and therapy of the xenografted human colonic carcinoma producing CEA since 1972 (Primus et al. 1973; Goldenberg et al. 1974b), including the use of hamster, monkey, and nude mouse models, we appreciate that a considerable number of questions still need to be resolved. These include the nature of the ideal antibody, the dose and dose schedule of antibody administered, the role of antibody mixtures, the site of tumor and its vascularization, the role of tumor antigen content and location, and the problems of circulating antigen and the patient's production of antibody against the injected antibody.

Factors Influencing Tumor-Targeting (Table 1)

The character of the antibody preparation continues to attract attention. The ideal tumor-targeting antibody should be directed against a target antigen that is tumor specific and abundantly available and accessible to the antibody. It should be selectively reactive with the tumor-specific antigen, nonimmunogenic in the patient, and abundantly available in an inexpensive and identically reproducible form. It should also have very high immunoreactivity, affinity, and avidity against the target antigen. Unfortunately, as yet no anticancer antibody has achieved these attributes. It is generally acknowledged that an antibody fragment, lacking the Fc portion of the immunoglobulin molecule, is preferred for imaging. In therapy, however, the fragment may show a decreased affinity and binding to tumor, as compared with whole immunoglobulin, and therefore may be less desirable than the latter unless given in high doses. The fragments clear more rapidly from background and nontarget tissues and are less immunogenic to

Table 1. Factors influencing radioimmunodetection

1. Character of radioantibody	4. Tumor antigen availability
Immunoreactivity	Density in tumor versus elsewhere
Isotype	Expression/modulation
Avidity	Cellular location
Affinity	5. Character of label
Specificity	Specific activity
2. Injection site	Linkage to antibody
Intravenous	Retention/degradation at site
Interstitial	Clearance/excretion
Intracavitary	Photon yield
3. Antibody availability	6. Target
Dose	Site of tumor/organ
Degradation	Distance from collimator
Binding to nontarget tissues	Size
Complexation to circulating antigen	Composition
Complexation with human antibody	Vascularization
	Vascular permeability

the recipient. Fragments may be rearranged to form hybrid antibody molecules, each end having a different target specificity, or re-engineered to form antibody chimers having a murine variable region and a human constant region, thus circumventing or mitigating a patient's immunological response to murine immunoglobulin. In addition to antibody form, isotype may also influence antibody targeting. Immunoglobulin-G preparations have been used most frequently for tumor-targeting, and would appear, because of the relatively low molecular size and ease of production, to be the preferred antibody isotype for use in isotope or drug immunoconjugates.

Monoclonal antibodies are directed against single antigen determinants, or epitopes. Although generally desirable from the aspects of purity, reproducibility, and production of antibody reagents, such monoclonals may not have the binding capacities of conventional or affinity-purified polyclonal antibodies. It has been proposed that mixtures of monoclonal antibodies may be preferred for radioimmunodetection or antibody therapy over single antibody preparations, since multiple antigen determinants would be targeted. Support for this view is found in experiments with purified polyclonal antibodies against CEA and colon-specific antigen-p (CSAp), which showed that the mixtures resulted in better tumor localization than with the single radiolabeled antibody preparations (Gaffar et al. 1981). Recent studies with monoclonal antibodies against different antigens have supported this observation (Munz et al. 1986), but other work involving mixtures of antibodies against different epitopes of the same antigen failed to show any significant localization advantage for the mixtures (Primus et al. 1984). Insufficient studies have been undertaken in this area, either for imaging or for therapy, so that the value of different antibody combinations needs to be assessed for each tumor and antibody system. It may well be that a complex mixture is needed in certain circumstances. The precise definition of such reagent mixtures can be considered the development of "engineered polyclonal antibodies."

Once the antibody enters the circulation, distribution and elimination kinetics are influenced by a number of factors, including vascularization and vascular permeability at the tumor and other sites of the body, complexation with circulating antigen, nonspecific binding to certain tissues and cells, binding to antigen in nontarget tissues when the antigen is not tumor specific, and accessibility and density of the target antigen sites. Finally, a number of still inadequately defined factors control the degradation and release (tumor residence) of the antibody from the tumor, as well as from other tissues.

Experiments in animal models rarely include repeated injections of xenogeneic immunoglobulins for imaging, and only short-term experiments for therapy. This explains why little attention was given to the production of anti-antibodies by the host animal. In humans, however, this has proved to be a major problem in the use of murine or other antibodies, since human antibodies against the foreign immunoglobulins result in rapid complexation, degradation, and clearance of these reagents, while presenting a real risk of hypersensitivity or anaphylactic reactions by the patient. We have also recently found that such anti-antibodies, such as against murine monoclonal antibodies, can result in a falsely elevated CEA blood titer when using current assay methods (Primus et al. 1987). This host sensitization to foreign immunoglobulins led Order (1984) to introduce the use of cyclic antibody therapy, where the antibody's host species would be varied in any therapy schedule. Others are attempting to develop human monoclonal antibodies, or chimeric antibodies involving the antigen-binding variable region of the murine monoclonal antibody and the constant region of a suitable human immunoglobulin.

Ultimately, the ability of a radiolabeled antibody to image a target lesion depends upon the ratio of counts in the area of interest to the counts in adjacent tissues. The absolute number of counts per collimator pixel influences image resolution. Not only does the antibody distribution determine such ratios, but also do the character of the radiolabel (photon yield), the size of the tumor, the organ involved, and the distance of the focus of radioactivity from the collimator.

Problems and Prospects of Clinical Cancer Radioimmunodetection

Imaging results with radiolabeled polyclonal or monoclonal antibodies have shown similar problems and successes, but the number of reports has flourished since the introduction of hybridoma technology for the production of murine monoclonal antibodies (Keenan et al. 1985; DeLand and Goldenberg 1986). Improvements have undergone a rapid progression, as reviewed recently elsewhere (Goldenberg et al. 1987). Suffice it to say that these advances have involved the nature of the antibody, the radionuclide, and the imaging process.

Antibodies for Radioimmunodetection

The first well-defined antibody system used for cancer radioimmunodetection in humans was for CEA, and showed a high rate of true-positive imaging, including the disclosure of occult lesions (Goldenberg et al. 1978). This involved the use of an affinity-purified goat antibody having an immunoreactivity with CEA of more than 70% and a very high affinity. The antibody was labeled with I-131 at a high specific activity (10-15 Ci/g IgG) without reducing CEA immunoreactivity. Images were made at 24 and 48 h after antibody administration, but these early scans required the use of a computer-assisted subtraction method for reducing nontargeted blood-pool and interstitial radioactivity, as discussed below. Following these encouraging results in CEA-producing tumors, other successful imaging studies were reported with polyclonal antibodies against other circulating tumor markers, such as AFP, human chorionic gonadotropin, and prostatic acid phosphatase (DeLand and Goldenberg 1986; Goldenberg et al. 1987). An intriguing and unexpected observation was that circulating levels of these antigens complexed with the injected antibody, yet tumor imaging was feasible (Primus et al. 1980). Murine monoclonal antibodies against these same tumor markers have also been tested clinically, and the results appear to correlate well with earlier findings involving polyclonal antibodies (Goldenberg, unpublished results). Monoclonal antibodies against a number of putatively new tumor-associated antigens have been developed in recent years and have been shown to be useful for disclosing tumors by radioimmunodetection, even when these antibodies do not appear to have application in immunoassays of blood and other body fluids (see reviews by Keenan et al. 1985; Begent 1985; DeLand and Goldenberg 1986). It is particularly interesting that there is considerable crossreactivity of tumor targets in different types of cancer even when the monoclonal was prepared against a specific tumor type, and with sufficiently little crossreactivity with normal tissues so as to permit tumor localization. Furthermore, a number of studies have shown that use of antibody fragments permits earlier imaging without background subtraction methods. Whether $F(ab')_2$ or Fab' fragments are preferred will be determined in part by the antibody/antigen system and the radionuclide used.

Radionuclides in Radioimmunodetection

Almost all of the initial imaging studies involved the use of I-131 attached to antibodies since this radionuclide is relatively inexpensive and the iodination of proteins, including antibodies, has been achieved in a simple and stable manner. However, iodinases in tissues result in deiodination of I-131 very rapidly, with accretion of free iodine in the thyroid and gut, and rapid excretion via the urine. Further, the high energy of I-131 (364 keV) necessitates the availability of a special high-energy collimator. From this vantage, I-123 is preferred, since its energy is in the medium range and thereby detectable by conventional gamma cameras. However, it is currently considerably more expensive than I-131. The other two radionuclides of choice for antibody imaging are In-111 and Tc-99m. After I-131, most antibody imaging studies have been undertaken with In-111, using a DTPA chelate for linkage to the antibody. It appears that most of these DTPA linkers release enough In-111 for deposition in RES organs, particularly the liver. This excess In-111 deposition makes it difficult to differentiate In-111 in tumor versus In-111 in liver, the major site of solid tumor metastasis. Therefore, methods are in development for improving the conjugation of In-111 to antibodies. Similarly, Tc-99m, perhaps the most desirable (low price and excellent imaging characteristics), requires improved chelation to antibody so as to achieve a very stable complex. It should be noted that the short half-lives of I-123 and Tc-99m require an antibody form that permits rapid localization and excretion of nontargeted radioactivity, such as is the case for Fab'.

Image Processing

We have found that tumor/nontumor ratios of an average of about 2.5 are found at 24–48 h after antibody administration (Goldenberg et al. 1980), increasing to more than 5:1 after about 5–6 days. Thus, planar imaging is first achieved at about a week without special image processing methods, such as computer-assisted background subtraction. At ratios of 2.5:1 or less, early imaging in the major blood pool regions, such as the chest and liver/spleen areas, is best achieved with background subtraction. This involves the preimaging injection of a blood pool/interstitial agent with a radionuclide of an energy that can be differentiated from that of the antibody's radionuclide, thus permitting computer-assisted subtraction of background nontargeted radioactivity, pixel-by-pixel, from antibody-associated radioactivity. The background reagent can be Tc-99m human serum albumin and Tc-99m pertechnetate, or I-123-labeled irrelevant immunoglobulin. If a region of interest is known or suspected, low tumor/nontumor ratios can still result in disclosure of the lesion if single-photon computed emission tomography (SPECT) is used, particularly with I-123, In-111, or Tc-99m.

Another approach to reducing background, nontargeted radioactivity so as to achieve early imaging is the use of second antibody, or antiantibody (Sharkey et al. 1984; Goldenberg et al. 1987). In order to rapidly reduce nontargeted antibody in the circulation and at certain tissues, an antibody made against the radiolabeled antibody is injected, resulting in complexes with nontargeted primary antibody. These complexes are localized in the RES organs, particularly liver and spleen. When I-131-labeled primary antibodies are used, the radioactivity of the complexes is cleared rapidly from the blood and most tissues, including the liver, thus achieving high early tumor/nontumor ratios without the use of computer-assisted subtraction methods. Whether this functions as well with radiometals attached to the primary antibody remains to be determined.

Current Results in Clinical Cancer Radioimmunodetection

Regardless of the antibody, antibody form, or imaging process used, the sensitivity of tumor detection is generally between 80% and 90% with I-131-labeled antibodies and between 50% and 60% for In-111 antibodies. The lower sensitivity for the latter is probably due to the high retention of In-111 in normal liver, the major site of tumor metastasis. However, when In-111 is deposited in peripheral tumors, including lymph nodes, the images appear superior to corresponding I-131 scans. It is interesting that with both I-131-labeled and In-111-labeled antibodies, occult tumor lesions have been described in many clinical studies of radioimmunodetection. Indeed, it has been our experience with CEA radioimmunodetection that about 20% of our case studies have occult sites first revealed by radioimmunodetection and confirmed up to 1 year later by conventional radiological methods or by surgery (Goldenberg et al. 1984).

The current resolution of radioimmunodetection, regardless of antibody, label, or imaging process, appears to be in the range of 1.5–2 cm. The smallest tumor lesions identified with radiolabeled antibodies are 0.4–0.5 cm, and this was achieved with Tc-99m-labeled antibodies in melanoma (Siccardi et al. 1986). Given the problems of circulating a foreign antibody in the body and targeting sufficient radioactivity counts for detecting by an external camera, it is impressive that tumors of such small dimensions can be imaged. Although neoplasms of 0.5 cm still contain a half-billion cells, this resolution is nevertheless encouraging that radioimmunodetection methods may indeed identify early and occult cancer sites. It is unlikely, however, than this will include incipient neoplasia, although the latter may indeed be a suitable target for antibody-mediated therapy if disclosed by other measures.

References

Begent RHJ (1985) Recent advances in tumor imaging: use of radiolabelled antitumour antibodies. Biochim Biophys Acta 780: 151–166

DeLand FH, Goldenberg DM (1986) Radiolabeled antibodies: radiochemistry and clinical applications. In: Freeman & Johnson's clinical radionuclide imaging. Grune and Stratton, Orlando, pp 1915–1992

Gaffar SA, Pant KD, Shochat D, Bennett SJ, Goldenberg DM (1981) Experimental studies of tumor radioimmunodetection using antibody mixtures against carcinoembryonic antigen (CEA) and colon specific antigen-p (CSAp). Int J Cancer 27: 101–105

Gold P, Freedman SO (1965) Specific carcinoembryonic antigens of the human digestive system. J Exp Med 122: 467–481

Goldenberg DM (1967) The use of several new human tumor lines in experimental cancer research, parts I and II. Arch Geschwulstforsch 29: 1–36

Goldenberg DM (1968) On the progression of malignancy: an hypothesis. Klin Wochenschr 46: 898–899

Goldenberg DM (1971) Stathmokinetic effect of colcemid on a presumptive human-hamster hybrid tumor, GW-478. Exp Mol Pathol 14: 134–137

Goldenberg DM (1979) CEA and other tumor-associated antigens in colon cancer diagnosis and management. In: Grundmann E (ed) Colon cancer. Fischer, Stuttgart, pp 163–168

Goldenberg DM, Gotz H (1968) On the "human" nature of highly malignant heterotransplanted human gastrointestinal tumors. Eur J Cancer 4: 547–548

Goldenberg DM, Hansen HJ (1972) Carcinoembryonic antigen present in human colonic neoplasms serially propagated in hamsters. Science 175: 117–118

Goldenberg DM, Pavia RA (1974) Role of somatic cell fusion in the progression of malignancy. In:

5th International Symposium on the Biological Characterization of Human Tumors, Bologna. Excerpta Medica, Amsterdam, pp 290-297

Goldenberg DM, Pavia RA (1981a) Malignant potential of murine stromal cells after transplantation of human tumors into nude mice. Science 212: 65-67

Goldenberg DM, Pavia R (1981b) Horizontal transmission of malignant conditions rediscovered. N Engl J Med 305: 283-284

Goldenberg DM, Pavia R (1982) In vivo horizontal oncogenesis by a human tumor in nude mice. Proc Soc Natl Acad Sci USA 79: 2389-2392

Goldenberg DM, Witte S, Elster K (1966) A new human tumor serially transplantable in the golden hamster. Transplantation 4: 760-763

Goldenberg DM, Bhan RD, Pavia RA (1970) Retention of human properties by a xenografted human colonic tumor, GW-77, propagated in unconditioned hamsters. Proc Soc Exp Biol Med 135: 657-659

Goldenberg DM, Bhan RD, Pavia RA (1971) In vivo human hamster somatic cell fusion indicated by glucose-6-phosphate dehydrogenase and lactate dehydrogenase profiles. Cancer Res 31: 1148-1152

Goldenberg DM, Pavia RA, Hansen HJ, Vandevoorde JP (1972) Synthesis of carcinoembryonic antigen in vitro. Nature [New Biol] 239: 189-190

Goldenberg DM, Pavia RA, Tsao MC (1974a) In vivo hybridization of human tumor and normal hamster cells. Nature 250: 649-651

Goldenberg DM, Preston DF, Primus FJ, Hansen HJ (1974b) Photoscan localization of human GW-39 tumors in hamsters using radiolabeled anti-CEA IgG. Cancer Res 34: 1-9

Goldenberg DM, Pant KD, Dahlman HL (1976) Antigens associated with normal and malignant gastrointestinal tissues. Cancer Res 36: 3455-3463

Goldenberg DM, DeLand F, Kim E, Bennett S, Primus FJ, van Nagell JR Jr, Estes N, DeSimone P, Rayburn P (1978) Use of radiolabeled antibodies to carcinoembryonic antigen for the detection and localization of diverse cancers by photoscanning. N Engl J Med 298: 1384-1388

Goldenberg DM, Primus FJ, DeLand F (1979) Tumor detection and localization with purified antibodies to carcinoembryonic antigen. In: Herberman RB, McIntire KR (eds) Immunodiagnosis of cancer, part 1. Dekker, New York, pp 265-304

Goldenberg DM, Kim EE, DeLand FH, Bennett SJ, Primus FJ (1980) Radioimmunodetection of cancer with radioactive antibodies to carcinoembryonic antigen. Cancer Res 40: 3008-3012

Goldenberg DM, Kim EE, Bennett SJ, Nelson MO, DeLand FH (1984) CEA radioimmunodetection in the evaluation of colorectal cancer and in the detection of occult neoplasms. Gastroenterology 84: 524-532

Goldenberg DM, Sharkey RM and Ford EH (1987) Anti-antibody enhancement of iodine-131-anti-CEA radioimmunodetection in experimental and clinical studies. J Nucl Med 28: 1604-1610

Keenan AM, Herbert JC, Larson SM (1985) Monoclonal antibodies in nuclear medicine. J Nuct Med 26: 531-537

Lampert F, Karsch P, Goldenberg DM (1968) Chromosomes of hetero- and homotransplanted human and hamster tumors. Arch Geschwulstforsch 32: 309-321

Munjal D, Goldenberg DM (1976) A study of carcinembryonic antigen and glucose phosphate isomerase in human colonic cancer and in the GW-39 human tumor model. Br J Cancer 34: 227-231

Munz DL, Alavi A, Koprowski H, Herlyn D (1986) Improved radioimaging of human tumor xenografts by a mixture of monoclonal antibody $F(ab')_2$ fragments. J Nucl Med 27: 1739-1745

Order SE (1984) Radioimmunoglobulin therapy of cancer. Compr Ther 10: 9-18

Primus FJ, Wang FH, Goldenberg DM, Hansen HJ (1973) Localization of human GW-39 tumors in hamsters by radiolabeled heterospecific antibody to carcinoembryonic antigen. Cancer Res 33: 2977-2982

Primus FJ, DeLand FH, Goldenberg DM (1984) Monoclonal antibodies for radioimmunodetection of cancer. In: Wright G (ed) Monoclonal antibodies in cancer. Dekker, New York, pp 305-323

Primus FJ, Kelley EA, Hansen HJ, Goldenberg DM (1987) Sandwich immunoassay for carcinoembryonic antigen in patients receiving murine monoclonal antibodies for diagnosis and therapy. Clin Chem 33

Primus FJ, Wang RH, Goldenberg DM, Hansen HJ (1973) Localization of human GW-39 tumors in hamsters by radiolabeled heterospecific antibody to carcinoembryonic antigen. Cancer Res 33: 2977-2987

Quinones J, Mizejewski G, Beierwalter WH (1971) Choriocarcinoma scanning using radiolabeled antibody to chorionic gonadotropin. J Nucl Med 12: 69-75

Sharkey RM, Primus DJ, Goldenberg DM (1984) Second antibody clearance of radiolabeled antibody in cancer radioimmunodetection. Proc Natl Acad Sci USA 81: 2843-2846

Siccardi AG, Buraggi GL, Callegaro L, Mariani G, Natali PG, Abbati A, Bestagno M et al (1986) Multicenter study of immunoscintigraphy with radiolabeled monoclonal antibodies in patients with melanoma. Cancer Res 46: 4817-4822

Therapeutic Consequences of Minimal Neoplasia of the Colon

J. W. Cole

Yale University School of Medicine, New Haven, CT, USA

The diagnosis of minimal neoplasia of the colon may pose difficult choices for the responsible clinician as well as the patient. As diagnostic techniques become more specific and more accurate, the decision to intervene therapeutically and what type of therapy to employ may become increasingly difficult.

It is imperative that, once detected, the focus or foci of malignant cells be eradicated and to do so with as little discomfort and disability to the host as possible. It is fortunate that the colon and rectum are expendable organs in the sense that many individuals can and do live long and productive lives following their removal. However, it is to be hoped that with newer and more precise diagnostic methods, earlier recognition of malignant lesions will allow therapeutic measures less radical than colectomy and proctectomy for cancer.

Substantial progress toward this goal has been made during the past decade and it is the purpose of this essay to review briefly some of these advances and how they are currently applied.

Perhaps the most dramatic of these newer therapeutic modalities is the colonoscope. The introduction and perfection of this instrument in our therapeutic armamentarium has truly revolutionalized the management of many patients with malignant and premalignant lesions of the bowel. The colonoscope in experienced hands serves not only in the diagnosis of colonic pathology but in the therapy as well.

If one subscribes to the theory that most adenocarcinomas of the colon arise from preexisting adenomas, then clearly adenomatous polyps should be sought out when suspected and excised when found. The colonoscopist can do both in the majority of cases.

The question that may arise clinically is what is the proper therapy when we are informed by the pathologist that the adenomatous polyp which has been removed contains a focus of malignant change - or minimal neoplasia. The issue briefly stated is - whether or not simple polypectomy with the colonoscope is adequate treatment?

In most instances, the problem is easily resolved. If the malignant focus is well differentiated histologically; if the muscularis mucosa has not been invaded; if there is no evidence of perineural or venous invasion and if the margins of the polyp are free of tumor, most pathologists and clinicians would agree that no further treatment is required. However, when all or several of these criteria do not obtain, differences of opinion may arise regarding the need for further treatment.

Most workers would agree that where the margins of the polyp are not free of tumor, indicating inadequate removal, further treatment is indicated. This can range from fulgu-

Recent Results in Cancer Research, Vol. 106

ration through the colonoscope of the excision site to laparotomy and segmental resection of the involved bowel.

Likewise, when an experienced pathologist reports the focus of malignant change to be highly undifferentiated with invasion of the muscularis mucosa, the risk of lymph node metastasis is substantially increased and additional surgery may be indicated. It should be pointed out, however, that this is a rare occurrence having been noted in only 4% of the cases of malignant polyps in Morson's et al. (1984) series from St. Marks Hospital in London.

The decision to resort to major surgery or not in any given case may be further tempered by other health-related conditions of the patients and their ability to withstand a major surgical procedure. In the very old patient with limited cardiorespiratory or renal reserve, conservatism may be in the patient's best interest.

In most institutions today where colonoscopy has become an integral part of therapeutic practice, the *need for surgery* in managing the problem of minimal neoplasia has been strikingly reduced.

In addition, colonoscopic polypectomy can be carried out with a much lower morbidity and mortality rate than that which accompanies surgical procedures.

One of the largest series of colonoscopic polypectomies is that reported by Shinya et al. (1982) and serves to reinforce the view that surgical intervention in the management of minimal neoplasia arising in an adenoma is seldom required.

In Shinya's series, 8753 polyps of the colon were removed colonoscopically, 6382 or 73% were completely benign, 888 or 10% were read as showing severe displasia, 1009 or 12% were interpreted as having carcinoma in situ, and 474 or 5% were reported as "malignant polyps".

Thus, 27% of the 8753 polyps removed had histological evidence of malignant change of varying degrees. It is noteworthy, however, that only 75 patients in this large series were thought to require colon resection for their disease and in only 3 patients was a focus of residual tumor found. In only one patient was a lymph node found with a metastatic deposit.

The experience at the Yale-New Haven Hospital (K. Barwick, personal communication) parallels that of Shinya and his group and the lesson seems clear that the early recognition of minimal neoplasia in polyps of the colon can be easily and effectively managed in the vast majority of cases with colonoscopic removal. This is particularly true in the case of *pedunculated* lesions where the task of complete excision is technically much easier. When dealing with *sessile* lesions not only is greater skill required in order to remove the lesion in its entirety but the risk of malignant change is statistically greater as well, particularly if the histological configuration is that of a villous adenoma. Under these circumstances close cooperation between the clinician and the pathologist is required if the proper choice of therapy is to be made. Fortunately, villous adenomas, which are more likely to harbor minimal neoplastic change, constitute only about 10% of the polypoid lesions encountered in the colon and rectum and only 16% of these will demonstrate minimal neoplasia or early invasive carcinoma (Morson et al. 1984).

While adenomatous polyps are the principal site of minimal neoplasia of the colon, other pathological conditions may show early malignant change that call for therapeutic intervention. One such disease is familial polyposis. An inherited disease, transmitted genetically as an autosomal dominant trait, it is manifest early in life, usually in the teens, by the appearance of multiple adenomas of the colon and rectum. If untreated, the patient can be expected to develop one or more adenocarcinomas in 100% of the cases.

Because of the inevitable outcome of the disease, and its multifocal nature, one seldom waits for a definitive diagnosis of minimal neoplasia before instituting therapy and preventive measures are usually instituted shortly after diagnosis. Until quite recently this meant subjecting the patient to a total coloproctectomy and the construction of a permanent abdominal ileostomy. While it is true that many patients have led and continue to lead full and productive lives with this artificial abdominal stoma, alternative therapies have continually been sought. One of the earliest attempts at maintaining intestinal continuity following removal of the colon and rectum was by Nissen of Berlin in 1933. He was the first to anastomose the terminal ileum to the anus. Since then, others have struggled to maintain the normal route of evacuation for these patients while at the same time removing the threat of colon cancer (Ravitch and Sabiston 1947). Their efforts have met with varying degrees of success. At the present time, the so-called Parks procedure (Parks and Nicholls 1978), named after the late Sir Alan Parks of St. Mark's Hospital, holds the most promise of not only preventing cancer development in the colon by total extirpation but maintaining the continent passage of feces through the anal canal as well. This is accomplished by the removal of the entire colon, followed by excision of the diseased rectal mucosa and the anastomosis of the ileum to anus within the muscular rectal cuff. In order to create a sufficiently large fecal reservoir in the terminal ileum, various pouches have been constructed – the so-called "J pouch" seems to be the most popular at the present time (Becker and Raymond 1986).

This is not an easy technical procedure and surgeons who choose to perfect this operation should be prepared to have discouraging results initially. However, with experience and meticulous attention to detail the results can be very gratifying.

A 2-year follow-up of a group of patients undergoing the procedure at the Mayo Clinic is summarized (Beart et al. 1984).

1. After 2 years, 7% of the patients required reoperation for a variety of reasons; 98% were satisfied and 6% noted no change.
2. Stool frequency averaged 5 during the daylight hours and once during the night; 67% reported no leakage while 33% had occasional spotting.

This procedure has also gained favor as a means of dealing with the problem of minimal neoplasia that may occur in conjunction with chronic ulcerative colitis.

Although the view that long-standing ulcerative colitis may undergo malignant change in a substantial percentage of cases has been called into question, the consensus still holds that these patients are at an increased risk of cancer (Riddle 1984). Efforts continue to find methods of determining at the earliest possible time when malignant change has occurred or is imminent. Thus far detection of minimal neoplasia remains difficult and the early report of Morson and Pang (1957) describing mucosal dysplasia in mucosal biopsies of chronic ulcerative colitis remains the best clue to the presence of incipient carcinoma. However, this is a highly subjective technique with significant observer error. If a diagnosis of minimal neoplasia is made, or the disability associated with long-standing disease is no longer acceptable, a colectomy and rectal mucosectomy with an ileal anal anastomosis may be a desirable option.

Ulcerative colitis is essentially a disease of the mucosa and the removal of the epithelial lining of the rectum along with the colon precludes the development of adenocarcinomas in these diseased organs.

The ileal pouch, anal anastomosis procedure therefore is equally appropriate in these two disease states both of which are known to be the forerunners of minimal neoplasias, and the results are encouraging in both. The frequency of stools is not appreciably different when the operation is performed for chronic ulcerative colitis or familial polyposis.

This operation continues to gain worldwide favor as a means of combatting not only established instances of malignancy but is particularly desirable when minimal neoplasia is diagnosed.

Thus today one can say with reasonable confidence that minimal neoplastic lesions of the colon and rectum presenting in adenomatous polyps can be successfully treated in the majority of cases by colonoscopic means by snare excision, fulgeration, or laser beam. Where the disease involves the entire colon and rectum and the risk of minimal or occult neoplasia is great as in ulcerative colitis or familial polyposis, colonoscopic treatment may not be feasible and a more extensive procedure may be indicated. Under these conditions, a colectomy, rectal mucosectomy, and ileal pouch anal anastomosis may be required.

This operation may also be considered should some of the as yet unproven diagnostic methods achieve a high degree of accuracy in detecting minimal neoplasia.

At the present time, one can only speculate about the impact that the monoclonal antibodies may have in identifying a cell or cluster of cells with the capacity for autonomous growth, or the use of supravital stains in uncovering alterations in the colonic mucosa which may be associated with malignancy (Isaacson 1982) and visualized with the techniques of chromoscopy. Recent interest in flow cytometry to quantify tumor DNA content may help in determining the biological behavior of a given lesion not otherwise predictable by standard histological features and thereby modify the therapeutic approach (Wolley et al. 1982; Goh and Jass 1986).

Still, other changes in some of the more newly recognized cellular proteins, i.e., villin, may foretell malignant change. This protein, a part of the cytoskeleton, is unique in brush border epithelium and is known to be altered when abnormal growth occurs. Similarly, there is evidence of certain increased enzyme activity (i.e., ornithine decarboxylase and polyamine levels) in neoplasms of the colorectal epithelium (LaMuraglia et al. 1986).

In brief, there continues to be many promising leads for ways of detecting the appearance of minimal neoplasia and the therapeutic consequences of these revelations must be such as to rid the body of the threat and to do so without disfiguring or disabling the host.

References

Beart RW, Metcalf AM, Dozois RR, Kelley KA (1984) The ileal pouch-anal anastomosis: the Mayo Clinic experience. In: Dozois RR (ed) Alternatives to conventional ileostomy. Yearbook Medical Publishers, Chicago, pp 384–397

Becker JM, Raymond JL (1986) Ileal pouch-anal anastomosis. A single surgeon's experience with 100 consecutive cases. Ann Surg 204: 375–381

Goh NS, Jass JR (1986) DNA content and the adenoma: carcinoma sequence in the colorectum. J Clin Pathol 39: 387–392

Isaacson PA (1982) Immunoperoxidase study of the secretory immunoglobulin system in colonic neoplasia. J Clin Pathol 35: 14–25

LaMuraglia GM, Lacaine F, Malt RA (1986) High ornithine decarboxylase activity and polyamine levels in human colorectal neoplasia. Ann Surg 204: 89–93

Morson BC, Pang LSC (1957) Rectal biopsy as an aid to cancer control in ulcerative colitis. Gut 8: 423–434

Morson BD, Whiteway JE, Jones EA (1984) Histopathology and prognoses of malignant colorectal polyps treated by endoscopic polypectomy. Gut 25: 437-444
Nissen R (1933) Demonstrationen aus der operativen Chirurgie. Zunächst einige Beobachtungen aus der plastischen Chirurgie. Zentralbl Chir 60: 883
Parks AG, Nicholls RJ (1978) Proctocolectomy without ileostomy for ulcerative colitis. Br Med J 2: 85-88
Ravitch MM, Sabiston DL Jr (1947) Anal ileostomy and preservation of the sphincter: a proposed operation in patients requiring total colectomy for benign lesions. Surg Gynecol Obstet 84: 1095-1099
Riddle RH (1984) Dysplasia and cancer in ulcerative colitis: a solvable problem? Scand J Gastroenterol 19 [Suppl 104]: 137-149
Shinya N, Cooperman A, Wolff WL (1982) A rationale for the endoscopic management of colonic polyps. Surg Clin North Am 62: 861-867
Wolley RC, Schneiber K, Kass LG, Karas M, Sherman A (1982) DNA distribution in human colon carcinomas and its relationship to clinical behavior. JNCI 69: 15-22

Early Cancer of the Lung

K.-M. Müller

Institut für Pathologie, Berufsgenossenschaftliche Krankenanstalten "Bergmannsheil Bochum", Universitätsklinik, Gilsingstraße 14, 4630 Bochum, FRG

Considering the early stages of lung cancer, we encounter numerous terms in the clinical and pathological-anatomical literature, such as: occult carcinoma, microcarcinoma, microfocally invasive carcinoma, miniature carcinoma, microscopic carcinoma, "minute" carcinoma, early cancer, tumorlets, stage 0 and 1 carcinoma, symptomless, and nearly invisible carcinoma (review of literature in Eck et al. 1969).

The first, mostly casuistic, reports in the literature microscopic carcinomas of the lung date back as early as 1925.

The terms used today in connection with minimal neoplasms and early stages of lung cancer are:

1. Occult carcinoma
2. Early carcinoma
3. Microcarcinoma
4. Tumorlets
5. T_1 carcinoma

Up to now, clinical, endoscopic, and morphological parameters were used simultaneously to define these terms for neoplasms of the bronchi and the lung. This results in understandable occasional difficulties in evaluation and interpretation of findings concerning clinical and prognostic consequences. From the morphological point of view, a clear demarcation of early neoplasms of the lung has to be made between the clearly defined preneoplasms (for review see Müller 1983; Gonzalez et al. 1986) and advanced stages of carcinomas, similar to corresponding findings in other organs.

Included in the preneoplasms are dysplasia and carcinoma in situ of the bronchial system. For these findings, defined clearly by histomorphological criteria, an own group B was established, which lies between the benign (group A) and malignant (group C) epithelial lung tumors of the Second Histological Classification of Lung Tumors by the WHO 1981.

Occult Lung Cancer

The term "occult lung cancer" was introduced as early as 1951 by Papanicolaou and Koprowska, meaning a carcinoma presenting with negative X-ray findings and positive cytology of sputum, and has gained wide acceptance in the clinical literature (for review

Recent Results in Cancer Research, Vol. 106

of the literature see Wilde 1985). To date, occult carcinomas of the bronchi have been observed in only 1-2‰. Generally, 10-18 months pass between the cytological diagnosis of the tumor and the first roentgenological findings. Some roentgenological occult carcinomas of the bronchi can today be detected by means of bronchoscopy. The symbol Tx has been established in the TMN system of the UICC (1979) for tumor diagnosis by demonstration of malignant tumor cells in the sputum only. Preoperative occult carcinomas can turn out as any tumor stage up to T3 tumor (Cortese et al. 1983; Kubik and Polak 1986).

Early Cancer

For the last few years, malignant tumors of the lung have been recognized in the minimal neoplasm stage by extended use of endoscopic-bioptic examinations. Corresponding to terms used with other organs, e.g., the stomach, a bronchial or pulmonary early cancer can be differentiated. The diagnosis of "early cancer of the bronchus" can only be obtained by examination of a surgically removed specimen. The decisive criterion for diagnosis is limitation of the local infiltrating growth of tumor to the different layers of the bronchial wall, which means the tumor tissue must not exceed the outer tunica fibrocartilaginea and the adjacent lung tissue must not be infiltrated. According to the definition, an invasion of lymph vessels or pleura and lymph node metastasis must be excluded (Brockmann and Müller 1986).

Macroscopically, a polypoid intraluminal and a superficially ulcerating type can be differentiated (Figs. 1, 2). The polypoid type can easily be found by means of bronchoscopy in the main and segmental bronchi and may lead to symptoms of local disturbance of ventilation with atelectasis or obstructive pneumonia in a relatively early stage. Concerning the differential diagnosis, rare bronchial papillomas or carcinoid tumors may cause similar symptoms. The superficially ulcerating type of early cancer macroscopically shows a granulated, irregular structure of the mucosa (Fig. 3).

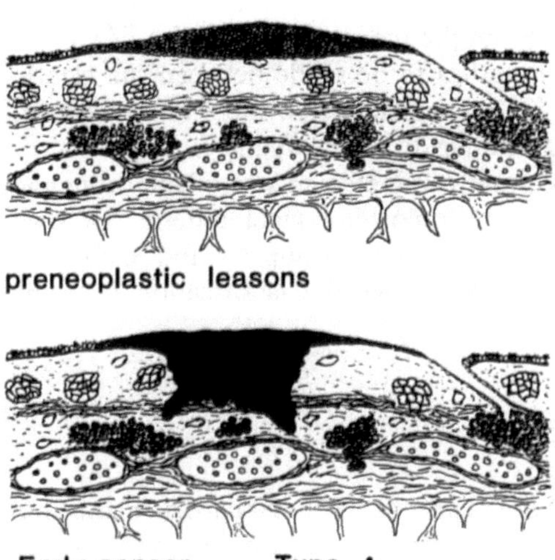

Fig. 1. Bronchial early cancer of the hilar type

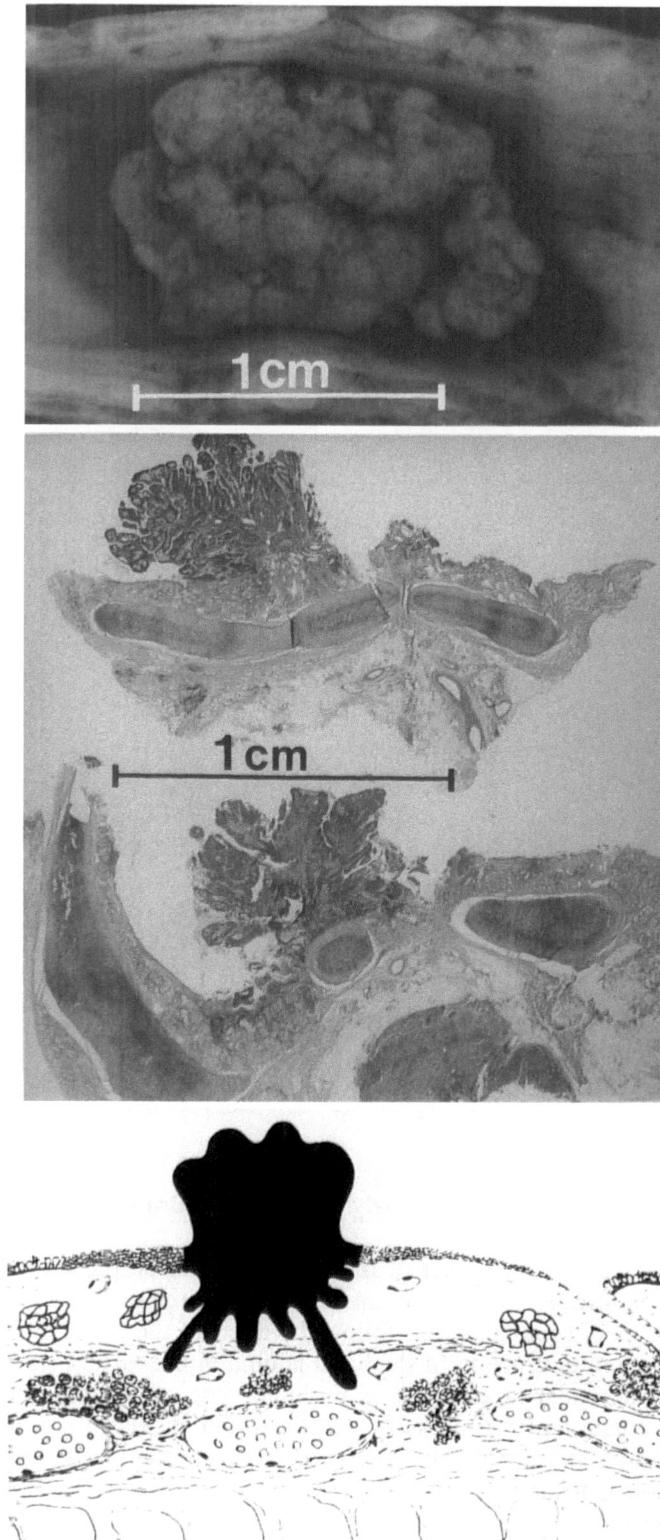

Fig. 2. Macroscopic and microscopic photographs and scheme of the polypoid type of central early cancer

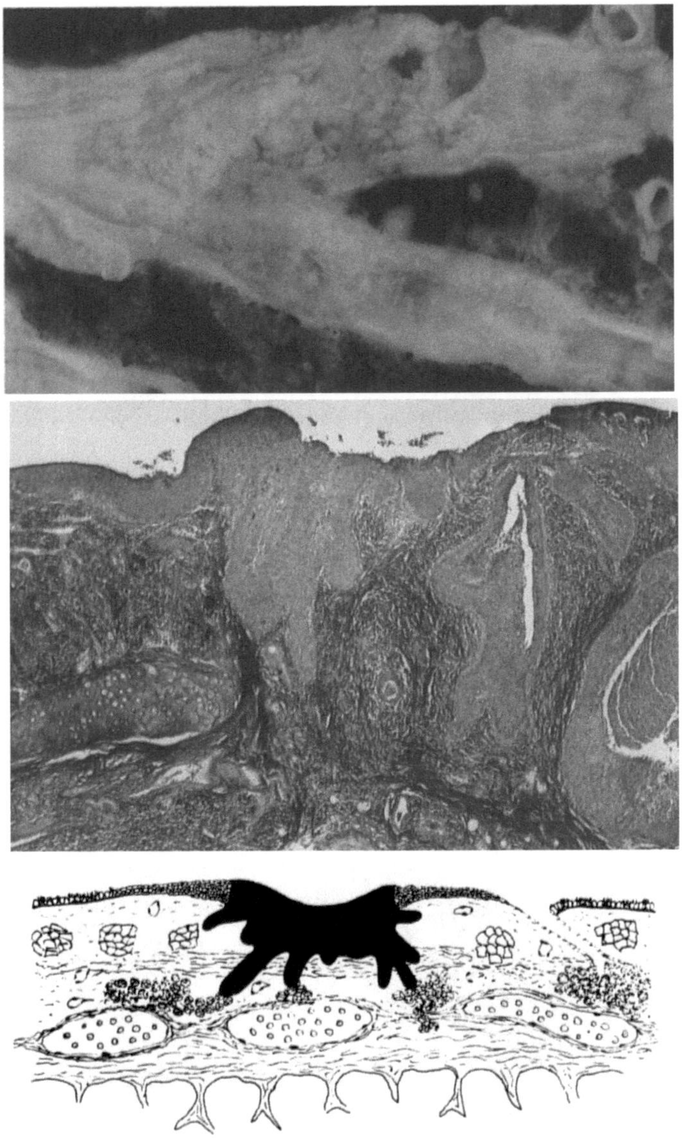

Fig. 3. Macroscopic and microscopic photographs and scheme of the superficially ulcerating type of central early cancer

Histological Findings of Early Cancer of the Bronchi

The term "early cancer of the bronchus" can be proved according to hitherto existing investigations in cases of squamous cell carcinomas only. Atypical proliferating complexes of squamous cells follow the ducts of the bronchial wall glands after disintegration and destruction of the basal lamina in the early stage of infiltration. Infiltration of the muscular layer as far as the inner side of the tunica fibrocartilaginea follows the destruction of the markedly developed lamina elastica, especially in the case of elderly men (2, 3). Lung tissue is reached after the outer layers of the bronchial wall have been passed, generally beginning between the cartilage of the bronchial wall, and so exceeding the morphological criteria for the diagnosis of early cancer.

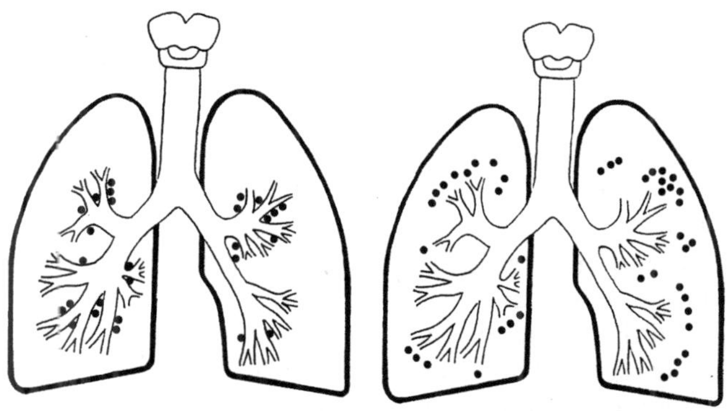

Early cancer of the lung	
► central type	► peripheral type
-segmental/ subsegmental area	-distal of subsegmental area
-limited to bronchial wall	-diameter of tumor max. 2 cm
no infiltration of pleura	
no metastasizion	

Early cancer of the lung		
	central type	peripheral type
♂ : ♀	9 :1	3 : 2
mean age :	59 Y.	56 Y.
histological type :	sqamous cell- CA	Adeno - CA 80% sqamous cell - CA 15%

Fig. 4. Comparison of morphclogical and clinical data of the cen:ral and peripheral types of early cancer of the lung

Among the clinical symptoms, hemoptysis (56%), cough (33%), and fever (22%) are the most common

- Mostly men
- Intensive smokers
- Hemoptysis, 56%
- Cough, 33%
- No symptoms, 11%
- X-ray of the lungs ↗ negative in 40% ↘ pneumonia/atelectasis 60%
- Cytology of sputum: positive in 90%

- Result of bronchoscopy: always positive findings
- Histology: nearly always squamous cell carcinoma

The diagnosis of early cancer of the bronchus, ascertained definitely by examination of surgical specimen or during necropsy, in termed the so-called hilar type of early cancer in contrast to early cancer in the periphery (peripheral early cancer) by Ikeda (1974, 1981).

In the study by Ikeda (1981), early cancer in the periphery of the lung is defined as a tumor of less than 2 cm in diameter, measured in the surgical specimen (Fig. 4). Infiltration of the pleura or lymph nodes as well as metastasis must also be excluded in a case of this type of early cancer. The tumor is localized distally of the subsegmental bronchi. In contrast to early cancer of the hilar type, peripheral early cancer presents histologically as an adenocarcinoma in most cases; a squamous cell carcinoma is observed only seldomly. From the morphological point of view, a strict demarcation of a peripheral early cancer is problematic, since the diagnosis is based on the morphological criterion of tumor diameter only. By means of serial sections of peripheral so-called early cancers up to 2 cm in diameter, we were able to prove that in these early stages of tumor development invasion of blood vessels, infiltration of lung tissue, and regressive changes of different degrees in the tumor can nearly always be observed, especially in cases of adenocarcinomas (Müller and Reitemeyer 1986). According to clinical observations, metastasis is to be expected in 1% of cases with an early cancer of the peripheral type with a tumor size of less than 2 cm. Metastasis can be observed in 35% of cases of tumors up to 3 cm in size. In our own group of 287 cases with malignant neoplasms of the lung, 6 cases (2%) fulfilled the morphological criteria for early cancer of the hilar type.

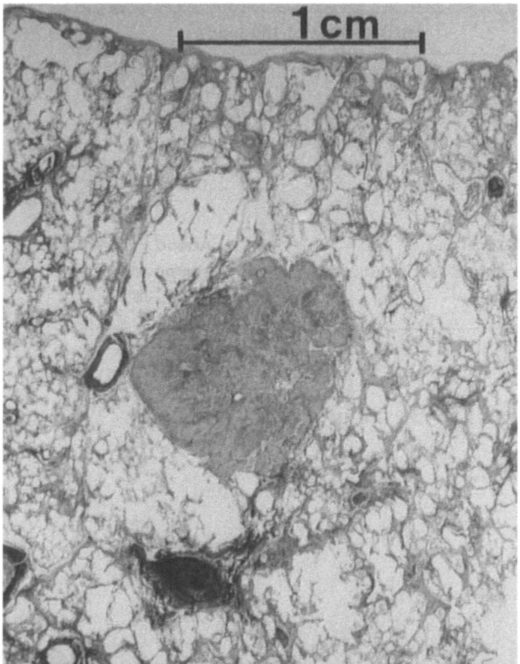

Fig. 5. Microscopic photograph of a small cell microcarcinoma of the lung verified during necropsy as the reason for extensive metastasis

Microcarcinoma

The term microcarcinoma of the lung has only been defined inaccurately up to now. This diagnosis must be considered in cases of already extensive metastasis without clinical demonstration of a primary tumor, which can be found only by extensive *microscopic* examination of lung tissue and generally have a size of 3-10 mm (Fig. 5). Among lung tumors, microcarcinoma is especially common in cases of small cell carcinomas. Well-differentiated squamous cell carcinomas or adenocarcinomas are found much more seldomly, presenting as clinically occult microcarcinomas with already extensive metastasis. A comprehensive characterization, orientated at definite morphological criteria, of the commonly used term "pulmonary micro- or miniature carcinomas" has not been possible so far (for review of the literature see Eck et al. 1969; Müller 1983, 1985).

Tumorlets

Tumorlets of the lung are defined as microscopic minimal neoplasms of the lung, mostly found occasionally and representing possible precursors of malignant lung tumors (Fig. 6). The term was introduced by Whitwell in 1955 for atypical epithelial proliferations of the terminal bronchioloalveolar segments. These cell proliferations, which can often be classified with respect to their uncertain biologic behavior only with difficulty, have to be considered as preneoplasms of an alveolar carcinosis (pulmonary adenomatosis), an especially rare type of a group of tumors classified with the adenocarcinomas. The development of alveolar carcinosis in advanced lung fibrosis confirms the hypothesis of development of carcinomas out of bronchioloalveolar tumorlets. Tumorlets of the squamous cell type can be demonstrated in a considerable number of cases with asbestosis of the lung. Here, continuous transitions from squamous cell tumorlets in areas of bronchioloalveolar fibrous reorganization to multifocal, only microscopically detectable microcarcinomas have been verified in advanced stages of asbestos-dust-induced fibrosis of the lung.

Tumorlets of the Carcinoid Type

The term pulmonary tumorlets is most often used today in the sense of the definition given by Churg and Warnock (1976) and Ranchod (1977) for "carcinoid tumorlets". In the literature, terms like carcinoid atypical proliferations, nodular epithelial hyperplasia, minute peripheral pulmonary tumors, microscopic oat cell carcinoma, basal-cell carcinoma, and microscopic multicentric carcinoma (for review of the literature see Carter and Egglestone 1983) are found. Tumorlets of the bronchial carcinoid type cause no symptoms in most cases. With a diameter of 3-10 mm, they cannot be demonstrated by means of radiology and are detected accidentally during necropsy or examination of surgical specimens. They are often combined with scars of the lung tissue (Fig. 7). The classification of this type of tumorlet with minimal neoplasms or possible precursors of small cell carcinoma of the lung results from the demonstration of multiple carcinoid tumorlets in lungs with already manifested small cell carcinomas of the oat cell type. According to results of immunohistochemical examinations, this type of tumorlet can be classified with the APUD cells of the lung similarly to carcinoid tumors and small cell carcinomas, especially of the oat cell type. In comparison to the high frequency of

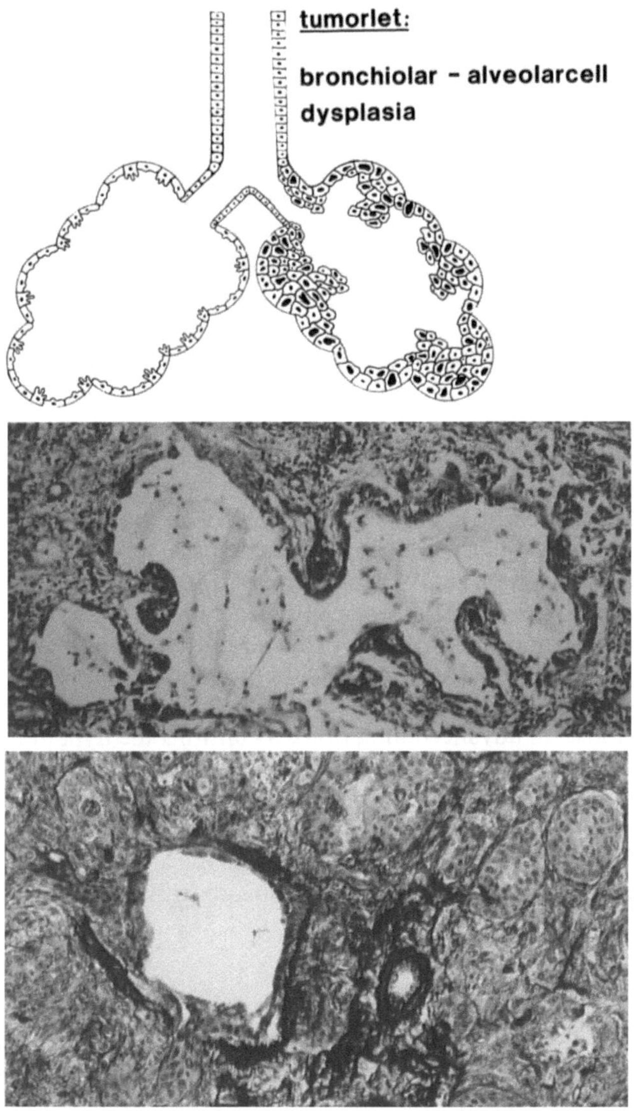

Fig. 6. Scheme and microscopic photographs of tumorlets of the bronchioloalveolar type

mostly far advanced small cell carcinomas of the bronchi at the time of diagnosis, the findings of minimal neoplasms of the tumorlet type can be regarded as an exception. A typical minimal neoplasm or an early cancer can not be differentiated on principle in the case of a small cell carcinoma, since at the time of diagnosis a far-advanced tumor stage is usually found.

Tumor Staging of Early Cancer of the Lung

In the staging of tumors according to the clinical TNM system, a relatively wide gap lies between the findings of a T_x tumor (cytological demonstration of cells of a malignant tumor in the sputum) and the group of T_1 tumors with a size of 3 cm at the most in the

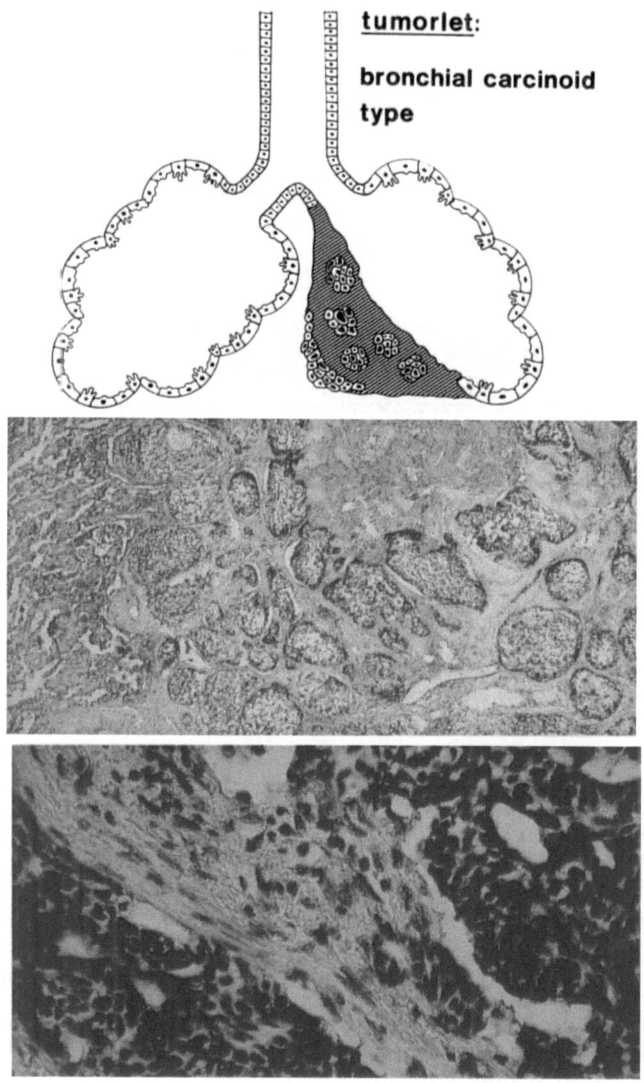

Fig. 7. Scheme and microscopic photograph of tumorlets of the bronchial carcinoid type

case of intrapulmonary localization (Fig. 8). From a clinical point of view, this definition of T_1 tumor is understandable, since the mostly roentgenological diagnosis of a tumor with a diameter of 1-3 cm in the early stages must still today be regarded as an accidental finding. The sole morphometric demarcation of T_1 tumors of the lung 3 cm at the most in diameter cannot be correlated with a definite morphological substrate. Histological typing is of outstanding importance for therapy and prognosis. Adenocarcinomas and squamous cell carcinomas are the most common tumor types in cases of roentgenological clearly defined T_1 stage coin lesions. We were able to find invasion of blood vessels in 70% and already advanced signs of regression with scarring and necrosis in more than 50% of 30 cases of well-differentiated adenocarcinomas in microscopically examined surgical specimens. These findings suggest that a morphologically very heterogeneous spectrum of tumors is hidden behind the clinical group of T_1 tumors. Hitherto,

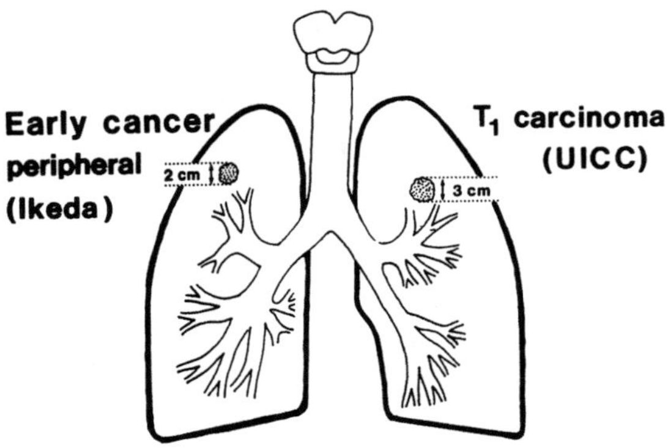

Early lung cancer

Staging		Survival following resection (5years from detection)
T_0	→ ca in situ → microfocally invasive carcinoma	100 %
T_1	carcinoma sized up to 3 cm Ø	70 %
T_{II-III}	>3 cm etc.	<10 %

Fig. 8. Scheme, staging, and 5-year survival rates of early and advanced stages of lung cancer

the definite demarcation of morphologically reproducible findings of early cancer has only been possible in the case of the hilar type of squamous cell carcinoma defined above, which also has to be included in the group of T_1 carcinomas according to the TNM classification, nevertheless. In the staging of tumors, Melamed and Zaman (1981) have suggested a staging of their own. Thus, preneoplasms of the degree of a carcinoma in situ and microscopically invasive carcinomas are classified together as T_0 tumors (Melamed et al. 1981). Carcinomas which are limited to the bronchial wall with a diameter of less than 1 cm, according to our own definition of early cancer type A, are called microfocally invasive carcinomas. The differentiation between this stage T_0 and stage T_1 is based mainly upon the observations of the clinical course of disease in only a few cases, with a 5-year survival rate of 100% after surgical resection. Also from our point of view, this group of minimal neoplasms has to be differentiated more clearly from the large group of T_1 tumors (up to 3 cm in diameter). In the case of small cell carcinoma, at the time of diagnosis, even with a very small primary tumor, a far-advanced stage of tumor metastasization (compare microcarcinoma) is found. This has led to the fact that today tumor staging is performed according to clinical symptoms in cases of small cell carcinoma (review of limited disease, extensive disease, and comprehensive stagings I–IV in review of the literature by Hermanek and Gall 1979; Austgen 1985).

Conclusions and Prospects

Morphologically detectable minimal neoplasms of the bronchial system and the lung of the early cancer type today are still very rare findings. Nevertheless, an increasing number of diagnoses of early stages of malignant lung tumor can be expected within the scope of the extension of endoscopic techniques. A common definition of early cancer, similar to the findings concerning other organs, is of outstanding importance also from a clinical point of view because of the extraordinary good prognosis following surgery of the tumor. Early cancer of the bronchus can easily be distinguished from preneoplasms of the bronchial mucosa and manifested, already transmurally advanced, and metastasizing bronchial carcinomas as a special type of tumor. This is reasonable especially with regard to the relatively long preclinical period of development of bronchial carcinomas. From observations of the clinical course of patients with carcinoma in situ of the lung, a latency period of 10-15 years can be expected until the development of a manifest carcinoma (Nasiell et al. 1982). The extraordinarily good prognosis after surgical treatment of bronchial carcinomas in the stage of morphologically verified early cancer also gives reason for a special classification of these minimal neoplasms of the lung with the relatively large, on the whole heterogeneous group of T_1 tumors according to the UICC (Spiessl et al. 1985) from the clinical point of view.

References

Austgen M (1985) Staging des Bronchialkarzinoms. In: Trendelenburg F (ed) Tumoren der Atmungsorgane und des Mediastinums. Springer, Berlin Heidelberg New York, pp 334-337 (Handbuch der Inneren Medizin, vol 4/4 A)

Brockmann M, Müller K-M (1986) Das Frühkarzinom des Bronchus. GBK-Mitteilungsdienst NF, H 49: 73-75

Carter D, Eggleston JC (1983) Tumorlets type bronchial carcinoid tumors. In: Tumors of the lower respiratory tract. Armed Forces Institute of Pathology, Washington, pp 181-188

Churg A, Warnock ML (1976) Pulmonary tumorlet. A form of peripheral carcinoid. Cancer 37: 1469-1477

Cortese DA, Pairolero PC, Bergstrahl EJ, Woolner LB, Uhlenkopp MA, Piehler IM, Sanderson DR et al. (1983) Roentgenographically occult lung cancer. A ten year experience. J Thorac Cardiovasc Surg 86: 373-380

Eck H, Haupt R, Rothe G (1969) Die gut- und bösartigen Lungengeschwülste. Springer, Berlin Heidelberg New York, pp 134-138 (Handbuch der speziellen pathologischen Anatomie und Histologie, vol 3/4)

González S, von Bassewitz DB, Grundmann E, Nakhosteen JA, Müller K-M (1986) The ultrastructural heterogeneity of potentially preneoplastic lesions in the human bronchial mucosa. Pathol Res Pract 181: 408-417

Hermanek P, Gall FP (1979) Lungentumoren. In: Hermanek P (ed) Kompendium der klinischen Tumorpathologie, vol 2. Witzstrock, Baden-Baden, pp 1-165

Ikeda S (1974) Atlas of flexible bronchofiberscopy. Thieme, Stuttgart

Ikeda S (1981) Die Effizienz der Fiberbronchoskopie bei der Früherkennung des Bronchialkarzinoms. In: Hamelmann H, Troidl H (eds) Die Behandlung des Bronchialkarzinoms: Resignation oder neue Ansätze? Thieme, Stuttgart

Kubik A, Polak J (1986) Lung cancer detection. Results of a randomized prospective study in Czechoslovakia. Cancer 57: 2427-2437

Melamed MR, Zaman MB (1982) Pathogenesis of epidermoid carcinoma of lung. In: Shimosato Y, Melamed MR, Nettesheim P (eds) Morphogenesis of lung cancer, vol 1. CRC, Boca Raton, pp 37-64

Melamed MR, Flehinger BJ, Zaman MB, Heelan RT, Hallerman ET, Martini N (1981) Detection of true pathologic stage I lung cancer in a screening program and the effect on survival. Cancer 47: 1182-1187

Müller K-M (1983) Praeneoplasien des Bronchialsystems. Pathologische Anatomie. Prax Klin Pneumonol 37: 644-648

Müller K-M (1985) Pathologie der Lungentumoren. In: Trendelenburg F (ed) Tumoren der Atmungsorgane und des Mediastinums. Springer, Berlin Heidelberg New York, pp 87-127 (Handbuch der inneren Medizin, vol 4/4 A)

Müller K-M, Reitemeyer E (1986) Lungentuberkulose und Lungenkrebs aus der Sicht des Pathologen. Öff Gesundheitswes 48: 481-487

Nasiell M, Sinner W, Tornvall G, Vogel B, Enstad T (1977) Clinically occult lung cancer with positive sputum cytology and primary negative roentgenologic findings. Scand J Respir Dis 58: 134-144

Nasiell M, Carlens E, Auer G, Hagata Y, Kato H, Konaka C, Roger V, Nasiell K, Enstad I (1982) Pathogenesis of bronchial carcinoma, with special reference to morphogenesis and the influence on the bronchial mucosa of 20-methylcholanthrene and cigarette smoking. Recent Results Cancer Res 82: 53-68

Papanicolaou GN, Koprowska (1951) Carcinoma in situ of the right lower bronchus. A case report. Cancer 4: 141-146

Ranchod M (1977) The histogenesis and development of pulmonary tumorlets. Cancer 39: 1135-1145

Spiessl B, Hermanek P, Scheibe O, Wagner G (eds) (1985) TNM-Atlas. Illustrierter Leitfaden zur TNM/pTNM-Klassifikation maligner Tumoren. Springer, Berlin Heidelberg New York

UICC (1979) TNM-Klassifikation der malignen Tumoren, 2nd edn. Springer, Berlin Heidelberg New York

Whitwell F (1955) Tumorlets of the lung. J Pathol 70: 529-541

WHO (1981) Histological typing of lung tumors, 2nd edn. WHO, Geneva (International histological classification of tumors, no 1)

Wilde J (1985) Das okkulte Bronchialkarzinom. In: Trendelenburg F (ed) Tumoren der Atmungsorgane und des Mediastinums. Springer, Berlin Heidelberg New York, pp 29-30 (Handbuch der inneren Medizin, vol 4/4 B)

Minimal Thyroid Neoplasia

W. Böcker, S. Schröder, and H. Dralle

Institut für Pathologie, Allgemeines Krankenhaus Altona, Universität Hamburg,
Paul-Ehrlich-Straße 1, 2000 Hamburg 50, FRG

Introduction

Every malignant tumor has its prestages; their earliest possible detection is of vital importance for the patient's prognosis (Grundmann 1979). Consequently, it is necessary to define these early lesions by exact morphologic criteria and to develop appropriate methods for clinical detection and treatment. In the thyroid, carcinoma pathology has many facets such as the different histologic types, stages of evolution, and correlation of morphology and prognosis. In contrast to the minimal cancers of other organs, it is important that some of the very early thyroid tumors are recognized clinically by the evidence of cervical lymph node metastases, and that this type of spread does not affect the generally favorable prognosis.

There are at least three distinct clinicopathologic types of thyroid cancer, which, on account of their good prognosis, may be defined as "minimal thyroid neoplasia": encapsulated follicular carcinoma, encapsulated papillary carcinoma, and occult papillary carcinoma. In the present study we have attempted to delineate the morphologic and clinical criteria of these lesions. The term "minimal thyroid neoplasia" was chosen in preference to "minimal invasive carcinoma" (Lang and Georgii 1982) because in some of these lesions invasiveness cannot be regarded as condition sine qua non for a diagnosis of malignancy (see below under "Encapsulated Papillary Carcinoma").

Classification of Thyroid Carcinomas

The thyroid gland contains two embryologically and functionally different cell types: the neuroendocrine calcitonin-producing *C-cell,* and the endodermally derived, thyroxin-secreting *follicular cell.* According to their histogenetic derivation from one of these cell types, two groups of carcinomas can be distinguished (Hedinger and Sobin 1974) (Table 1).

1. The *C-cell carcinoma* (Williams 1985); since it has not been possible so far to define a minimal C-cell neoplasia by morphologic criteria of the primary, this group will be left aside in our analysis.
2. The other group, derived from follicular cells, comprises the different types of *follicular cell carcinoma,* which are subdivided into follicular, papillary, and anaplastic tumors. The latter are always well advanced with poor prognosis (Schröder et al.

Recent Results in Cancer Research, Vol. 106

Table 1. Classification of 433 thyroid malignancies

Tumor type	*n*	%
Follicular	95	21.9%
Papillary	202	46.7%
Squamous	2	0.5%
Anaplastic	63	14.5%
C-Cell carcinoma	31	7.2%
Sarcoma	1	0.2%
Malignant lymphoma	14	3.2%
Metastases	25	5.8%
	433	100.0%

Institute of Pathology, University of Hamburg (1963-1983).

1987), whereas the differentiated carcinomas show a much more favorable prognosis. Recent analyses have shown that both types of differentiated carcinoma correlate with distinct patterns of clinical behavior and that, in addition to histology, their macroscopic growth is of relevance to prognosis. This report summarizes our experience of 80 cases of minimal thyroid neoplasia found in the files of the Department of Pathology of Hamburg University in a 20-year period (1963-1983).

Minimal Thyroid Neoplasia, Follicular Type

Data from several analyses of follicular carcinoma have shown the outstanding importance of the macroscopic aspect for prognosis. Two follicular subtypes can be distinguished on this basis:

1. Grossly invasive follicular carcinoma (GIFC)
2. Encapsulated follicular carcinoma (EFC)

Grossly invasive follicular carcinoma is an advanced tumor with poor prognosis. On the other hand, certain tumors are totally encapsulated and thus hardly distinguishable from benign lesions by the mere macroscopic aspect. Since Cohnheim's first description (1876) it was known that encapsulated follicular tumors are able to metastasize. The importance of vascular and/or capsular invasion as a criterion of malignancy was outlined later by Graham (1924) and Warren (1931, 1956). Since the study of Hazard and Kenyon (1954a, b), invasion of the capsule or the blood vessels was regarded as prerequisite for a diagnosis of malignancy in encapsulated follicular tumors. These lesions had been originally described as "malignant or angioinvasive adenomas" (Graham 1924; Hazard and Kenyon 1954), but by now the term "encapsulated follicular carcinoma" (EFC) is generally accepted (Crile 1968; Selzer et al. 1977; Franssila 1971; Lang and Georgii 1982; Kahn and Perzin 1983; Schröder et al. 1984a). It is still a point of controversy whether angioinvasion (Lang and Georgii 1982) and capsular infiltration/penetration can be used as equivalent diagnostic proofs of malignancy.

In our retrospective study of 40 cases of EFC the main preoperative presentation was that of a cold nodule, less frequently of goiter; in only one case was a bone metastasis the primary clinical manifestation (Table 2). In contrast to papillary carcinoma, only 2 of

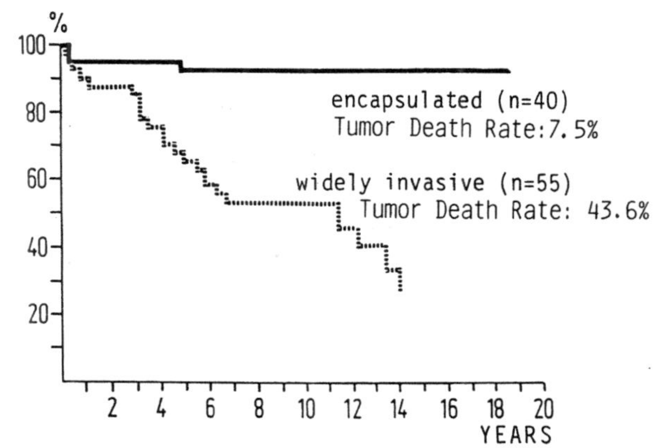

Fig. 1. Follicular carcinoma. Relative survival rates of grossly invasive follicular carcinoma and encapsulated follicular carcinoma. For corresponding tumor death rates, see Table 2

Table 2. Characteristics of 95 follicular carcinomas

Criterion	Encapsulated	Grossly invasive
Number	40 (42.1%)	55 (57.9%)
Age	46.5 years	58 years
Initial LN metastases	2 (5.0%)	6 (10.9%)
Initial distant metastases	2 (5.0%)	14 (25.5%)
Tumor death rate	3 (7.5%)	24 (43.6%)

Institute of Pathology, University of Hamburg (1963–1983).

40 EFCs had cervical node enlargement which was histologically recognized as metastatic spread. The macroscopic diameters of totally encapsulated lesions ranged from 2 to 10 cm, with a mean diameter of 4.1 cm. The histologic picture of these lesions varied from trabecular to follicular patterns; nine of them displayed an oxyphilic cell type.

Of our 40 EFC cases nearly 80% showed histologic evidence of vascular invasion; in 20% the diagnosis was based only on the evidence of capsular infiltration or, less often, penetration. The appraisal of capsular infiltration as a criterion of malignancy is confirmed by Kahn and Perzin (1983) and Evans (1984).

It has been shown by other authors (Crile 1968; Woolner 1971) that there are grave differences of prognosis between EFC and grossly invasive follicular carcinoma (GIFC). In our material the death rate from GIFC was six times that of EFC (Table 2, Fig. 1). Our death rate of 7.5% for EFC is somewhat lower than the figures of 11.8% and 15.6% given by Beaugie et al. (1976) and Crile (1968), respectively. Data from the literature on the course of the disease (Beaugie et al. 1976; Hirabayashi and Lindsay 1961; Woolner 1971) and from our own series (Schröder et al. 1984b) reveal that death as a result of hematogenous spread will often occur as late as 10–22 years after surgery.

A comparison of morphological and clinical parameters from EFC cases with benign and those with fatal outcome gives some indication that the size of the primary, the age of the patient, and the presence of oxyphilic metaplasia are of prognostic significance. Figure 2 shows the correlation between tumor size and age at the time of surgery in patients with EFC. It becomes evident that tumor diameters were always over 5 cm in patients with poorer prognosis. No patients with EFC under 5 cm were recorded as dying from the disease, whereas 25% of those with EFC over 5 cm did eventually die of it. In

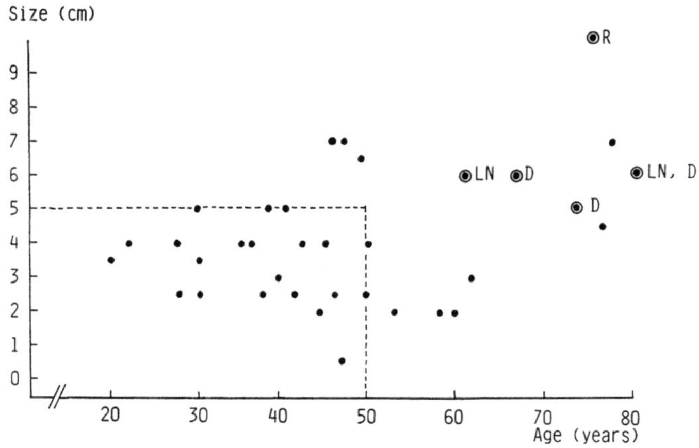

Fig. 2. Encapsulated follicular carcinoma. Correlation between tumor size and age of patients at the time of surgery. Cases of cervical lymph node metastases *(LN)*, local recurrence *(R)*, and death due to carcinoma *(D)*

addition we are able to confirm Crile's evidence that the prognosis of EFC will be worse in patients over 50 years of age. Contradictory observations have been presented by several authors on the biologic significance of oxyphilic metaplasia (Schäffer et al. 1983; Ruchti et al. 1976). In our material 25.7% of EFC showed oxyphilic metaplasia, 66.7% of these oxyphilic tumors showing fatal outcome. In contrast to other authors we were unable to confirm the correlation between prognosis and the amount of capsular and/or vascular invasions as published by Hofstädter and Unterkircher (1980).

In conclusion our findings indicate that prognosis worsens if the patient is over 50, if the tumor is greater than 5 cm, and/or if it shows oxyphilic metaplasia (Fig. 2). Consequently the group of EFC should be subdivided into a low-risk and a high-risk group by the above criteria. The recommendation of surgical intervention in the form of subtotal lobectomy of the affected side as an adequate treatment for EFC (Crile 1968, and other authors) should be restricted to EFC of low-risk type. In patients with high-risk EFC a primary total thyroidectomy appears necessary to ensure adequate postoperative radioiodine therapy.

Minimal Thyroid Neoplasia, Papillary Type

In accordance with the WHO criteria (Hedinger and Sobin 1974), all differentiated thyroid tumors that demonstrate papillary excrescences have to be classified as papillary carcinomas. In addition, carcinomas of follicular structure with the cytologic hallmark of clear nuclei ("alveolar variant of papillary carcinoma" according to Crile and Hazard 1953; "nonpapillary, papillary carcinoma" according to Rosai et al. 1983) were found to behave like papillary carcinomas (Lindsay 1960; Schröder et al. 1984b).

In analogy to follicular tumors, papillary carcinomas can be subdivided into three groups:

1. Grossly invasive papillary carcinoma (GIPC)

Table 3. Characteristics of 202 papillary thyroid carcinomas

Criterion	Encapsulated	Occult	Grossly invasive
Number	28 (13.9%)	34 (16.8%)	140 (69.3%)
Initial LN metastases	7 (25.0%)	19 (55.9%)	70 (55.0%)
Initial distant metastases	–	–	18 (12.9%)
Tumor death rate	–	–	31 (22.1%)

Institute of Pathology, University of Hamburg (1963–1983).

(The following two are recognized as minimal thyroid neoplasias of the papillary type):

2. Encapsulated variant = encapsulated papillary carcinoma (EPC)
3. Occult papillary carcinoma (OPC), including occult sclerosing carcinoma (OSC) = Graham tumor and papillary microcarcinoma

The latter two have an unusually good prognosis even for papillary carcinoma in general, despite the relatively high frequency of cervical lymph node metastases in this tumor group (cf. also Table 3).

Encapsulated Papillary Carcinoma

It has been said that encapsulated papillary carcinoma (EPC) has now achieved the status of a genuine variant (Vickery 1983; Schröder et al. 1984b). Its preoperative symptoms are uni- or bilateral goiter (75%) with a cold nodule or cervical lymph node metastases (25%). Common to all tumors of this group is total encapsulation. In our own material of 28 EPCs, the mean diameter was 3.3 cm (range: 0.2–7.5 cm, Table 4). The rate of papillarity varied over a broad spectrum from purely papillary lesions to entirely follicular tumors with the typical cytologic hallmark of ground glass nuclei. Capsular and even more important, vascular, invasion is, in contrast to EFC, not a prerequisite for this diagnosis. Judging by the coexistence of adenomatous tissue and papillary carcinoma, Vickery et al. (1985) suggested that papillary carcinoma might develop from

Table 4. Characteristics of 28 encapsulated papillary carcinomas

Age	48.2 years (range 21–84)	
Preoperative findings	Goiter	75%
	Cold nodule	64%
	LN metastases	25%
Tumor size	Mean 3.3 cm (range 0.2–7.5)	
Histology	Papillary	2%
	Follicular	24%
	Mixed	64%
Intraglandular spread		2.5%
Survival without disease		100%

Institute of Pathology, University of Hamburg (1963–1983).

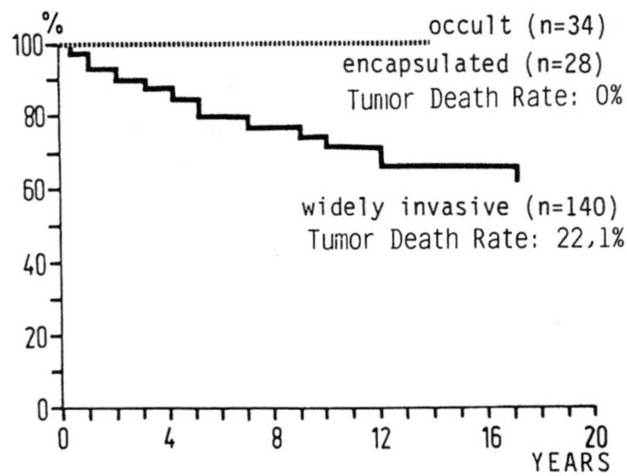

Fig. 3. Papillary carcinoma. Relative survival rates of occult papillary carcinoma, encapsulated papillary carcinoma, and grossly invasive papillary carcinoma. For corresponding tumor death rates see Table 3

preexisting adenoma. However, our immunhistochemical studies rather support the theory that even colloid follicles do represent an integral part of papillary carcinoma.

Through a prolonged follow-up (1–15 years, mean period 7 years) a favorable prognosis could be ascertained for each of our 28 patients with EPC (Figs. 3, 4).

Occult Papillary Carcinoma

The most important lesion of the occult papillary carcinoma (OPC) type is *occult sclerosing carcinoma* (OSC), a relatively small lesion of up to 1.5 cm. Its incidence among all the papillary carcinomas of biopsy material lies between 13% and 34%. The predominant clinical presentation of OSC is a cervical enlargement of lymph nodes by metastatic spread (Table 5); its percentage in the literature ranges from 7.1% to 76.9%. In more comprehensive studies, however, the rate settles at 40% (Hubert et al. 1980; Patchefsky et al. 1970). Distant metastases of such lesions are extremely rare (Frauenhoffer et al. 1979; Laskin and James 1983; Patchefsky et al. 1970). On the other hand, these lesions may be detected as an incidental finding in thyroid surgical specimens excised for goiter or other causes. The great majority of OSCs are less than 1 cm in diameter.

A second type of OPC is the *papillary microcarcinoma,* a lesion of some 0.1 cm in diameter detectable only by histology. In our own material the percentage of papillary microcarcinoma among OPC was 11%, which is somewhat higher than the figures usually given for microcarcinomas in the literature. Sixty-six percent of our microcarci-

Table 5. Characteristics of 34 occult papillary carcinomas

Age	42.5 years (range 22.1–80.9)	
Preoperative findings	LN metastases	55.9%
	Goiter	35.3%
	Cold nocule	8.8%
Tumor size	Mean: 1.1 cm (6 microcarcinomas)	
Survival without disease	100%	

Institute of Pathology, University of Hamburg (1963–1983).

nomas were clinically manifested by cervical lymph node metastases; the remainder were found incidentally in resected thyroid specimens.

Recent studies have shown that there is a great difference between the estimated incidence of occult papillary carcinomas as based on autopsy studies, and the actual incidence of clinically detected cases (Williams 1980). The percentage of OSC was put at some 20% in autopsy studies (Sampson et al. 1974), while circumscribed microcarcinomas with a diameter of less than 1 cm were recorded at a high 61% (Sampson et al. 1971). To date, it is still an open question why the vast majority of papillary carcinomas will neither progress to a clinically detectable stage nor actually metastasize.

References

Beaugie JM, Brown CL, Doniach I, Richardson JE (1976) Primary malignant tumours of the thyroid: the relationship between histological classification and clinical behaviour. Br J Surg 53: 173-181

Cohnheim J (1876) Einfacher Gallertkropf mit Metastasen. Virchows Arch [Pathol Anat] 68: 547-554

Crile G (1968) Treatment of carcinomas of the thyroid. In: Young S, Inman DR (eds) Thyroid neoplasia. Academic, New York, pp 39-47

Crile G Jr, Hazard JB (1953) Relationship of the age of the patient to the natural history and prognosis of carcinoma of the thyroid. Ann Surg 138: 33-38

Evans HL (1984) Follicular neoplasms of the thyroid. A study of 44 cases followed for a minimum of 10 years, with emphasis on differential diagnosis. Cancer 54: 535-540

Franssila KO (1971) Value of histologic classification of thyroid cancer. Acta Pathol Microbiol Scand [A] [Suppl] 225

Frauenhoffer CM, Patchefsky AS, Cobanoglu A (1979) Thyroid carcinoma. A clinical and pathologic study of 125 cases. Cancer 43: 2414-2421

Graham A (1924) Malignant epithelial tumors of the thyroid. With special reference to invasion of blood vessels. Surg Gynecol Obstet 39: 781-790

Grundmann E (1979) Histopathologie früher neoplastischer Veränderungen. Verh Dtsch Krebsges 2: 27-39

Hazard JB, Kenyon R (1954a) Encapsulated angioinvasive carcinoma (angioinvasive adenoma) of thyroid gland. Am J Clin Pathol 24: 755-766

Hazard JB, Kenyon R (1954b) Atypical adenoma of the thyroid. Arch Pathol 58: 554-563

Hedinger C, Sobin LH (1974) Histological typing of thyroid tumours. WHO, Geneva (International histological classification of tumours, vol 11)

Hirabayashi RN, Lindsay S (1961) Carcinoma of the thyroid gland: a statistical study of 360 patients. J Clin Endocrinol Metab 21: 1596-1610

Hofstädter F, Unterkircher S (1980) Histologische Kriterien zur Prognose der Struma maligna. Pathologe 1: 79-85

Hubert JP, Kiernan PD, Beahrs OH, McConahey WM, Woolner LB (1980) Occult papillary carcinoma of the thyroid. Arch Surg 115: 394-398

Kahn NF, Perzin KH (1983) Follicular carcinoma of the thyroid: an evaluation of the histologic criteria used for diagnosis. Pathol Annu 18/1: 221-253

Lang W, Georgii A (1982) Minimal invasive cancer in the thyroid. In: Burghardt E, Holzer E (eds) Minimal invasive cancer (microcarcinoma). Saunders, London, pp 527-537

Laskin WB, James LP (1983) Occult papillary carcinoma of the thyroid with pulmonary metastases. Hum Pathol 13: 83-85

Lindsay S (1960) Carcinoma of the thyroid gland. A clinical and pathologic study of 293 patients at the University of California Hospital. Thomas, Springfield

Patchefsky AS, Keller IB, Mansfield CM (1970) Solitary vertebral column metastasis from occult sclerosing carcinoma of the thyroid gland: report of a case. Am J Clin Pathol 53: 596-601

Rosai J, Zampi G, Carcangiu ML (1983) Papillary carcinoma of the thyroid. A discussion of its

several morphologic expressions, with particular emphasis on the follicular variant. Am J Surg Pathol 7: 809-817
Ruchti C, Komor J, König MP (1976) Großzellige Tumoren (sog. Hürthle-Zell-Tumoren) der Schilddrüse. Helv Chir Acta 43: 129-132
Sampson RJ, Key CR, Buncher CR, Jijima S (1971) Smallest forms of papillary carcinoma of the thyroid. A study of 141 microcarcinomas less than 0.1 cm in greatest dimension. Arch Pathol 91: 334-339
Sampson RJ, Woolner LB, Bahn RC, Kurland LT (1974) Occult thyroid carcinoma in Olmsted county/Minnesota: prevalence at autopsy compared with that in Hiroshima and Nagasaki, Japan. Cancer 34: 2072-2076
Schäffer R, Reiners C, Reimann J, Börner W (1983) Das onkozytäre Schilddrüsenkarzinom: Klinisch-pathologische Renaissance einer Tumorform? Tumordiagn Ther 4: 161-168
Schröder S, Pfannschmidt N, Dralle H, Arps H, Böcker W (1984a) The encapsulated follicular carcinoma of the thyroid. A clinicopathologic study of 35 cases. Virchows Arch [A] 402: 259-273
Schröder S, Böcker W, Dralle H, Kortmann KB, Stern C (1984b) The encapsulated papillary carcinoma of the thyroid. A morphologic subtype of the papillary thyroid carcinoma. Cancer 54: 90-93
Schröder S, Baisch H, Rehpennig W, Müller-Gärtner HW, Schulz-Bischof K, Sablotny B, Meiners I, Böcker W, Schreiber HW (1987) Morphologie und Prognose des folliculären Schilddrüsencarcinoms - Eine klinisch-pathologische und DNS-cytophotometrische Untersuchung an 95 Tumoren. Langenbecks Arch Chir 370: 3-24
Selzer G, Kohn LB, Albertyn L (1977) Primary malignant tumors of the thyroid gland. A clinicopathologic study of 254 cases. Cancer 40: 1501-1510
Vickery AL (1983) Thyroid papillary carcinoma. Pathological and philosophical contriveries. Am J Surg Pathol 7: 797-807
Vickery AL, Carcangiu ML, Johannessen JV, Sobrinho-Simoes M (1985) Papillary carcinoma. Semin Diagn Pathol 2: 90-100
Warren S (1931) The significance of invasion of blood vessels in adenomas of the thyroid gland. Arch Pathol 11: 255-257
Warren S (1956) Invasion of blood vessels in thyroid cancer. Am J Clin Pathol 26: 64-65
Williams ED (1980) Pathology and natural history. In: Duncan W (ed) Recent results in cancer research: thyroid cancer. Springer, Berlin Heidelberg New York, pp 47-55
Williams ED (1985) Medullary carcinoma of the thyroid. In: Polak JM, Bloom SR (eds) Endocrine tumours. Livingstone, Edinburgh, pp 229-240
Woolner LN (1971) Thyroid carcinoma: pathologic classification with data on prognosis. Semin Nucl Med 1: 481-502

Minimal Thyroid Cancer: Clinical Consequences

I. G. Böttger

Klinik und Poliklinik für Nuklearmedizin, Westfälische Wilhelms-Universität Münster, Albert-Schweitzer-Straße 33, 4400 Münster, FRG

The definition and histology of minimal thyroid cancer has been discussed by Böcker et al. in this meeting. The paper presented here will, therefore, deal with the clinical consequences of minimal thyroid carcinoma, i.e., diagnosis, therapy and follow-up. However, a few additional data of general interest are included.

The incidence of thyroid carcinoma is 30/1000000 inhabitants in the Federal Republik of Germany (FRG) and 28 in the United States of America (USA). The mortality is 5/1000000 in the FRG, 4 in the USA (Bretzel and Schatz 1985). Thyroid carcinoma is shown by autoptic thyroids in up to 20% of cases, and by surgical specimens in between 1% and 16% of cases. It is found in 0%-11% of goitrous patients with multiple nodules, in 3%-33% of cases of solitary thyroid nodules, and in 2%-20% of cases of cold nodules.

The histological classification (Hedinger and Sobin 1974) of 358 patients with thyroid carcinoma seen in the in- and outpatient clinic of nuclear medicine of the Technical University of Munich between 1972 and 1982 showed the following distribution:

most frequent was follicular carcinoma at 44.7%, then papillary carcinoma with 32.1%, followed by anaplastic carcinoma at 11.2%, oncocytic carcinoma at 7.8%, medullary (C-cell) carcinoma at 2.5%, and others at 1.7%.

Minimal thyroid carcinoma is practically identical to minimal papillary carcinoma. Papillary carcinoma is the most common type in nonendemic areas, in contrast to our area southern Bavaria. It is about twice as frequent in females as in males.

The *classification* of minimal thyroid (papillary) cancer is not done uniformly. Its definition and histology have been outlined in the previous communication by Böcker. Minimal thyroid carcinoma comprises papillary microcarcinoma, occult carcinoma detected secondary to lymph node metastasis, and latent carcinoma, i.e., neoplasms diagnosed postmortem (Schäffer 1986).

However, there is obviously no generally accepted upper limit for the size of papillary microcarcinoma. As in our study, a diameter of 1 cm has been accepted for occult papillary microcarcinoma, which is attributed to T_1-pT_1 by the Thyroid Gland Section of the German Society for Endocrinology (Krüskemper et al. 1985). This is in accordance with the postoperative histopathological UICC classification (T_1, 1 cm) and has also been adopted by the Arbeitsgemeinschaft Schilddrüse (Thyroid Work Group) of the German Society for Nuclear Medicine (Heinze et al. 1986). However, many authors consider 1.5 cm as the upper limit of diameter (Mazzaferri and Young 1981; Schäffer 1986), or even diameters up to 3 cm (Reinwein, 1984). As specified elsewhere (Schäffer 1986),

Recent Results in Cancer Research, Vol. 106

the term "minimal thyroid cancer" not only applies to the size of the papillary carcinoma, but also to other criteria. Since this tumor is hormone dependent, age is a very important factor. Thus, especially females aged less than 40–45 years at the time of diagnosis have a very good prognosis even in the presence of lymph node metastasis.

Diagnosis

History and clinical findings are obviously of little help in the detection of minimal thyroid carcinoma, since all of the clinical symptoms relevant to thyroid carcinoma in general are rather unlikely to appear in this early stage. Nevertheless, besides the occult type, minimal thyroid carcinoma may be present in comparably small thyroid nodules. As mentioned above, especially solitary thyroid nodules are suspicious. Due to their decreased or absent capability to accumulate radioiodine, even differentiated thyroid carcinomas, in general, reveal decreased or absent radioiodine uptake. Therefore, those nodules have to be examined by nuclear medicine techniques. Principally due to its higher specificity, iodine-123 should be preferred. However, as used in our clinic, technetium-99m-pertechnetate will generally be sufficient. The respective nuclear medicine finding is a cold or partially cold thyroid nodule or, if there is no nodule present, an area of decreased or absent iodine-123 (or technetium-99m) accumulation. The likelihood that such a cold thyroid nodule consists of a minimal thyroid carcinoma is considerably higher than in the case of a warm or hot nodule (e.g., in the case of autonomous adenoma) as cited above. When using technetium-99m it has to be remembered that in rare instances, technetium-99m accumulation may be present in a nonfunctioning thyroid nodule, just reflecting uptake, which on the use of iodine-123 would be cold.

Nowadays thyroid scintigraphy is best done by using a gamma camera, although employing a rectilinear scanner cannot be regarded as obsolete. With the latter the marking of findings on palpation is easier to perform.

When such a nodule has been recognized as cold, interest focuses on its morphology. Whereas scintigraphy reveals functional morphology, ultrasonography using a 5-MHz detector permits the analysis of structural morphology. Therefore, a solitary cold nodule should be further investigated by ultrasound examination in order to determine whether it is cystic or solid. Especially cold nodules that are solid on ultrasound, yet demonstrate reduced echogenicity, or are complex (mixture of solid and liquid echo pattern), will carry the highest risk of malignancy.

Thus, in a selected group of patients, about 9% of solitary cold nodules were found to be thyroid carcinomas. This probability increased by a factor of 3 to about 25% in the case of an additional presence of a hypodense echo pattern (Baum et al. 1983). Therefore it is essential in the case of even small solitary thyroid nodules (which may represent minimal thyroid carcinoma) to employ both imaging techniques, scintigraphy and ultrasonography, optimally to be performed by the same person.

A third established and extremely useful diagnostic tool is fine needle biopsy, as already outlined by Dr. Böcker. In our patients (Kempken 1985), fine needle biopsy, not guided by ultrasonography, directly established the diagnosis of carcinoma in 61.4% of cases, and yielded equivocal (suspicious) findings in another 31.6% ($n=329$ patients with goiter). The sensitivity in experienced hands is therefore above 90%. Even in the case of minimal thyroid carcinoma, fine needle biopsy may be guided by ultrasonography, as is routinely done in our clinic. All three diagnostic techniques have increasingly improved thyroid diagnostics during recent years, and led to a significant reduction in the percentage of patients with thyroid nodules who have to be operated on for suspected or unexcludable thyroid carcinoma (Spiegel et al. 1986). All these procedures have to be considered complementary. By no means will either of them be able to replace the other(s).

Therapy

Operative Strategy

The term minimal thyroid carcinoma certainly does not apply to anaplastic thyroid carcinoma and medullary (C-cell) carcinoma. Differentiated thyroid carcinoma, whatever its extent at the time of diagnosis, used to be managed rather aggressively in the past (Ng et al. 1983). Thus, also all of our patients with thyroid carcinoma underwent total or near-total thyroidectomy.

Since the interdisciplinary discussion during the German Cancer Congress of 1982 in Munich, there is now general agreement that the clinically unsuspected microcarcinoma in the form of occult papillary carcinoma of the thyroid, pT_1, found in thyroid tissue resected for benign conditions, does not require reoperation, since curative resection has already been accomplished (Edis et al. 1984). It is generally agreed that the occult papillary carcinoma of the thyroid, with or without local metastasis, can by cured by conservative surgical treatment, which means less than total thyroidectomy. These authors usually perform total lobectomy on the side of the lesion with a contralateral subtotal lobectomy and, on the presence of any palpably enlarged metastatic lymph nodes, a "modified" neck dissection. It is felt that long-term follow-up studies indicate that more extensive surgery with the concomitant increase in potential morbidity is unnecessary for cure. For intrathyroidal papillary carcinoma over 1.5 cm in diameter, however, total or near-total thyroidectomy with modified neck dissection on the presence of metastatic lymph nodes is favored.

A recent meeting on differentiated thyroid carcinoma and the aggressiveness of the therapeutic strategy (Reinwein 1984) revealed the absence of extremely controversial views. Therapy nowadays is performed in a more differentiated and less aggressive way. In the case of papillary carcinoma, it was outlined that the TNM system, as used in the earlier literature, is not suitable for the evaluation of prognosis, and that, e.g., the prognostic EORTC index, which is based on age but also considers sex, tumor type, spread and distant metastases, but not lymph node metastases, is clearly superior. Concerning tumor size, four out of six groups present suggest in the case of tumors 2–3 cm in diameter in a patient under 40 years a one-sided lobectomy with resection of the isthmus. The other two groups favor subtotal resection and total thyroidectomy. In a patient aged over 40 years, at least a subtotal resection of the contralateral side with or without dissection of the lymph nodes is generally proposed. The occult papillary thyroid carcinoma detected in the course of goiter resection is generally treated by a lobectomy on the side of the tumor.

In the case of an encapsulated follicular carcinoma (T_0, T_1), one group has moved away from the principle of aggressiveness. The other authors, however, prefer total or near-total thyroidectomy in follicular thyroid carcinoma, regardless of its size (Edis et al. 1984).

Our patients with papillary thyroid carcinoma, classified according to the postoperative histological findings, belonged to tumor stage pT_1 in 14% (pT_0 in another 5%), and to pT_2 in 37%, of cases. During the follow-up over up to 25 years, patients with pT_1 papillary (and follicular) carcinoma ($n=15/n=11$), originally without distant metastases, failed to show any local recurrence and/or distant metastases. pT_2 papillary carcinomas, however, demonstrated metastatic complication in 5.4% ($n=37$). The respective percentage for follicular carcinoma ($n=39$) was 15.4%. In the case of papillary carcinoma we consider only those patients with a contralateral, median, or bilateral lymph node metastasis (pN_2 stage expressing lymphogenous spread to the other side) and those with fixed regional lymph nodes (pN_3 stage expressing infiltration of the overlaying tissue) as high-risk patients.

Radioiodine Therapy

Differentiated carcinoma and in part its metastases will accumulate radioiodine, though to a lesser extent than functioning normal thyroid tissue. Therefore, the uptake of radioiodine by papillary and follicular thyroid carcinoma can be increased by reducing the amount of functioning normal thyroid tissue. This is one of the arguments for elimination of residual thyroid tissue in the case of total or near-total surgery. Radioiodine therapy is not appropriate in all cases of minimal thyroid carcinoma not treated by near-total or total thyroidectomy.

In contrast, radioiodine therapy should be performed in those patients with minimal thyroid cancer which have been treated by total or near-total thyroidectomy with the aim of removing as much of the thyroid tissue as possible. Radioiodine therapy is then used to eliminate the residual thyroid tissue.

In order to promote radioiodine uptake and to optimize radioiodine therapy, treatment should be performed after endogenous TSH has risen to more than 30 mU/liter, which is generally not earlier than 4–5 weeks postoperatively. A test activity of 74 MBq (2 mCi) iodine-131 is then administered orally; thyroid uptake is measured beginning 6 h after the administration. Thyroid scintigraphy is performed 2 days later together with whole-body scintigraphy. The volume of residual thyroid tissue is calculated scintigraphically (planimetry) and/or by ultrasonography. It is essential, however, to establish the clinical findings. In ablative radioiodine therapy of postoperative residual thyroid tissue, we have generally tried to achieve a dose of 1000 Gray (100000 rad). Radioiodine therapy was only performed if at least 3% of the administered iodine-131 was taken up by the residual thyroid tissue. Other authors prefer a dose 500 Gray (50000 rad) with a mean activity of 1.7 GBq (45 mCi) and never more than 3 GBq (80 mCi), whereas others apply 3.7–5.55 GBq iodine-131 (Reinwein 1984). If there is still significant radioiodine uptake 3 months later under deficient endogenous TSH stimulation, the treatment may be repeated. Moreover, rather small areas within the original thyroid bed with only insignificant radioiodine uptake do not necessarily require further iodine-131 treatment.

Thyroid-Stimulating Hormone-Suppressive Thyroid Hormone Therapy

Thyroid-stimulating hormone-suppressive therapy with either T4 (generally about 200 µg/day) or T3 (generally about 60 µg/day) aims at suppression of possibly remaining tissue of differentiated thyroid carcinoma following surgical and (if appropriate) nuclear medicine therapy. The TRH test used to be the tool of choice for monitoring complete TSH suppression, and still is in spite of the availability of supersensitive immunoradiometric assays for TSH based upon monoclonal antibodies. Those facilitate discrimination between basal TSH levels in the reference range, in a "grey zone," and suppressed TSH concentrations below the lower detection limit, which is only 0.02 mU/liter. In general, a supersensitively determined basal TSH level below the detection limit will indicate complete suppression. However, there are cases which despite basal TSH levels below the detection limit do show some TSH stimulation following TRH administration (Böttger et al. 1987). We have observed this phenomenon especially in a few patients with thyroid carcinoma under TSH-suppressive thyroid hormone therapy. Thus, it is safer to continue the TRH test even despite the availability of the new supersensitive TSH assays.

Thyroid-stimulating hormone-suppressive thyroid hormone medication is generally used in differentiated thyroid carcinoma. Therefore it also concerns minimal thyroid (papillary) cancer. In the case of less than total or near-total thyroidectomy, in the presence of a significant amount of residual thyroid tissue, suppressive therapy is begun directly following surgery. In the case of near-total or total thyroidectomy, thyroid hormones are administered following radioiodine therapy after the maximal uptake has been reached.

Follow-up

Although minimal thyroid (papillary) carcinoma, once surgically removed by subtotal (lobectomy) or near-total/total thyroidectomy, will only rarely recur locally or metastasize, careful follow-up is indicated.

In the case of less than near-total or total thyroidectomy we do not favor the use of radioiodine whole-body scanning in order to detect metastasis, which is at variance with other opinions (Heinze et al. 1986). In our opinion, due to a significant amount of residual functioning thyroid tissue leading to reduced radioiodine uptake, no significant additional information can be obtained by the radioiodine whole-body scan. Furthermore, according to our own results, the potency for radioiodine accumulation of papillary carcinoma metastases (in the whole) is only approximately 40%. In the case of near-total or total thyroidectomy in minimal papillary thyroid carcinoma, a group which, according to our follow-up scheme, is considered to be "low risk," we suggest performing one radioiodine whole-body scan 12 months after surgery and radioiodine therapy, together with history, physical examination, determination of FT3 and FT4 or another indirect parameter for free thyroid hormones, TRH test, serum thyroglobulin (hTg) concentration, chest X-ray, skeletal scintigraphy, sonography of the neck, erythrocyte sedimentation rate and blood cell counts. Part of this procedure, up to the determination of the hTg level, but without a radioiodine whole-body scan, is performed after 2–6 months (Kanitz et al. 1987). Ultrasonography of the neck is particularly useful in papillary thyroid carcinoma. Similar follow-up schemes (for near-total or total thyroidectomy and radioiodine therapy) and for lobectomy in the case of papillary microcarcinomas with the inclusion of a radioiodine whole-body scan 3 months after surgery, and facultatively later, have been published recently (Heinze et al. 1986).

Besides the individual follow-up of papillary microcarcinomas, the introduction of hTg as a very valuable tumor marker for differentiated thyroid carcinoma, and of basal TSH, supersensitively determined (vide supra), have improved the follow-up procedure. hTg has been found to be of such a high clinical value that, in general, its determination even during TSH-suppressive thyroid hormone medication can substitute for the routinely performed whole-body radioiodine scan. In order to do so, it is essential to use the entire diagnostic potential of the hTg determination. This is only feasible if indeed all of the residual thyroid tissue has been eliminated so that the patient is virtually athyrotic. The situation is a little bit different in minimal (papillary) thyroid carcinoma treated with less than near-total or total thyroidectomy without subsequent radioiodine therapy. The remaining thyroid tissue will by itself generate near-normal hTg serum levels. Recurrence/metastasis-induced hTg stimulations will, therefore, further elevate the hTg level, whereas in athyrotic patients, in general, nondetectable hTg will rise to significant levels of over 20 μg/liter ("grey zone", 10–20 μg/liter), indicating tumor growth. In our hands the tumor marker hTg, even under TSH-suppressive thyroxin medication, is at 97.9% vs. 83% clearly more sensitive in the detection of metastases of differentiated thyroid carcinoma, compared with the radioiodine whole-body scan. Its specificity was found to be 93.6% (Böttger et al. 1985). Including the data of 14 European Centers with a total of 2193 patients who had hTg determinations, 795 patients with recurrences/metastases revealed a sensitivity of hTg of 86% under hormone replacement, and of 94% after hormone withdrawal, despite a constant specificity of 96% (Hüfner and Reiners 1986).

References

Baum K, Reiners C, Wiedemann W, Müller HA, Böcker W (1983) Differentialdiagnose von Schilddrüsenknoten. Sonographie als Ergänzung der Szintigraphie und Punktionszytologie. Dtsch Med Wochenschr 108: 1359–1364

Böttger I, Kanitz W, Pabst HW (1985) Klinische Reevaluierung der radioimmunologischen Thyreoglobulin(hTg)-Bestimmung in der Nachsorge des differenzierten Schilddrüsenkarzinoms. Nucl Compact 16: 182–190

Böttger I, Pabst HW, Bienhaus G, Seidel C (1987) Non-linear correlation of basal serum TSH and TRH-stimulated TSH response: new aspects in pituitary thyroid regulation. Nucl Med Commun (in press)

Bretzel RW, Schatz H (1985) Prognose bei Schilddrüsenkarzinom. Lebensversicherungsmedizin 37: 172–179

Edis AJ, Grant CS, Egdahl RH (1984) Surgery of the thyroid. In: Edis AJ, Grant CS, Egdahl RH (eds) Manual of endocrine surgery. Springer, Berlin Heidelberg New York, pp 71–150

Hedinger C, Sobin LH (1974) Histological typing of thyroid tumours. WHO, Geneva, p 22 (International histological classification of tumours, vol 11).

Heinze HG, Reiners C, Becker W, Börner W (1986) Tumornachweis beim Schilddrüsenmalignom. Nuklearmediziner 9: 193–207

Hüfner M, Reiners C (1986) Bericht über den internationalen Workshop "Thyreoglobulin und Thyreoglobulin-Antikörper in der Nachsorge des differenzierten Schilddrüsenkarzinoms und der endemischen Struma". In: Pfannenstiel P, Emrich D, Weinheimer B (eds) Schilddrüse 1985. 7. Konferenz über die menschliche Schilddrüse, Homburg/S., Thieme, Stuttgart, pp 2–9

Kanitz W, Böttger IG, Pabst HW, Heidenreich P, Dirr W (1987) Nachsorge des differenzierten Schilddrüsenkarzinoms unter spezieller Berücksichtigung des Serum-Thyreoglobulin(hTg)-Spiegels. Fortschr Röntgenstr 147 (3): 282–287

Kempken K (1985) Diagnostik des Schilddrüsenkarzinoms. Nuklearmediziner 8: 315–326

Krüskemper HL, Joseph K, Köbberling J, Reinwein D, Schatz H, Seif FJ (1985) Klassifikation der Schilddrüsenkrankheiten. Intern Welt 8: 47–49

Mazzaferri EL, Young RL (1981) Papillary thyroid carcinoma: a 10 year follow-up report of the impact of therapy in 576 patients. Am J Med 70: 511–518

Ng TF, Maisey MN, Howorth PJN (1983) Thyroid disease. In: Maisey MN, Britton KT, Gilday DL (eds) Clinical nuclear medicine. Saunders, Philadelphia, pp 213–247

Reinwein D (1984) Differenzierte Schilddrüsenkarzinome. Radikalität der therapeutischen Strategie. Dtsch Med Wochenschr 109: 626–634

Schäffer R (1986) Aktuelle Gesichtspunkte zur histologischen Klassifikation, Verlauf und Prognose der Struma maligna. Nuklearmediziner 9: 73-96

Spiegel W, Baum K, Reiners C, Börner W, Müller HA (1986) Die Operationsindikation szintigraphisch kalter Strumaknoten in Abhängigkeit vom klinischen, szintigraphischen, sonographischen und zytologischen Befund. Dtsch Med Wochenschr 111: 173-176

Cryptic Gliomas

F. Gullotta

Institut für Neuropathologie, Westfälische Wilhelms-Universität Münster, Domagkstraße 17, 4400 Münster, FRG

The central nervous system's highly specialized functions, complicated structures, and complex metabolism illustrate and confirm its distinctive place in clinical medicine and pathology. The very topic of minimal neoplasia and early cancer on which this meeting is focused tends to emphasize this special role: Although we do know quite a catalogue of gliomas, paragliomas, meningeomas, and other brain tumors, safely discernible precancerous lesions ("minimal neoplasias" or "early cancer lesions") like those identified and adequately characterized in many other organs are practically unknown in the human CNS.

This point was stressed as early as 1956 by Zülch in his monograph on brain tumors. The following 3 decades have seen many new developments in the field of neurooncology. Nothing has changed, however, with regard to precancerous conditions in the human brain, a fact emphasized a new by Zülch (1986) in his latest publications. He is by no means alone in his ideas. The general opinion was expressed by Weller (1980) with typical British laconism: "The question that arises, however, is whether (in CNS) truly neoplastic or premalignant lesions really exist".

In fact, it is only in experimental brain tumors induced, e.g., by methylnitrosourea, that we may occasionally detect small cellular foci in the CNS of carcinogen-treated animals, foci that show the morphologic features of incipient autonomous growth, and might therefore be appraised as "early" gliomas. We do know, however, that these foci are *even then* genuine gliomas. Any comparison with the human brain is impracticable here, since all types of experimentally induced brain tumors do show a biological behavior that is entirely different from that of spontaneous human brain tumors. Experimental gliomas are always malignant, whereas human neoplasm are not necessarily so; even in repeated recurrences the malignant transformation of a benign glioma is not an obligatory biological phenomenon.

The discovery of "progressive multifocal leukoencephalopathy" and its identification as an opportunistic infection provoked by oncogenic viruses (papova) leading to neoplastoid transformation of the affected astrocytes has evoked, quite understandably, a number of speculative hypotheses about cerebral carcinogenesis. Nevertheless, solid proof is lacking to this day for the induction of gliomas in man by papova viruses. Such a possibility is not to be excluded on principle, but it would be incorrect or at least precipitate to interpret PML as a precancerous condition of the CNS.

The striking fact was duly stressed by Zülch (1986) that the enormous wealth of worldwide macroscopic and microscopic postmortem studies of brains from patients

Recent Results in Cancer Research, Vol. 106

with a great variety of diseases has never led to the detection of any "minimal lesions" - of posttraumatic, postinflammatory, or any other nature - which could be safely appraised as preneoplastic.

Some authors want to regard as CNS preneoplasias the tissue alterations that appear in so-called "dysontogenetic syndromes with blastomatous involvement" (i.e., neurocutaneous blastodermoses or phacomatoses: von Recklinghausen, von Hippel-Lindau, Sturge-Weber, tuberous sclerosis). These syndromes, however, represent a separate group of diseases which, in my opinion, should be distinguished from the brain tumor group on account of their genetic factors, and of the potential, often obligatory, metachronous involvement of several different organs.

In clinical neuropathology, the term "miniglioma" is applied to dysontogenetic lesions of very low growth rate, and which will provoke cerebral symptoms merely on account of their localization. The term thus has not so much a strictly oncological meaning, but rather defines, in a wider clinicomorphological sense, certain microscopic tumor-like cell aggregates (dysplastic lesions) occurring mostly in the temporal lobe or fourth ventricle. For these lesions Cavanagh (1958) coined the term "cryptic gliomas," meaning occult, undetectable lesions. He wanted to apply this name exclusively to dysplasias of the temporal lobe; I prefer to enlarge its meaning so as to cover certain neoplastic formations of extremely low growth tendency which may occur in the third or fourth ventricle.

The *first group,* Cavanagh's (1958) cryptic gliomas sensu strictu, are located in the temporal lobe, particularly in the hippocampus or in the nucleus amygdalae, usually causing temporal lobe epilepsy (Figs. 1, 2). Their nosological classification by mere morphological criteria is often far from easy. Some authors want to see them as pure hamartomas, others as dysplasias. Stochdorph (1963a) described them as "tumors of arrested growth"; Courville (1931) called them "gangliogliomas." The morphologic spectrum of these lesions is indeed rather wide: Some cryptic gliomas consist of a small aggregation

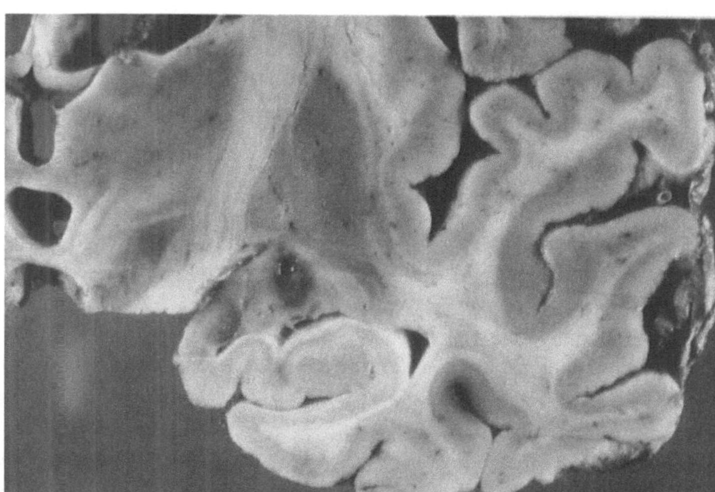

Fig. 1. In this 79-year-old woman with genuine epilepsy, who died suddenly from heart failure, autopsy disclosed a small cryptic glioma involving the nucleus amygdalae and extending between the hippocampus and capsula interna. No signs of brain edema or a local space-occupying lesion were found

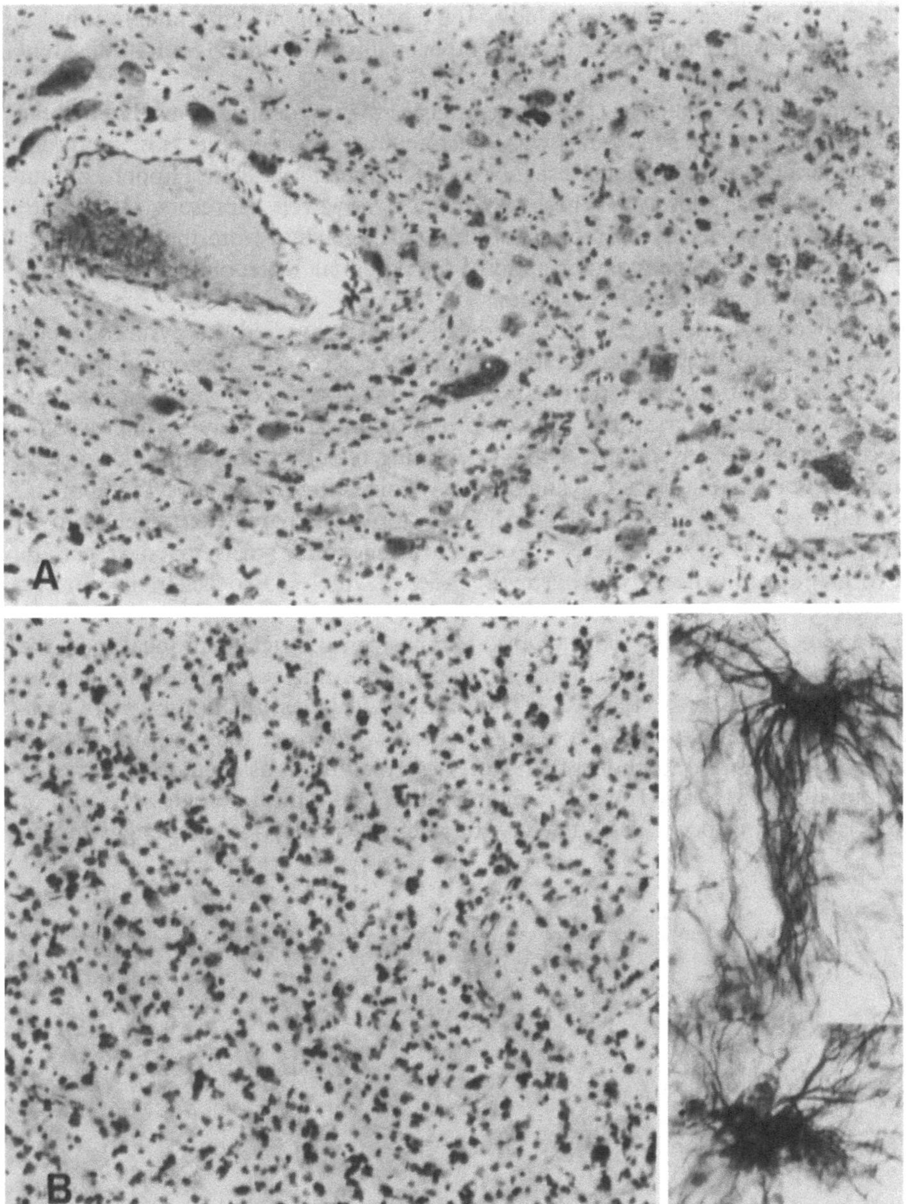

Fig. 2 A, B. Same case as in Fig. 1. The tumor is built up partly of large neuron-like elements (**A**), partly of oligodendroglia (**B**) intermingled with some large fibrillary astrocytes *(inset)*. (Dill and Gullotta 1970) Celloidin, van Gieson (*inset,* Kanzler). All magnifications 40: 1

of atypical ("exotic") ganglion cells, others are made up of different gliomatous components (astrocytic, ependymal, oligodendroglial, etc.), and still others are even mixed gliovasal dysplasias. The often heterogeneous structure of these lesions can be assessed exactly only by synoptic comparison of several parallel cases (Dill and Gullotta 1970; Gullotta et al. 1970). In this respect Courville's (1931) "ganglioglioma" as a general morphologic term appears not inadequate.

The frequent occurrence of cryptic gliomas in the temporal lobe may be explained by embryologic factors. According to Jacob (1966), the *carrefour temporo-insulino-hippocampique* is a poliomyelencephalic border region and, as such, particularly exposed to many different noxae during its complicated evolution. Findings like micro- or macroangioma, or telangiectasia, are in fact not rare in this area.

These occult gangliogliomas of the temporal lobe are, as a rule, absolutely benign; they are relatively well circumscribed without any growth potential. Only a few of them will increase in size over the years (thereby manifesting themselves as genuine gliomas). Malignant transformation is an absolute rarity. Only one case was described by Russell and Rubinstein (1962); even these authors cannot exclude that in their "gangliocytoma plus glioblastoma" (developing 23 years after the first operation) malignant transformation affected only the glial, but not the neuronal, compartment.

The *second group* of cryptic gliomas consists of so-called subependymomas, a term coined by Scheinker (1945) for tumor-like neoplasms of the subependymal region. They are poorly cellular, fibrillary "gliomas" bearing the morphologic characteristics of ependymoma, but also of pilocytic astrocytoma. The tumors are often called "ependymospongioblastomas"; American authors prefer the term "subependymal glomerulated astrocytomas." In my opinion we are dealing with ependymoastrocytic mixed gliomas, which was confirmed by investigations of in vitro-cultured subependymomas performed together with Casentini et al. (1981).

Macroscopically, subependymomas appear as small or medium-sized subependymal nodules protruding polyp-like into the ventricular system. They are often detected incidentally at autopsy in the cerebral ventricles as well as in the fourth ventricle, where they manifest themselves as pure hyperplasia of the subependymal glial plate without causing any symptoms, as a rule (Wüllenweber and Gullotta 1986). They are occasionally found after sudden death in cases where even the most meticulous necropsy discloses only this tumor "infiltrating" (or arising from) the floor of the fourth ventricle. This raises the problem whether in such conditions these tumors could be considered as the actual cause of death due to infiltration and at least functional impairment of the medullary cardiorespiratory centers (Völpel 1983). Obviously, the tumor size is not relevant, since bean-sized tumors causing subtotal occlusion of the foramen of Magendie are not infrequent incidental findings (Fig. 3). Any evaluation of the potential role of these "neoplasms" in terms of fatality would therefore require a very careful histopathologic examination of the medulla oblongata and the safe exclusion of any other cause of death.

The very low growth tendency of these subependymomas is confirmed by the absence of the common general symptoms evoked by a space-occupying process. Evidence of hydrocephalus is very rare. It is, however, one of the special features of these dysplasias that they may often turn into "genuine" tumors (especially in cerebellar localizations) with clinical manifestations. The histologic picture of these cases, however, will in no way differ from that of nonproliferating, asymptomatic subependymomas, a fact that may underline the difficulty and even impossibility of diagnosing an "early cancer" or a "preneoplastic lesion" in the presence of glial "dysplasias."

From the large group of dysontogenetic tumors I finally want to pick out a curious neoplasm that I feel inclined to classify among the cryptic gliomas on account of its biological behavior. This intraventricular formation may also appear as an occasional finding at autopsy, as in the case of the neurosurgeon Harvey Cushing.

I am speaking of the *colloid cysts of the third ventricle,* peculiar formations of so far unknown origin. Their old hypothetical interpretation as remnants of the paraphysis was

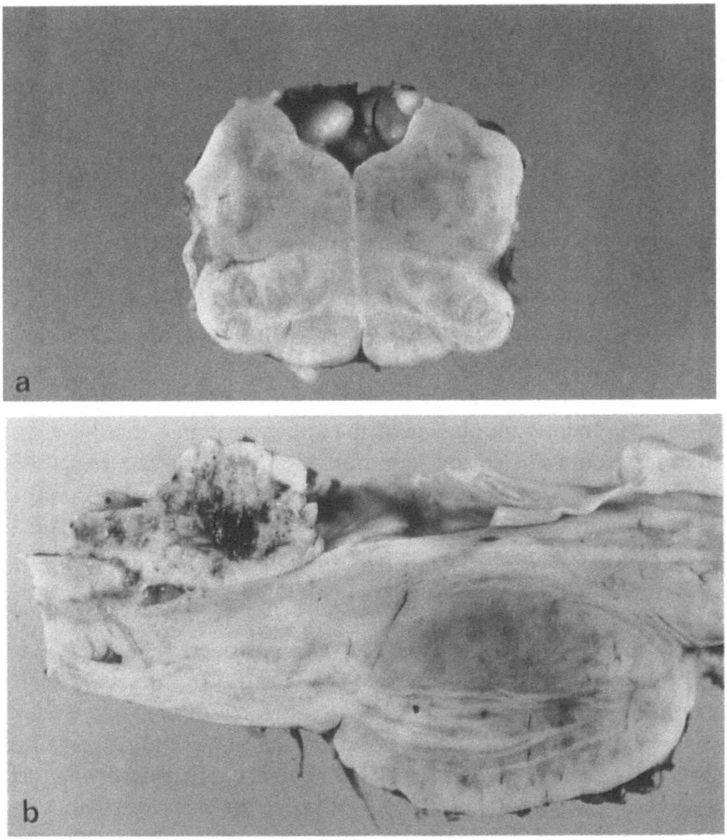

Fig. 3 a, b. Subependymomas of the fourth ventricle, incidentally detected at autopsy. In the patient in **a** an almost complete occlusion of the foramen of Magendie was evident, but neither hydrocephalus nor any clinical signs had ever been observed. The patient in **b** had suffered of unexplained respiratory arrests. Histologically the floor of the fourth ventricle was "infiltrated" by tumor cells

rejected long ago, and is of merely historical interest. Some authors regard them as ependymal cysts (which is not always correct), others prefer the noncommittal term of neuroectodermal cysts. Stochdorph (1963b) suggested that they might represent dislodged remnants of bronchial epithelium, being thereby related to Rathke's cyst of the hypophysis. These colloid cysts, localized below the columnal fornices, may finally provoke a blocking of the foramina Monroi by their progressive, though not obligatory expansion. This, in turn, leads to biventricular hydrocephalus and sudden death (Fig. 4). The main symptoms, if any, would be headaches, syncopal attacks, and chronic seizures in some instances.

In conclusion, morphological alterations that could be appraised as "early cancer" within the terminology of general pathology are practically unknown in the human central nervous system. The term "minimal or cryptic glioma" has rather a clinical and descriptive meaning for some dysontogenetic formations (microdysplasias of blastomatous appearance) that are found in some patients as the potential or actual cause of chronic cerebral disease (such as epilepsy) or of sudden death.

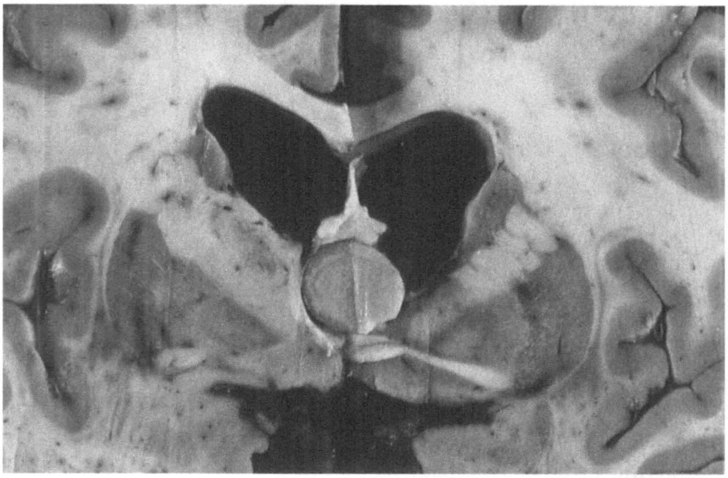

Fig. 4. Colloid cyst of the third ventricle detected in a 39-year-old woman who had suffered from increasing headaches for 10 days. She was found dead in bed. The cyst has produced a blocking of both foramina Monroi with hydrocephalus. Similar cysts, without Monroi-blocking, may be found incidentally at autopsy

References

Casentini E, Möhrer U, Gullotta F (1981) Clinical and morphological investigations on ependymomas and their tissue cultures. Neurochirurgia (Stuttg) 24: 51-56

Cavanagh JB (1958) On certain small tumours encountered in the temporal lobe. Brain 81: 389-405

Courville CB (1931) Gangliogliomas. A further report with special reference to those occurring in the temporal lobe. Arch Neurol Psychiatry 25: 309-326

Dill R, Gullotta F (1970) Pathomorphologische Befunde bei Temporallappenepilepsien. Ein Beitrag zur Frage des "Ganglioglioms". Schweiz Arch Neurol Neurochir Psychiatr 106: 241-255

Gullotta F, Cervós Navarro J, Puig Serra J (1970) Istologia ultrastruttura e comportamento in vitro di un gangliocitoma cerebrale. Acta Neurol (Napoli) 25: 188-192

Jacob H (1966) Zur Verlaufspathologie und zur Korrelation zentralnervöser Dysgenesien (Poliomyeloenzephale Dysgenesien). In: Lüthy P, Bischoff A (eds) Proceedings of the 4th International Congress on Neuropathology, Zürich 1965. Excerpta Medica, Amsterdam

Russell D, Rubinstein LJ (1962) Ganglioglioma, a case with long history and malignant evolution. J Neuropathol 21: 185-193

Scheinker IM (1945) Subependymoma. A newly recognized tumor of subependymal derivation. J Neurosurg 2: 232-240

Stochdorph O (1963a) Epileptogene Schläfenlappenveränderungen mit strittiger Einordnung. Zentralbl Gesamte Neurol Psychiatr 177: 195

Stochdorph O (1963b) Zur Abkunft der Foramen-Monroi-Cysten. Nervenarzt 34: 226-229

Völpel M (1983) Kleine Subependymome des IV. Ventrikels. Harmloser Nebenbefund oder Todesursache? 2nd Meeting der Niederländischen und Nordrhein-Westfälischen Neurochirurgen und Neuropathologen, Jan. 28-29, Bonn

Weller RO (1980) Perspectives in neuro-oncology. In: Thomas DGT, Graham DI (eds) Brain tumours. Butterworth, London

Wüllenweber R, Gullotta F (1986) Subependymomas. Morphological and clinical validity. Neurosurgical Symposium on Low Grade Gliomas of the Brain, Aug. 28-30, Budapest

Zülch KJ (1956) Hirntumoren. In: Olivecrona H, Tönnis W (eds) Handbuch der Neurochirurgie, vol 3. Springer, Berlin Göttingen Heidelberg

Zülch KJ (1986) Brain tumours. Springer, Berlin Heidelberg New York

Cytogenetics of Preleukemic Stages in Experimental and Human Leukemogenesis

H.J. Seidel[1], F. Carbonell[2], H. Hameister[3], and J. Eul[3]

[1] Abteilung für klinische Physiologie, Institut für Arbeits- und Sozialmedizin, Universität Ulm, Oberer Eselsberg M 24, 7900 Ulm, FRG
[2] Hospital Clinico Universitario, Facultad de Medicina, Av. Blasco Ibañez, 17, 46010 Valencia, Spain
[3] Abteilung für klinische Genetik, Institut für Arbeits- und Sozialmedizin, Universität Ulm, Oberer Eselsberg M 24, 7900 Ulm, FRG

Introduction

The accessibility of tissue material for diagnostic purposes is an important factor in the early diagnosis of cancer. The human bone marrow as the site of interest in leukemia research is generally considered as accessible. Nevertheless, our knowledge about the early stages of leukemia is sparse. This has several reasons: One is that leukemia is a rare disease; another is that symptoms can develop rather late after the manifestation of the disease; finally, screening programs for populations at risk are nonexistent and even the definition of populations at risk is an unsolved problem. These populations are rather large in view of the expense of the studies needed, and the final incidence of leukemia is too low - benzene-exposed people, patients after Thorotrast (see Seidel 1978), now the population exposed at Chernobyl. For the study of early phases of the leukemogenic process animal models have to be used; they are readily available. A further consideration has to be that leukemic cells, at least in small numbers, are not easy to identify. A proper marker would help and many workers in immunology or molecular research are investigating this problem. We will discuss the presence of abnormal karyotypes in hemopoietic cells as markers of an abnormal cell proliferation which may be itself leukemic or on the way to an expanding malignant population.

We have carried out cytogenetic studies in man in those rare syndromes with a high potential for leukemia development and in mice after leukemogenic treatment - in a model where all mice develop leukemia after a single injection of the chemical leukemogen.

Materials and Methods

The studies in patients (Fundacion Jimenez Diaz, Spain, and University of Ulm, FRG) were performed as described by Benitez et al. (1985). Chromosome analysis was made on direct bone marrow samples; banding was carried out using Giemsa-Trypsin (GTG) and Quinacrin-fluorescence (QFQ) techniques. Chromosome identification and nomenclature were in accordance with the recommendations of the International System for Human Cytogenetic Nomenclature (1978). The clinical diagnosis followed the French-American-British (FAB) criteria (Bennett et al. 1982; see also Hoelzer et al. 1984).

Recent Results in Cancer Research, Vol. 106

The animal studies were carried out in BDF_1 mice after i.v. injection of 50 mg/kg methylnitrosourea (MNU), as described in detail recently (Seidel 1986). The chromosome analysis was performed after i.p. injection of colchicine 2 h prior to killing. Chromosome preparations were carried out using standard techniques (see Carbonell et al. 1982) and classified according to the criteria of the Committee on Standardized Genetic Nomenclature for Mice (1979).

Results and Discussion

In man, the term preleukemia (Block et al. 1953) has to be defined whenever it is used. We are interested in the early developmental stages of leukemias, when they have less than 10^{11} cells and cannot be detected with the microscope. These stages could be found in Thorotrast-exposed patients, but this population is too large for serial bone marrow aspiration and chromosome analysis, as are other populations also at risk. It is for only this reason that we study patients with myelodysplastic syndromes (Bennett et al. 1982), which is a summary of disease states in the hemopoietic system in the marrow and in the peripheral blood, further classified as refractory anemia (RA), refractory anemia with ring sideroblasts (RAS), refractory anemia with excess of blasts (RAEB), and described in many reviews, e.g., by Hoelzer et al. (1984) (Table 1). Patients with these diseases are a population at risk for leukemia development. This is where chromosomal analysis comes into consideration. Would the presence of cytogenetic changes be of any help for diagnosis and prognosis, especially for the prediction of clinical transformation. At present, the answer is no. This statement is based on the following facts:

1. Even in frank leukemias only about 50% of cases have abnormal karyotypes with present technology. This at least suggests that 50% of leukemias have no cytogenetic marker in the preclinical phase.
2. In the group of myelodysplastic syndromes, about 50% - with exceptions (5q-syndrome) - have a normal karyotype. The proportion with progression to leukemia is somewhat higher in patients with an abnormal karyotype (Second International Workshop on Chromosomes in Leukemia 1980).

Cytogenetic abnormalities are often used as a marker for the cell population under study. The presence of a marker is suggestive of clonality, and clonality has always been very attractive in ideas about the origin of cancer cells. Another marker, often used in leukemia research, is glucose-6-phosphate-dehydrogenase in heterocygotic women, appearing in two forms, A and B. The presence of one type in a specific cell population,

Table 1. Myelodysplastic syndromes

Refractory anemia (RA)
Sideroblastic anemia (RAS)
Refractory anemia with excess of blasts (RAEB)
5q-Syndrome (5q-S)
Abnormal cell clones, 50%
Most frequent aberrations:
monosomy 7 or 7q-
trisomy 8, or trisomy 8 and additional aberrations
monosomy 5 or 5q-

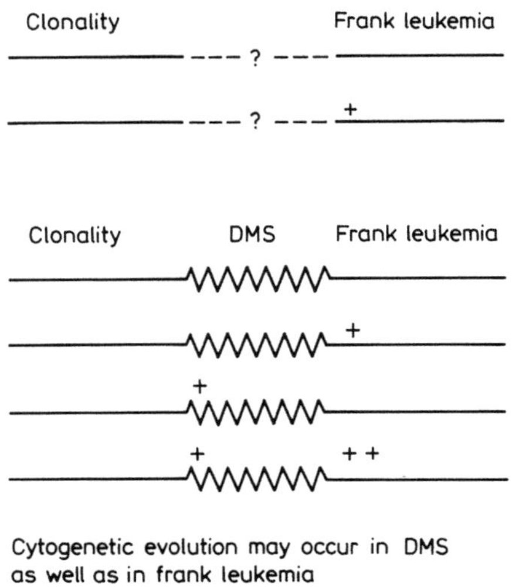

Fig. 1. Chromosome abnormalities and clonality in leukemia development: hypothetical model

with both enzyme types in, e.g., skin fibroblasts, is indicative of clonality. Using this method, clonality has been described in a 61-year-old woman with myelodysplastic syndrome (Raskind et al. 1984), as in all forms of classical leukemias (see Fialkow and Singer 1985).

With this in mind, the following hypothesis can be raised (Fig. 1):

1. A single clone of cells comes into the feeding position of the hemopoietic system, leukemic cells are generated in the clone, and leukemia develops - with or without cytogenetic marker.
2. A single clone of cells expands and for an unknown period a leukemic population is not generated. During this period various defects in cell production and maturation are present - one of the dysmyeloplastic syndromes, again with or without cytogenetic marker. This stage may persist as long as the patient is observed or develop further to frank leukemia, again with or without marker, with a new marker just in the transitional stage, with the same marker as during the dysplastic phase, or with additional ones.

Unfortunately nature has realized all possibilities. Tables 2 and 3 illustrate several pathways. The whole series has been published (Benitez et al. 1985).

Table 2 gives four examples of stable karyotypes during the observation period of 2-3 years: normal karyotypes, one with leukemia development, and two abnormal karyotypes, again one with leukemia.

Probably more interesting are those cases with unstable karyotypes (Table 3). The question arises whether the development of a new karyotype is associated with a change in the clinical picture, e.g., clinical transformation. Case No. 1 in Table 3 shows the appearance and loss of a new clone (+8) without clinical correlation. Case No. 2 shows the outgrowth of a clone, present after 5 months of observation, to the single, and then leukemic, clone 6 months later.

The conclusion from this part of the study must be that the cytogenetic approach certainly is a useful tool to study and document clonal growth patterns and the sequence of clones during the preleukemic and leukemic phase, but so far the technology is not suitable for any prediction.

Table 2. Stable karyotypes

Patient		Diagnosis	Karyotype	n	Observation time
52 yrs	M	RAS	N	43/23/37	13/39 months
47 yrs	F	RAEB	N/+8	23/7 17/18	35 months
62 yrs	M	RAEB	−7, del(3)(p21)/N	14/3 50/4	19 months - leukemia
16 yrs	F	RA	N	47/41/42/34	3/11/22 months - leukemia

Table 3. Unstable karyotypes

Patient	Diagnosis	Karyotype	n	Observation time
69 yrs F	RA	N/del(5)(q13q33)	3/3	
		↓		
		del(5)(q13q33)	40	18 months
		↓		
		del(5)(q13q33)/+8	33/4	24 months
		↓		
		del(5)(q13q33)	42	42 months
62 yrs F	RAS	N/+8	16/14	
		↓		
		−10, del(5)(q13q31)	2	
		−10, del(5)(q13q31), del(12)(p11)	12	
		↓		
		del(5)(q13q31)	4	5 months
		del(5)(q13q31), del(12)(p11)	5	
		↓		
		−10, del(5)(q13q31), del(12)(p11)	19	11 months - leukemia

As already mentioned in the "Introduction," we have available a mouse model of chemically induced T-cell lymphoma (Seidel 1986). Since all mice will develop leukemia, each observation made during the latency period of at least 12 weeks can be related to the final outcome - thymic lymphoma. Problems in the definition of the preleukemic state in mice, in comparison with man, have been discussed by Block (1966). With respect to cytogenetics, this model seems to be unique, since all mice with leukemia show trisomy 15, some also further abnormalities (Table 4). There is obviously chromosomal evolution and progression, as also observed previously (Carbonell et al. 1982; Haas et al. 1984; Newcomb et al. 1985).

Obviously trisomy 15 is a marker for the leukemic cell population. We wanted to know whether trisomy 15 is associated with minimal disease, whether it can be used to detect leukemic cells very early after transformation, whether trisomy 15 and the leukemic nature of the leukemic cells are associated from their very beginning? The results of a study during the latency period are given in Table 5. Trisomy 15 is seen 6–9 weeks after the injection of the leukemogen, while no frank leukemia is observed. These and additional data led to the hypothesis on the clonal evolution in the thymus, described in Table 6. The early appearance of trisomy 15 also in the bone marrow has to be con-

Table 4. Methylnitrosourea-induced T-cell leukemias, cytogenetic analysis and G-banding: % hyperploid karyotypes and definition of the predominant clone

	Thymus	Bone marrow	Spleen	Lymph node
1	90% +15	7 normal	10 normal	-
2	85% +15	5 normal	-	-
3	87% +15	4 normal	17 normal	29 normal
4	96% +15, +marker	80 =	66 =	92 =
5	94% +15	10 normal	84 =	-
6	72% +14, +15	91 =	-	-
7	86% +14, +15	24 normal	14 normal	-
8	85% +14, +15	96 =	98 =	-
9	100% +15/+14, +15	0 normal	-	-
10	90% +15/inv(x)	28 =	56 =	-
11	100% +15/t(2/15)	0 normal	58 =	7 normal
12	94% +1, +14, +15, +marker	7 normal	11 normal	64 =
13	93% +4, +14, +15	60 +14, +15	16 normal	90 +6, +14, +15
14	85% +4, +14, +15	81 =	28 normal	87 =
15	54% +marker	5 =	-	-
16	35% +marker	37 =	40 =	58 =

firmed by further studies. Possibly the cells with trisomy 15 originate there and migrate to the thymus.

From this we conclude that the presence of trisomy 15 is a more sensitive parameter for the detection of the new and most probably transformed cell clone, better than, e.g., the transplantation of cell suspensions (Seidel and Kreja 1985). We can further conclude that more emphasis has to be given to the bone marrow. Although the question is not yet answered of whether trisomy 15 is something like an epiphenomenon with respect to the

Table 5. Methylnitrosourea-induced T-cell leukemogenesis: cytogenetic analysis and G-banding

Weeks after MNU	Chromosome number		Predominant clone
	Bone marrow	Thymus	
6	40	40	t(4, 15)
	40	40/41 (70%)	+15
	40	40/41 (50%)	+15, −12, marker
	40	40	–[a]
9	40	40	–
	40	40	–
	40	40/41 (40%)	–
	40	40/41 (8%)	–
	40	–	–
	40/41 (7%)	40/41 (12%)	–
	40/41 (7%)	–	–
	40/41 (5%)	–	–
12	40	40/41 (70%)	+15
	40	40/41 (90%)	+15
	40	40/41 (8%)	–
	40/41 (20%)	40/41 (6%)	+14

[a] Not enough metaphases and/or insufficient resolution.

Table 6. Clonal evolution (karyotype) during MNU-induced T-cell leukemogenesis (thymus)

	→ – – – – – – – – – – – – – – – – – – →				
N	100%	50	–	–	–
+15	–	50	100	50	–
+15, +6[a]	–	–	–	50	100

[a] Or +14, +6, +19, +1, +4.

leukemogenic process - we now have a good opportunity to trace the clone, its origin, and its evolution in the various organ sites.

Both models show that the cytogenetic technique is useful for study of cellular clonality and evolution. In principle, however, the presence of a marker must be classified as an epiphenomenon associated with the leukemic nature of the cells.

References

An International System for Human Cytogenetic Nomenclature. (1978) Cytogenet Cell Genet 21: 313-405

Benitez J, Carbonell F, Fayos JS, Heimpel H (1985) Karyotypic evolution in patients with myelodysplastic syndromes. Cancer Genet Cytogenet 16: 157-167

Bennett J, Catovsky D, Daniel M, Flandrin G, Galton D, Gralnick M, Sultan C (1982) Proposal for the classification of the myelodysplastic syndromes. Br J Haematol 51: 189-199

Block M (1966) Prelymphomatous or preleukemic state in mice: relation to human preleukemia. Natl Cancer Inst Monogr 22: 559-570

Block M, Jacobson LO, Bethard WF (1953) Preleukemic acute human leukemia. JAMA 152: 1018-1028

Carbonell F, Seidel HJ, Saks S, Kreja L (1982) Chromosome changes in butylnitrosourea (BNU)-induced mouse leukemia. Int J Cancer 30: 511-516

Carbonell F, Heimpel H, Kubanek B, Fliedner TM (1985) Growth and cytogenetic characteristics of bone marrow colonies from patients with 5q-syndrome. Blood 66: 463-465

Committee on Standardized Nomenclature for Mice (1979) New rules for nomenclature of genes, chromosome anomalies and inbred strains. Mouse News Lett 61: 4-16

Fialkow PJ, Singer JW (1985) Tracing development and cell lineages in human hemopoietic neoplasia. In: Leukemia, ed. I.L. Weissmann, pp 203-222, Dahlem Konferenzen 1985, Berlin, Springer-Verlag

Haas M, Altman A, Rothenberg E, Bogart MH, Jones OW (1984) Mechanism of T cell lymphomagenesis: transformation of growth-factor-dependent T-lymphoblastoma cells to growth-factor-independent T-lymphoma cells. Proc Nat Acad Sci USA 81: 1742-1746

Hoelzer D, Ganser A, Heimpel H (1984) Atypical leukemia: preleukemia, smoldering leukemia and hypoplastic leukemia. Rec Res Cancer Res 93: 69-101

Newcomb EW, Binaru R, Fleissner E (1985) A comparative analysis of radiation- and virus-induced leukemias in Balb/C mice. Virology 140: 102-112

Raskind WH, Firumali N, Jacobson R, Singer J, Fialkow PJ (1984) Evidence for a multistep pathogenesis of a myelodysplastic syndrome. Blood 63: 1318-1323

Second International Workshop on Chromosomes in Leukemia 1979 (1980) Chromosomes in preleukemia. Cancer Genet Cytogenet 2: 108-113

Seidel HJ (1978) Ätiologie der Leukämien. In: Begemann H (ed) Leukämien. Springer, Berlin Heidelberg New York (Handbuch der inneren Medizin, vol 2/6)

Seidel HJ (1986) Die Entwicklung von T-Zell-Leukämien. Untersuchungen an der Maus nach einmaliger Gabe von Methylnitrosoharnstoff. Thieme, Stuttgart

Seidel HJ, Kreja L (1985) Leukemia induction by methylnitrosourea in BDF_1 mice. The origin of transplantable cells and the activity of the natural killer cells during the preleukemic period. Nat Immun Cell Growth Regul 4: 163-201

Preleukemia: Bone Marrow Histopathology in Myelodysplasia and Preleukemic Syndrome

A. Georgii, K. F. Vykoupil, and T. Buhr

Pathologisches Institut, Medizinische Hochschule Hannover, Gutschow-Straße 8, 3000 Hannover 61, FRG

Introduction

Precursors of leukemia have been widely discussed since the term "preleukemia" was introduced by Hamilton-Peterson (1949) and Block et al. (1953). Characteristic cytological features in blood and bone marrow have been defined as common precursors of acute nonlymphocytic leukemia (ANLL) by Saarni and Linman (1973), also termed hemopoietic dysplasia by Linman and Bagby (1978) and preleukemic syndrome (PLS) by Bagby (1985). The occurrence of blasts preceding the clinical symptoms of overt ANLL has long been recognized, with the introduction of various terms such as "smouldering" or "oligoblastic" leukemia, which are also used to designate preleukemic conditions (Rheingold et al. 1963; Seauer et al. 1974; Izrael 1975). The terminology has thus become confused, with many ambiguities and synonyms (Bagby 1985).

A morphological approach has been used to classify the variety of clinical conditions comprising the myelodysplastic syndrome (MDS) according to the FAB system (Bennett et al. 1976, 1982). A histological approach, comparable to Saarni and Linman's method, revealed a peculiar pattern seen in bone marrow preceding leukemia; this was termed myeloid dysplasia (Thiele et al. 1980; Georgii et al. 1981). The histological approach was extended by Tricot et al. (1984, 1986) with particular referral to the occurrence of immature cells to help explain the great variation in clinical course within the categories of the FAB system. As well as efforts to classify the various preleukemic conditions and define the prognosis of each, the question of neoplastic cellular transformation has also been widely emphasized (Greenberg and Bagby 1983; Bagby and Magenis 1985; Tricot et al. 1986a, b). Last but not least, the problem of cytogenetic alterations in preleukemia must be addressed. A great variety of karyotypic abnormalities have been reported (Magenis et al. 1985). Moreover, abnormal karyotypes occur during the preleukemic phase and are related to leukemic transformation (Miller et al. 1985; Tricot et al. 1986; Mecucci et al. 1986). Other primary conditions with an increased risk of acute leukemic transformation are, by definition, not classified as preleukemia or myelodysplasia at present, since they are generally not accompanied by hematological dysplasia.

The discussion of preleukemic conditions has focused upon the variance in clinical outcome among patients with conditions of this type. This is presumed to be due to imprecise nosological definition and the relative difficulty of achieving diagnostic reproducibility using the FAB classification system (Tricot et al. 1984; Bagby 1985). Since bone marrow biopsies greatly improve cytomorphological definition beyond that

Recent Results in Cancer Research, Vol. 106

achieved using bone marrow aspirates alone (Thiele et al. 1980; Tricot et al. 1986) the topic of histopathology will be emphasized within the text. The purpose of this article, therefore, is to critically review the results of studies applying the FAB classification. An alternative system, Bagby's PLS classification, is proposed in the light of our experience with bone marrow histopathology.

Terminology

Preleukemia is a very complex term which is not frequently used at present. One of the major terms used is "myelodysplasia" (MD) - or "myelodysplastic syndrome" (MDS) - which is among the few terms that will be discussed in detail here since it is widely applied in the current literature. This applies to MDS as defined by the FAB group (Bennett et al. 1976, 1982), PLS (Bagby 1985), and MD (Thiele et al. 1980). The present definitions of preleukemia and MDS do not include certain primary diseases and conditions that show a high risk of transformation into leukemia. Among such primary diseases are Fanconi's anemia, Down's syndrome, Bloom's syndrome, and Kostman's syndrome. Neither drug-induced myelodepression following intensive chemotherapy for cancer or lymphoma is regarded among preleukemias; moreover they are not accompanied by typical cytomorphological changes of MDS, although they have a high risk of transformation to ANLL.

Chronic myeloproliferative disorders (CMPD) have been designated secondary preleukemias, since they display myelodysplastic hematological findings, and in chronic myelocytic leukemia (CML) acute leukemia often develops (Mayer and Canellos 1983).

Refractory anemia with an excess of blasts (RAEB) has been described as a characteristic precursor of ANLL that shows the occurrence of ringed sideroblasts (Dreyfus et al. 1970). This represents the most common preleukemia now included in the FAB classification.

Smoldering leukemia is a rather old term designating a benign clinical course that is not really accompanied by clinical markers of ANLL, although an increase of blasts can be observed in bone marrow and blood (Rheingold et al. 1963; Knospe and Gregory 1971). Thus it represents real leukemia at a slowly proliferating stage beyond preleukemia. The term designates a special clinical condition and course and should therefore be applied carefully.

Oligoblastic leukemia, as described by Izrael et al. (1975), displays more than 5% blasts in blood and bone marrow, and therefore represents leukemia, either at a very early or at a very slowly proliferating stage; this will be discussed in the context of PLS.

Hemopoietic dysplasia represents the preleukemic features which were detected by Saarni and Linman (1973) in their retrospective analysis of patients with acute leukemia (Linman and Bagby 1978). It seems to be synonymous with the term PLS.

FAB classification of MDS

When the difficulties of distinguishing very early leukemia from advanced preleukemia first became apparent, the FAB group had already established a system of classification primarily based on the classification of acute leukemia. The FAB nomenclature (Table 1) comprises the old terms RA, RARS - or its synonym "acquired idiopathic sideroblastic anemia," (AISA) - and RAEB (Dreyfus et al. 1970). Chronic myelomonocytic leukemia

Table 1. FAB classification of the myelodysplastic syndromes (MDS) according to Bennett et al. (1982)

Category	Acronym	Maximal percentage of blasts	
		Peripheral blood	Bone marrow
Refractory anemia	RA	1	5
RA with ringed sideroblasts	RARS	1	5
RA with excess blasts	RAEB	5	20
Chronic myelomonocytic leukemia	CMML	5	5
RAEB in transformation to ANLL	RAEB/T	5	30

Table 2. Distribution of MDS patients within the five FAB categories, comparing results from five different studies

FAB	Coiffier et al.		Mufti et al.		Foucar et al.		Vallespi et al.		Tricot et al.	
	n	%	*n*	%	*n*	%	*n*	%	*n*	%
RA	60	31	53	37	13	12	32	32	25	30
RARS	20	11	21	15	22	20	15	15	12	14
RAEB	97	50	25	18	41	38	21	21	14	16
CMML	15	8	31	22	11	10	12	12	11	13
RAEB/T	0	0	11	8	22	20	21	21	23	27
Totals	192	100	141	100	109	101	101	101	85	100

(CMML) (Seauer et al. 1974; Geary et al. 1975; Zittoun 1976) has been classified as MDS, because it is a slowly progressive leukemia terminating in ANLL, although it does not really display the hematological findings of preleukemia, e.g., dyserythropoiesis and dysmegakaryopoiesis.

The revised FAB classification includes the category RAEB/T, which marks the borderline between MD and ANLL (Bennett et al. 1982). The definition of acute leukemia has been altered by this addition, since the limiting value for blasts in bone marrow films has been lowered from 50% to 30% (Table 2).

The FAB classification is based on cytomorphology of smears from peripheral blood and bone marrow aspirates (Table 1). In RA, there are serious cytological abnormalities which may predominate in one, but basically concern all three series of hematopoietic cells. Hence, the terms "dyserythropoiesis" and "dysmyelopoiesis" have evolved, and the abnormalities are now classified as myelodysplasia (Bennett et al. 1976). The reliability of the FAB classification has become the subject of discussion, since it is imprecise and diagnoses are not reproducible, although it is widely applied in hematology (Spitzer and Goldsmith 1982; Greenberg and Bagby 1983; Bagby, 1985; Tricot et al. 1986). Some, however, have found it useful in understanding and treating dysplasia (Economopoulos et al. 1981; Vallespi et al. 1985). Others have pointed out that neither frequency of leukemic transformation nor survival time can be predicted reliably using the FAB classification (Coiffier et al. 1983; Foucar et al. 1985; Tricot et al. 1986a, b).

We have compared reports from five different authors with respect to: first, the spectrum of diagnoses; second, the frequency of leukemic transformation; and third, the duration of disease. Considering the distribution of the five FAB categories among patients studied in these five different reports, conspicuous differences are observed (Table 2). Even between RA and RARS, great variation occurs since the percentages of patients within the categories vary widely. We decided to consider RAEB and RAEB/T under one heading, since these entities are difficult to distinguish from one another; this group occurred in 36%-58% of patients. Moreover, ringed sideroblasts were found in all categories, and the limit of 30% blasts in aspirates may be difficult to reproduce, since the distribution of blasts among hemopoietic cells is quite different in different regions of bone marrow.

The percentage transformation of MDS into acute leukemia reported by different authors also varies considerably (Table 3), with ranges of 8%-18% for RA, 0%-20% for RARS, and 28%-50% for RAEB suggesting that these categories comprise different entities. Although reported survival times have also varied widely, it is possible to roughly compare results from the three authors who have presented evaluable data (Table 4). From comparison of results from different authors who have applied the FAB classification to patients with myelodysplastic conditions, it must be concluded that either the diagnostic criteria of MDS are not sufficient to define comparable conditions or hematological disorders or the diagnostic criteria of the classification itself are not concise enough to distinguish comparable issues.

Table 3. Transformation of MDS into acute leukemia according to the five FAB categories, comparing results from five different studies

FAB category	Coiffier et al. (1983)		Vallespi et al. (1985)		Mufti et al. (1985)		Foucar et al. (1985)		Tricot et al. (1984)	
	Ratio	%	Ratio	%	Ratio	%	Ratio	%	Ratio	%
RA	9/60	14	5/27	18.5	6/53	11	2/13	15	2/25	8
RARS	4/20	20	1/11	9	1/21	5	0/22	0	1/12	8
RAEB	32/97	44	8/19	42	7/25	28	13/41	32	7/14	50
CMML	6/15	40	0/8	0	4/32	13	3/11	27	6/11	55
RAEB/T	0	0	10/14	71	6/11	55	11/22	50	14/23	61
	62/192	32	24/79	30	24/141	17	29/109	27	30/85	35

Table 4. Survival of all patients with MDS according to the five categories of FAB classification; medians and days. Comparison of results from three different studies

FAB	Coiffier et al. (1983)		Mufti et al. (1985)		Foucar et al. (1985)	
	n	Days	*n*	Days	*n*	Days
RA	60	1223	53	960	11	2220
RARS	20	1581	21	2280	21	930
RAEB	97	319	25	315	23	240
CMML	15	340	31	660	6	240
RAEB/T	0		11	150	16	150
	192		141		77	
Mean length		636		873		756

Table 5. The FAB categories of MDS versus Bagby's preleukemic syndrome (PLS) as an approach to distinguishing oligoblastic and smoldering leukemias from the complex of preleukemias

	PLS	Bagby classification	
		Oligoblastic or smoldering leukemia	ANLL
Blasts in bone marrow (%)	5	5–30	30
FAB category of MDS	RA RARS	RAEB RAEB/T CMML	ANLL M1–M6

Preleukemic Syndrome

As a result of the difficulties in clearly distinguishing between different preleukemic conditions, e.g., myelodysplasias, Bagby and others (Bagby 1985) have proposed the PLS classification system (Table 5). The system is based upon the simple criterion of blast distribution; more than 5% blasts, even in bone marrow smears, indicates real leukemia, e.g., oligoblastic disease. Only myelodysplasias having less than 5% blasts are considered as PLS (Table 5). An approach simplifying the FAB term MDS to denote Bagby's PLS seems quite convincing considering the great variations in results between authors regarding criteria such as distribution, life expectancy, and leukemic transformation.

Histopathology of Myelodysplasia or Myelodysplastic Syndromes

Retrospective analysis of bone marrow (BM) biopsy specimens obtained before definitive diagnosis of ANLL has revealed the histological pattern of MD (Thiele et al. 1980; Georgii et al. 1981). This approach has also revealed the following histopathological features of MD which are similar to smears of BM aspirates:

1. Hyperplasia of the hematopoietic tissue is a common feature in the great majority of biopsies of these cases and not only found in cases with increase of blasts, however normocellularity may occur to some extent, whereas hypocellularity is rarely found.
2. Erythropoietic hyperplasia occurs, with macrocytic or megaloblastoid inhibition of maturation (Fig. 1); binucleated cells and pyknotic or fragmented nuclei are rarely found.
3. Histiocytes and erythropoietic cells generally stain more intensely for siderin; ringed sideroblasts can be recognized, but are more difficult to identify than in BM smears from the same patient.
4. Megakaryocytes are more abundant and smaller, representing dwarfed or micromegakaryocytes (Figs. 1a and 2). Nuclei are often roundish, since their lobulation is reduced. Grouping or clustering of the increased megakaryocytes is found in some cases.
5. Granulopoietic tissue may be hyperplastic, but is generally reduced in quantity. There is little disturbance of maturation, and an increase in the number of immature cells is rarely observed in real MD. However, the site of granulopoiesis is displaced from the

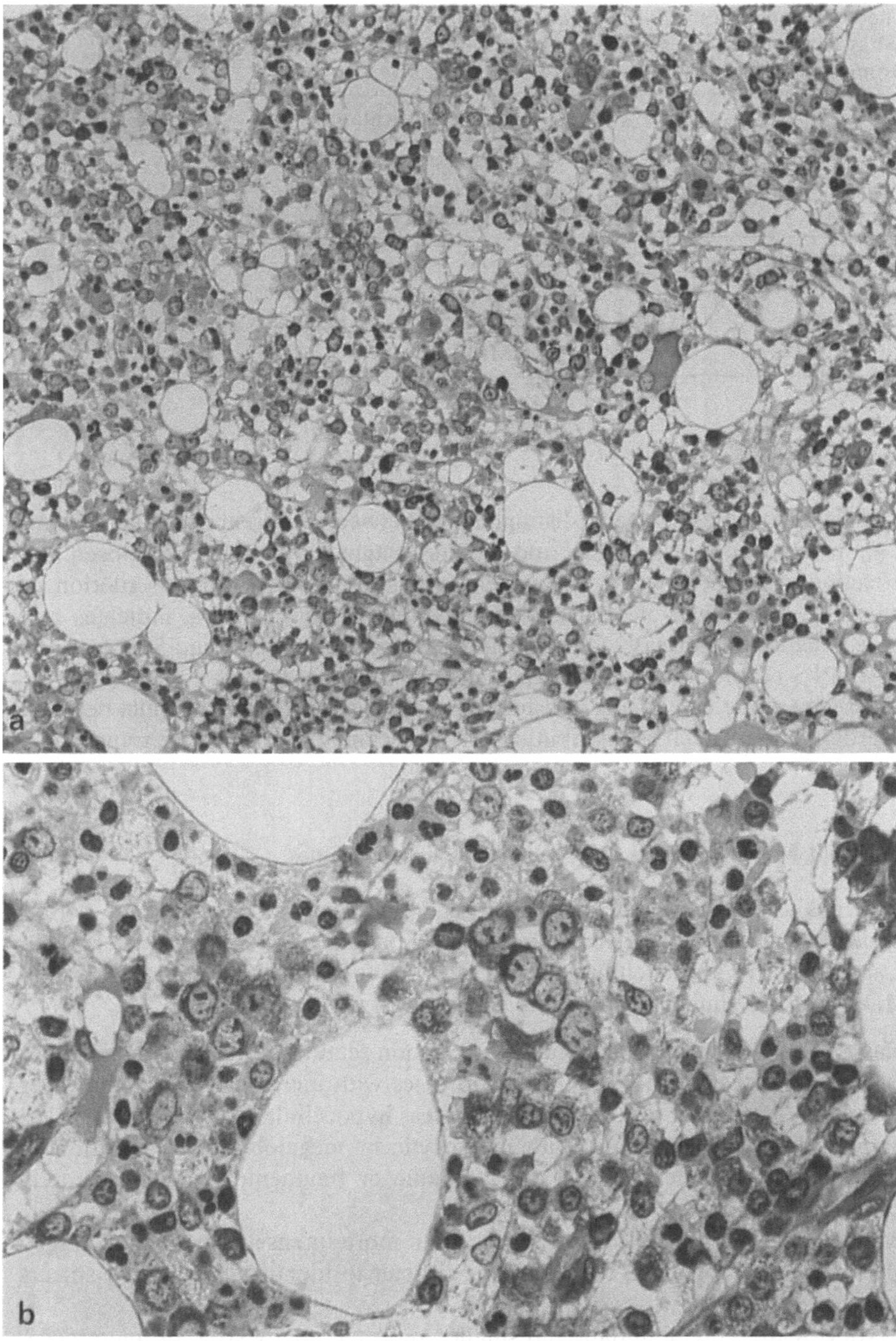

Fig. 1 a, b. Myelodysplasia with predominant erythropoiesis which can be misinterpreted as blasts because of poor technical preparation. The megakaryocytes are not very numerous and are dwarfed or micromegakaryocytes. Conspicuous inflammation with patchy edema can be seen. ×12

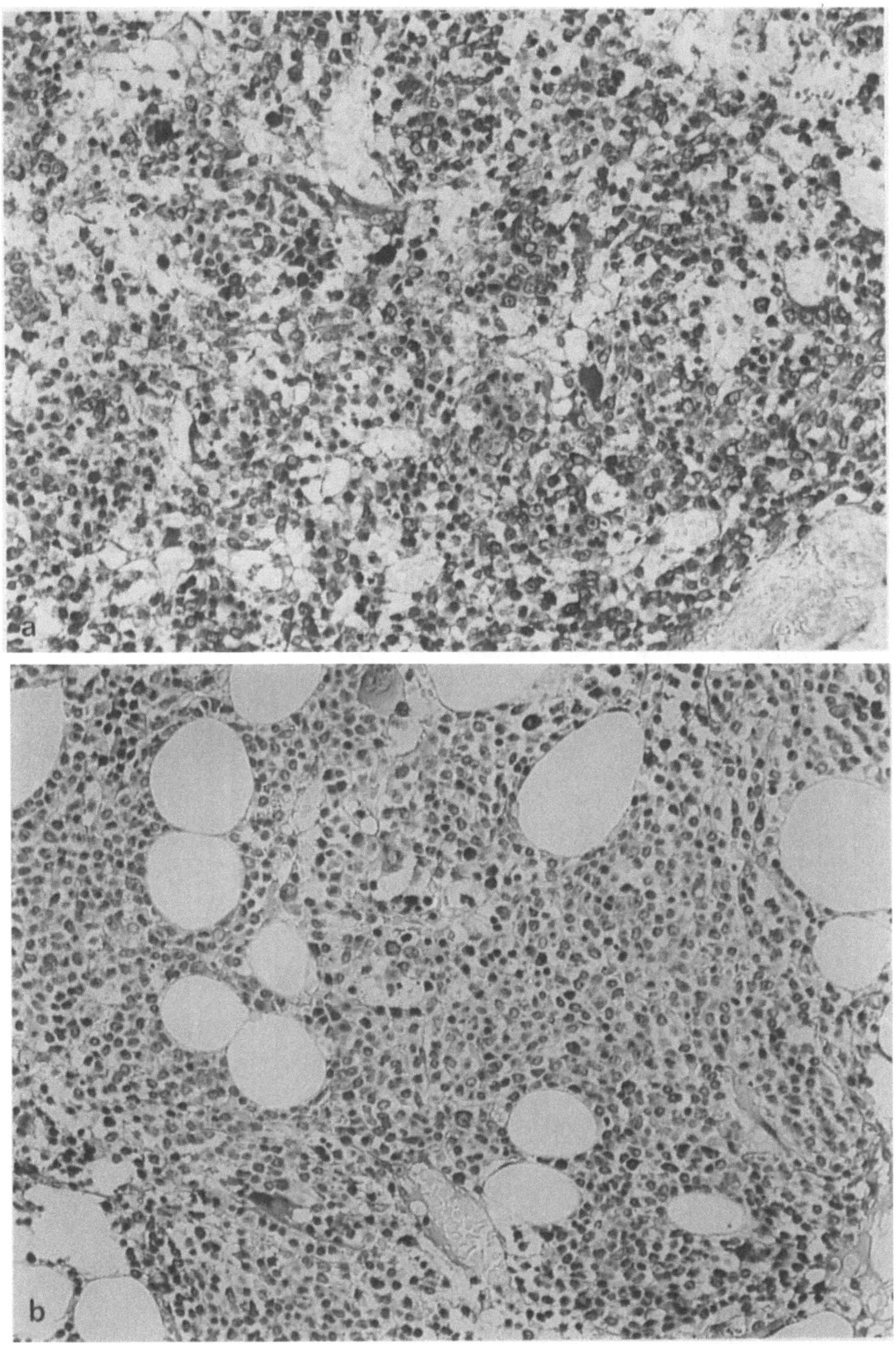

Fig. 2a, b. Myelodysplasia versus early ANLL. **a** Myelodysplasia with numerous proerythroblasts and small megakaryocytes but without increase in nonerythropoietic immature or blast cells. This may correspond with RA and RARS of the FAB classification. **b** Early ANLL with fields of blasts distant from the original location of granulopoiesis. This is more than RAEB/T, although remnants of MD with hyperplastic erythropoiesis and micromegakaryocytes can be recognized

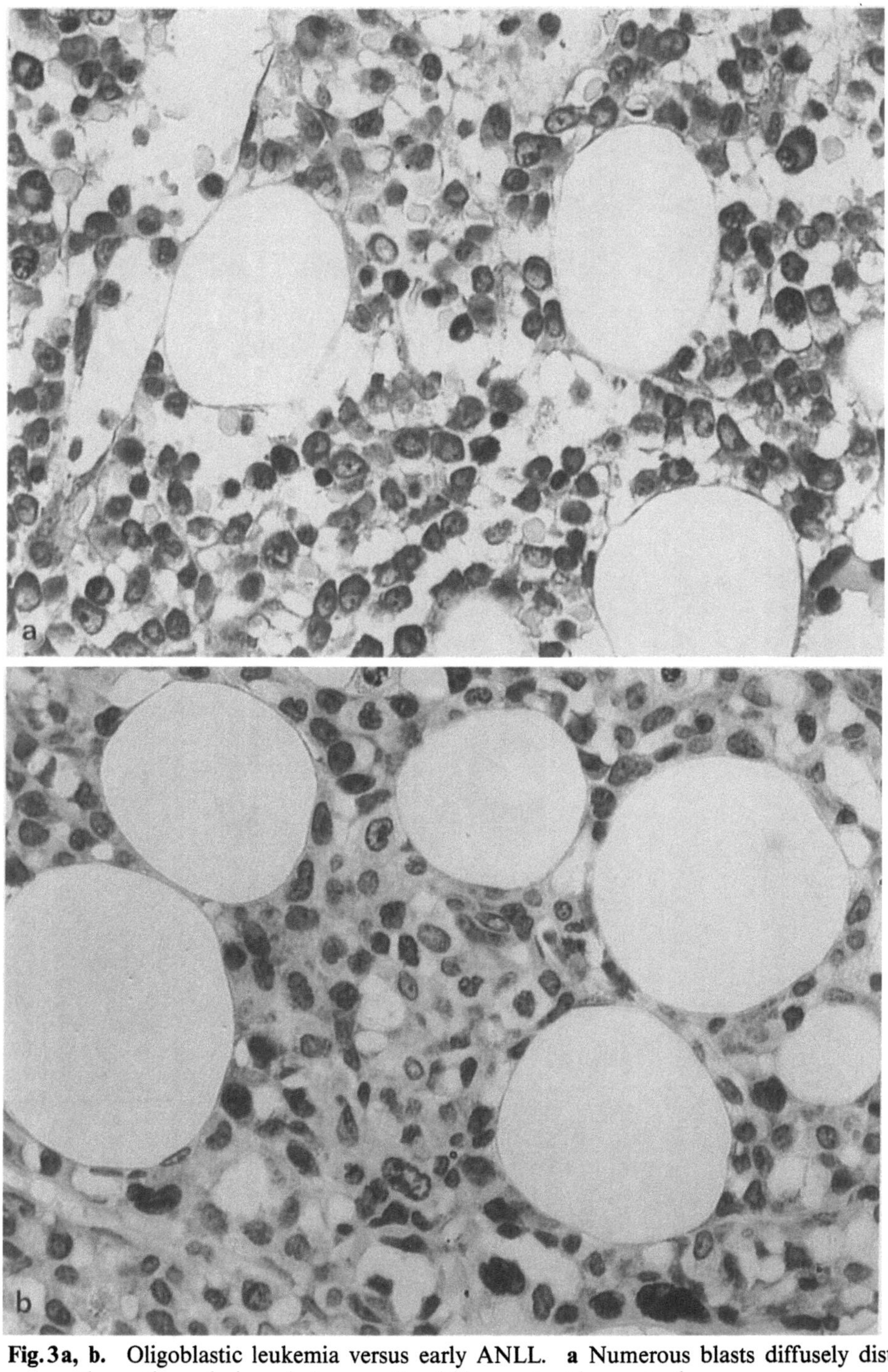

Fig. 3 a, b. Oligoblastic leukemia versus early ANLL. **a** Numerous blasts diffusely distributed among the erythropoiesis and plasma cells within a not yet hyperplastic marrow represent an oligoblastic leukemia or RAEB/T. **b** Early ANLL reveals higher cellularity with numerous blasts but not yet the packed marrow as in overt leukemia. ×300 in both

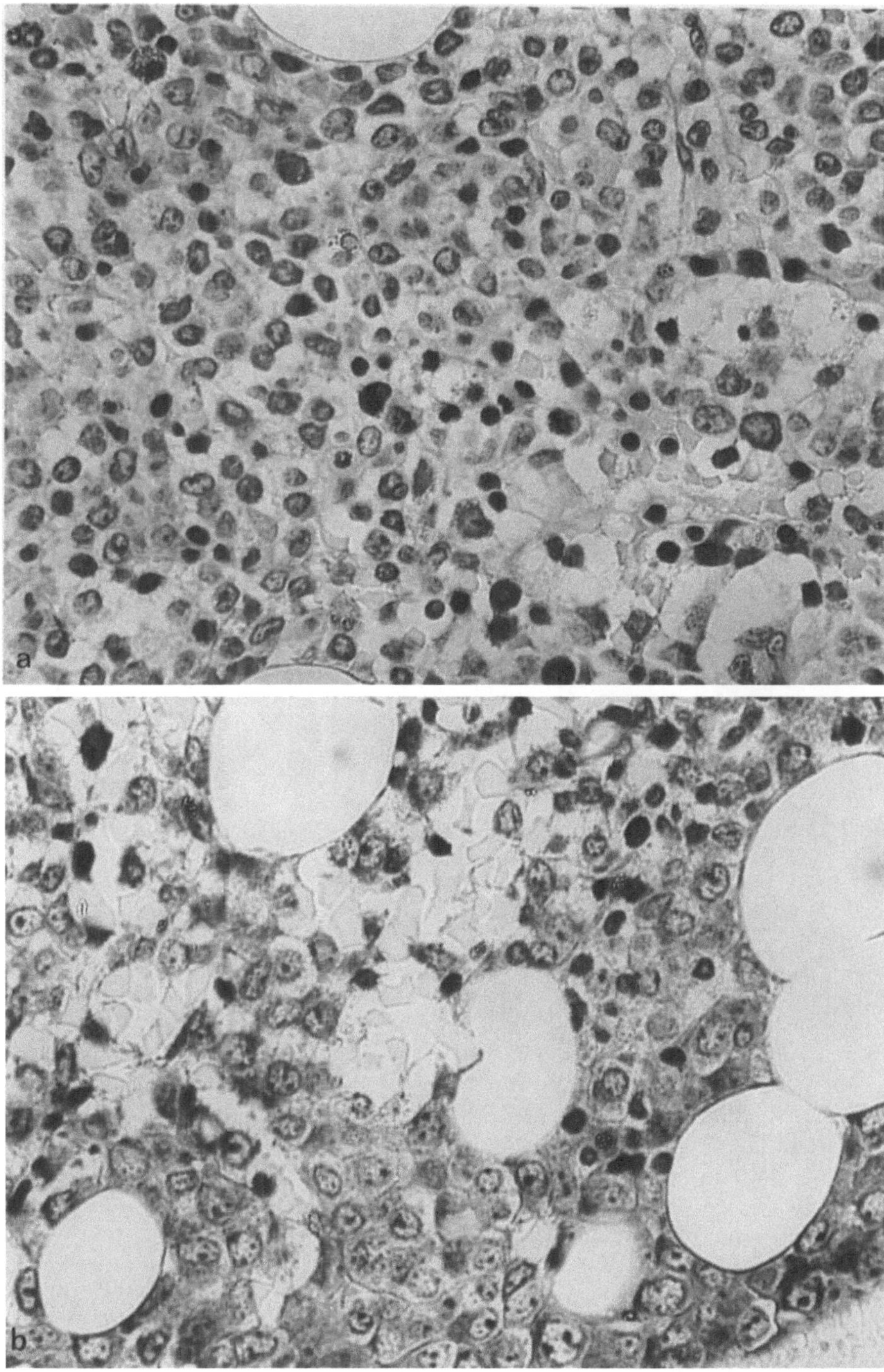

Fig. 4 a, b. Oligoblastic leukemia versus complete ANLL. **a** Loosely intermingled blasts with hyperplasia of erythropoietic and hemopoietic tissue. **b** Dense blastic transformation adjacent to a bone trabeculum; marker analysis of BM smears revealed erythroleukemia of the FAB type M6. ×300 fold in both

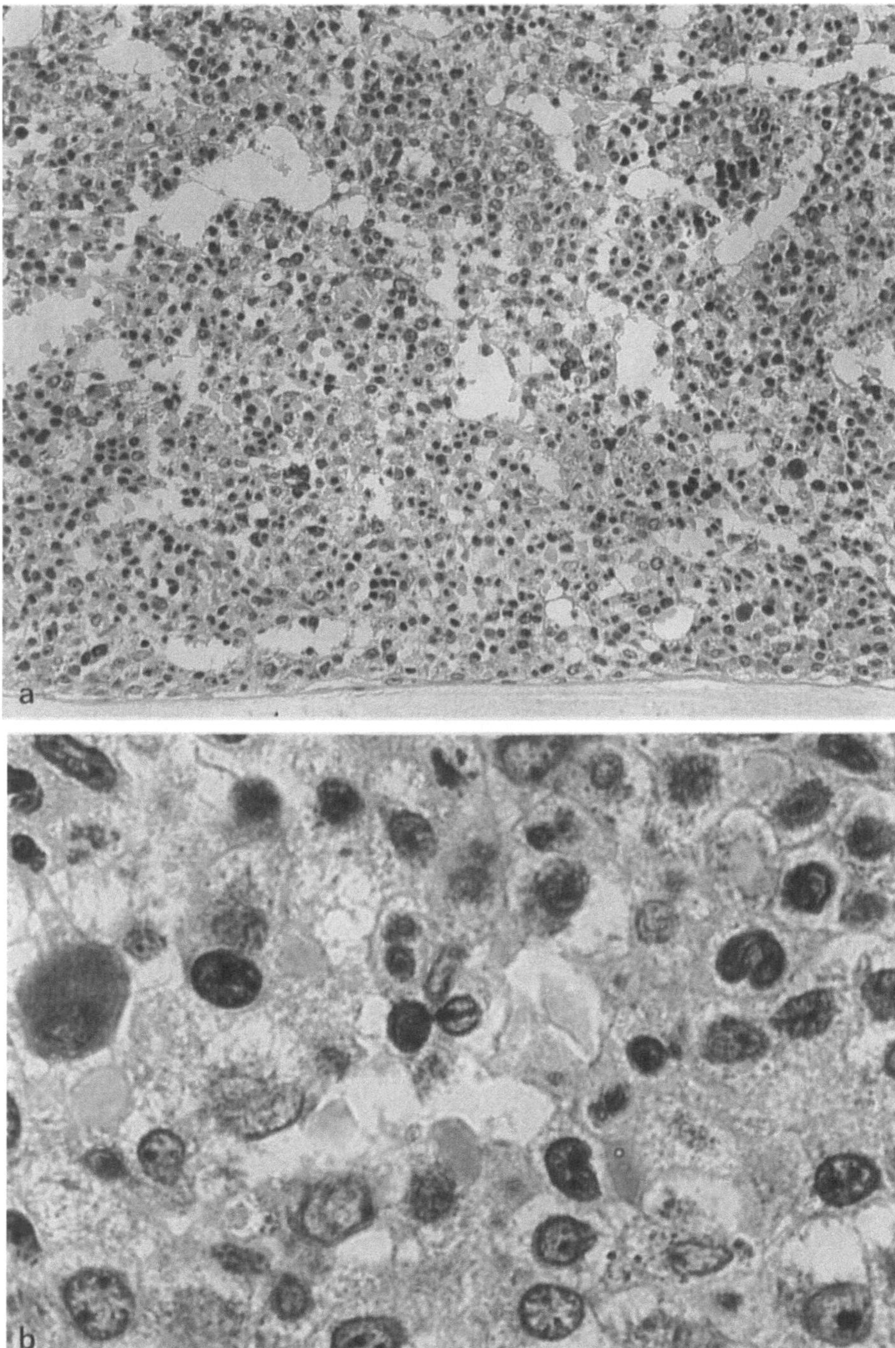

Fig. 5 a, b. Chronic myelo-monocytic leukemia. **a** Mixed population of monocytes, monoblastic cells, and micromegakaryocytes. **b** Higher magnification of *bottom right* of **a**. Magnifications: **a** approximately × 120, **b** approximately × 500

endosteal region toward the center of the marrow. This is described as atypical localization of immature precursor cells (the ALIP phenomenon) (Tricot et al.); the displacement is not necessarily accompanied by proliferation of immature cells. Inhibition of nuclear segmentation, resulting in pseudo-Pelger forms, is another possible feature.

6. There is often mesenchymal involvement, with inflammation characterized by plasma- and mast-cell increases, patchy edema and capillary dilatation (Fig. 1a). The number of reticulin fibers is only rarely increased. Tricot et al. (1984, 1986a) described similar features using a comparable technique, and employing undecalcified methacrylate embedding. The ALIP phenomenon was shown to be a reliable prognostic indicator (Tricot et al. 1986b).

The important question as to whether the changes seen with histopathology of BM biopsies correspond to the cytological criteria of the FAB classification, as determined from BM smears, still remains unanswered. The first two groups - RA and RARS - are easily classified, although a high percentage of ringed sideroblasts is more difficult to demonstrate in sections than in smears. However, histopathology of core biopsies can reliably exclude an increase in numbers of immature or blast cells of granulopoiesis, apart from megaloblastoid erythropoiesis. The distinction between RAEB and RAEB/T may be clarified by intensively evaluating the course and outcome of a sufficient number of MDS patients. Besides comparing the histopathological findings with the clinical course, an attempt to distinguish between oligoblastic leukemia and early ANLL should also be made, since these histological categories may correspond to RAEB and RAEB/T, at least in cases which rapidly progress to overt leukemia. ALIP-positive histology presumably corresponds to RAEB or RAEB/T.

Since megaloblastoid erythropoiesis, sideroblasts, and pseudo-Pelger cells do not occur in CMML, this condition belongs to a different category than MD. In CMML, monocytoid elements and granulopoietic hyperplasia are found (Fig. 5). The finding of micromegakaryocytes is the only feature common to CMML and MD.

Occurrence of MD in BM Biopsies

The histopathological changes of MD are not frequently observed among large numbers of randomly referred BM biopsies (Table 6). In our own material the percentage was approximately 1.43%. The great majority of these biopsies were performed following a

Table 6. Frequency of occurrence of myelodysplastic syndrome among routine bone marrow biopsies

Year	Total number of biopsies	MDS among the total	
		No.	Percent
1979	2915	34	1.16
1980	3297	44	1.33
1981	3447	36	1.04
1982	3970	62	1.56
1983	5295	68	1.28
1984	5895	111	1.88
	24819	355	1.43

clinical diagnosis of RA or MDS. A clinical diagnosis of leukemia was only rarely made; in contrast, myeloproliferative disorders were often detected when MDS was presumed by hematologists.

Discussion

Several aspects of the classification of MDS or PLS should be considered. The reliability with which the clinical outcome can be evaluated and decisions regarding therapeutic consequences are the two important issues. Finally, the question as to the level of cellular proliferation at which leukemic transformation occurs is of importance in these clinically very different conditions. It has been proposed that all of these conditions are based upon neoplastic transformation at the stem cell or progenitor level, since the Fialkow phenomenon, the loss of one isoenzyme from glucose-6-phosphate dehydrogenase (G6PD), can be observed in all cases of MDS (Tricot et al. 1986a, b). It is not clear at present whether this hypothesis can be widely accepted.

The FAB classification offers a reasonable instrument for diagnosis and subtyping of MDS patients. However, inadequacies of this system must be admitted since a variety of survival times and rates of leukemic transformation have been reported by various authors who applied this classification system.

The main problem underlying the difficulties in obtaining reproducible results may be found in a kind of over-classification inherent in the five categories of the FAB typing. One could argue that a simpler way of classifying the two entities could avoid those conspicuous differences in the courses and outcome of the course of these patients, since the term "PLS" would comprise the first three of the five FAB categories, whereas the "oligoblastic leukemia" would cover the RAEB and the RAEB/T categories. So, the comparison of those two different classification systems could offer a way to avoid the impediment of unreliable classification with considerable variation between observers.

The histopathology of BM biopsies is an additional way to distinguish MD from preleukemic conditions. It not only reveals features which correspond to those found in smears of BM aspirates but also increases the relevance of such findings since hemopoiesis is observed intact in large fields. Bone marrow aspiration, by contrast, results in a degree of selection of the cells drawn for analysis.

References

Bagby GC (ed) (1985) The preleukemic syndrome (hemopoietic dysplasia). CRC, Boca Raton

Bagby GC, Magenis RG (1985) Clonal evolution in the preleukemic syndrome. In: Bagby GC (ed) The preleukemic syndrome (hemopoietic dysplasia). CRC, Boca Raton, pp 127-134

Bennett JM, Catovsky C, Daniel MT, Flandrin G, Galton DAG, Gralnick HR, Sultan C (1976) Proposals for the classification of the acute leukaemias. Br J Haematol 33: 451-458

Bennett JM, Catovsky D, Daniel MT, Flandrin G, Galton DAG, Gralnick HR, Sultan C (1982) Proposals for the classification of the myelodysplastic syndromes. Br J Haematol 51: 189-199

Block M, Jacobson LO, Bethard WF (1953) Preleukemic acute human leukemia. JAMA 152: 1018-1028

Coiffier B, Adeleine P, Viala JJ, Bryon PA, Fiere D, Gentilhomme O, Vuvan H (1983) Dysmyelopoietic syndromes. A search for prognostic factors in 193 patients. Cancer 52: 83-90

Economopoulos T, Stathakis N, Maragoyannis Z, Gardikas E, Der Venoulas I (1981) Myelodysplastic syndrome. Clinical and prognostic significance of monocyte count, degree of blastic infiltration, and ring sideroblasts. Acta Haematol (Basel) 65: 97-102

Foucar K, Langdon RM II, Armitage JO, Olson DB, Carroll TJ Jr (1985) Myelodysplastic syndromes. A clinical and pathologic analysis of 109 cases. Cancer 56: 553-561

Geary CG, Catovsky D, Wiltshaw E, et al. (1975) Chronic myelomonocytic leukaemia. Br J Haematol 30: 289

Georgii A, Thiele J, Vykoupil KF (1981) Myeloid dysplasia: the histopathology of preleukemia. In: Neth R, Gallo RG, Mannweiler K, Graf T, Winkler K (eds) Modern trends in human leukemia IV. Springer, Berlin Heidelberg New York, pp 34-37

Gralnick HR, Galton DAG, Catovsky D, Sultan C, Bennett JM (1977) Classification of acute leukemia. Ann Intern Med 87: 740-753

Greenberg P, Bagby G (1983) Biologic rather than morphologic markers in myelodysplastic syndromes. Br J Haematol 53: 532-534

Hamilton-Paterson JL (1949) Preleukemic anemia. Acta Haematol (Basel) 2: 309

Heimpel H, Drings P, Mitrou P, Quisser W (1979) Verlauf und prognostische Kriterien bei Patienten mit Präleukämie. Klin Wochenschr 57: 21-29

Izrael V, Jacquillat C, Chastaing G, Weil M, Deheaulme M, Boiron M, Bernard J (1975) Données nouvelles sur les leucémies oligoblastiques. A propos d'une analyse de 120 cas. Nouv Presse Med 4: 947

Knospe WH, Gregory SA (1971) Smoldering acute leukemia. Arch Intern Med 127: 910-917

Linman JW, Bagby GC Jr (1978) The preleukemic syndrome (hemopoietic dysplasia). Cancer 42: 854-864

Magenis RE, Yoshitomi M, Smith L, Bagby GC (1985) Cytogenetic studies on marrow cells from patients with the preleukemic syndrome. In: Bagby GC (ed) The preleukemic syndrome (hemopoietic dysplasia). CRC, Boca Raton, pp 103-126

Mayer RI, Canellos GP (1983) Preleukemic syndromes and other myeloproliferative disorders. In: Gunz FW, Henderson ES (eds) Leukemia. Grune and Stratton, New York, p 741

Mecucci C, RegeCambrin G, Michaux J-L, Tricot G, van den Berghe H (1986) Multiple chromosomally distinct cell populations in myelodysplastic syndromes and their possible significance in the evolution of the disease. Br J Haematol 64: 699-706

Miller BA, Weinstein HJ, Neil M, Henkle CT, Dillon PL, Tantravahi R (1985) Sequential development of distinct clonal chromosome abnormalities in a patient with preleukaemia. Br J Haematol 59: 411-418

Mufti GJ, Stevens JR, Oscier DG, Hamblin TJ, Machin D (1985) Myelodysplastic syndromes: a scoring system with prognostic significance. Br J Haematol 59: 425-433

Rheingold JJ, Kaufman R, Adelson E, Lear A (1963) Smoldering acute leukemia. N Engl J Med 268: 812-815

Saarni MI, Linman JW (1973) Preleukemia. The hematologic syndrome preceding acute leukemia. Am J Med 55: 38-48

Seauer J, Kass L, Schnitzer B (1974) Subacute myelomonocytic leukemia. Am J Med 57: 853

Spitzer TR, Goldsmith GH (1982) Myelodysplastic syndromes: is another classification necessary? Br J Haematol 52: 343

Thiele J, Vykoupil K-F, Georgii A (1980) Myeloid dysplasia (MD): a hematological disorder preceding acute and chronic myeloid leukemia. Virchows Arch [A] 389: 343-367

Tricot G, de Wolf-Peeters C, Hendricks B, Verwilghen RL (1984) Bone marrow histology in myelodysplastic syndromes. I. Histological findings in myelodysplastic syndromes and comparison with bone marrow smears. Br J Haematol 57: 423-430

Tricot G, Mecucci C, van den Berghe H (1986a) Evolution of the myelodysplastic syndromes. Br J Haematol 63: 609-614

Tricot G, Vlietinck R, Verwilghen RL (1986b) Prognostic factors in the myelodysplastic syndromes: a review. Scand J Haematol [Suppl 45] 36: 107-113

Vallespi T, Torrabadella M, Julia A, Irriguible D, Jaen A, Acebedo G, Triginer J (1985) Myelodysplastic syndromes: a study of 101 cases according to the FAB-classification. Br J Haematol 61: 83-92

Zittoun R (1976) Subacute and chronic myelomonocytic leukaemia: a distinct haematological entity. Br J Haematol 32: 1-7

Cytobiology and Clinical Findings of Myelodysplastic Syndromes

D. Hoelzer

Abteilung für Hämatologie, Zentrum der Inneren Medizin, Johann-Wolfgang-Goethe-Universität, Theodor-Stern-Kai 7, 6000 Frankfurt 70, FRG

The term preleukemia introduced by Hamilton-Paterson in 1949 and Block et al. in 1953 described any syndrome which precedes the onset of acute leukemia but in which the criteria for the diagnosis of acute leukemia are not fulfilled. Later preleukemia was considered as peripheral pancytopenia with hyperplastic bone marrow due to ineffective hemopoiesis.

The main symptoms of preleukemia are a bi- or tricytopenia in the peripheral blood, a normal or more often a hypercellular bone marrow, qualitative changes in erythro-, granulo- and megakaryopoiesis, and leukemic blast cells in bone marrow and/or blood. The involvement of all three myeloid cell series suggests that there is a somatic mutation at the level of the hemopoietic stem cell common for the erythro-, granulo-, and megakaryopoiesis. Thus preleukemia, as acute leukemia, can be considered a clonal disease.

The typical morphological alterations in the granulopoietic series are hyposegmentation resulting in pseudo-Pelger cells and hypogranulation, both probably contributing to the loss of function and thereby leading to increased risk of infection. Changes in the erythropoietic series include multinucleated precursors, karyorrhexis, and ringed sideroblasts. Dyshemoglobinization as well as aniso- and poikilocytosis can also be observed. Notable abnormalities in the megakaryopoiesis are hyper- or, more often, hyposegmentation leading to the typical micromegakaryocytes.

Myelodysplastic Syndrome - FAB Classification

The qualitative and quantitative hemopoietic changes are not solely characteristic of preleukemia but a variety of other syndromes, such as smoldering leukemia and subacute myeloid leukemia. di Guglielmo's syndrome and hypocellular leukemia show similar alterations. Therefore a uniform classification according to morphological criteria was introduced, as for the acute leukemias. This French-American-British (FAB) classification (Bennett et al. 1982) assembles all these diseases under the term myelodysplastic syndromes (MDS). The division into five subtypes is made according to (Table 1) the proportion of blast cells in the bone marrow and in the blood, the presence of Auer rods, the absolute monocyte count, and the percentage of ringed sideroblasts in the bone marrow. Refractory anemia (RA) is characterized by having less than 5% blast cells. The same is true for acquired idiopathic sideroblastic anemia (AISA), which typically also has over 15% ringed sideroblasts in the bone marrow. Refractory anemia with excess of

Recent Results in Cancer Research, Vol. 106

Table 1. FAB classification of myelodysplastic Syndromes

	% blasts in the bone marrow	% blasts in the peripheral blood	Monocytes 1×10^9/liter	Ringed sideroblasts >15% in bone marrow
RA Refractory anemia	[<5%]	<1%		
AISA Acquired idiopathic sideroblastic anemia	<5%	⩽1%		[+]
RAEB RA with excess of blasts	[5%–20%]	<5%	−/+	−/+
CMML Chronic myelo-monocytic leukemia	<20%	<5%	[+]	−/+
RAEBT RAEB in transformation	[>20%–30%]	⩾5%	−/+	−/+
AML	>30%			

Table 2. Frequency of different FAB types in MDS. (Data from Teerenhovi and Lintula 1986; Todd and Pierre 1986; Tricot et al. 1986b)

FAB	Teerenhovi (N=162)	Todd (N=326)	Coffier/Mufti/Tricot (N=418)	Total[a] (N=906)
RA	28%	39%	33%	34%
AISA	26%	17%	13%	17%
RAEB	29%	8%	33%	23%
CMML	11%	9%	13%	11%
RAEBT	5%	1%	8%	5%

[a] Weighted mean.

blasts (RAEB) is defined by a blast cell content of 5%–20%. In chronic myelomonocytic leukemia (CMML) there is in addition an absolute monocyte count of over 1×10^9/liter. The newly defined subgroup RAEBT, i.e., RAEB in transformation, has a blast cell content of between 20% and 30%. Acute myeloid leukemia is distinguished by having a blast cell content of more than 30% in the bone marrow. Everyone who deals with the evaluation of bone marrow histology and aspirates knows that it is difficult to distinguish between a blast cell content of 19% and 21% or between 29% and 31%. This becomes evident when the frequency distribution of FAB subtypes in the three largest published series of patients with myelodysplastic syndromes is considered (Table 2). There is quite good agreement with respect to the frequency of RA and CMML; however, quite large differences appear in the assessment of RA, RAEB, and RAEBT. These disagreements arise from the fact that morphological criteria form the only basis for classification and probably additional parameters, such as cytogenetic analysis and growth pattern of hemopoietic stem cells, should be included. Despite these limitations, the FAB classification for MDS is a useful instrument for comparing different therapeutic modalities in this heterogeneous group of diseases.

Frequency

The myelodysplastic syndromes are apparently increasing. In the United States the incidence is 1 per 100000 inhabitants and for Belgium a threefold increase was seen in recent years. The probable reasons for the higher frequency of MDS are firstly wider recognition due to better knowledge of the disease, secondly an absolute rise with higher age due to increased life expectancy, and thirdly the effect of environmental factors. Thus, for example, secondary leukemias after treatment of neoplastic disease with alkylating agents and radiation are mostly preceded by a myelodysplastic phase.

Clinical Findings

Myelodysplastic syndrome is a disease found principally in the higher age group (Table 3). The average age is 65 years and male sex is predominant. About 10%–15% of patients with MDS are below the age of 50 years and myelodysplastic syndromes are even diagnosed in children. Anemia is the change found most frequently at diagnosis. About half of the cases have a thrombocytopenia or a leukopenia. Only a minority of patients show a leukocytosis at presentation. Of organ involvement, only splenomegaly is noticeable.

Course of MDS

The major risk in myelodysplastic syndromes is the transition to an overt acute leukemia. The risk for leukemic transformation, as can be seen from a series of large and well-documented studies (Table 4), is increasing from 15% for refractory anemia to about 60% for RAEBT. Correspondingly, the median survival decreases. For the subtypes RA and AISA a wide range of survival times is evident. The very short survival time for RAEBT, which is even shorter than that for acute myeloid leukemia, demonstrates the difficulties involved in treating this advanced form of myelodysplastic syndrome.

Table 3. Clinical findings in patients with MDS ($N = 814$). (Data from Hoelzer et al. 1984)

Age (years)	65 (16–92)
Sex (m:f)	1.6:1
Anemia	83%
Thrombocytopenia	54%
Leukopenia	48%
Leukocytosis	15%
Splenomegaly	15%

Table 4. Clinical outcome according to FAB types

FAB	Risk of leukemic transformation	Survival time (median)
RA	5%–15%	17–52 months
AISA	15%–20%	16–76 months
RAEB	20%–40%	11–17 months
CMML	30%	2–22 months
RAEBT	60%	2–11 months

Pooled data from the literature.

The major causes of death in patients with myelodysplastic syndromes are a transformation into acute leukemia in about one-third and death occurs in the same proportion due to infections and bleeding. The causes of death are clearly related to age and in patients above 70 years, deaths due to infections or bleeding amount to 59% compared with 24% for patients less than 50 years of age (Tricot et al. 1986b). About 10% of patients die of age-related causes not associated with the underlying disease.

Prognostic Factors

For a therapeutic decision it would be helpful if a transformation of MDS into an acute leukemia could be foreseen. From the published data several criteria arise which can predict such a transformation within 2 years with a probability of more than 50% for preleukemia (Heimpel and Hoelzer 1982). Such parameters are (1) involvement of all three cell lines, (2) a high percentage of micromegakaryocytes, (3) a high content of blast cells in bone marrow, (4) the emergence of chromosomal abnormalities, and (5) atypical growth pattern of hemopoietic stem cells. In several studies it has been demonstrated (Table 5) that the risk of leukemic transformation is clearly increased in patients with an abnormal clone, with 43% compared with only 21% for those patients with MDS who have a normal karyotype. Chromosome abnormalities are now believed to be an independent prognostic factor for myelodysplastic syndromes (Yunis et al. 1986). Similarly, there is a higher transformation rate in those patients where the growth pattern of hemopoietic stem cells in agar culture is leukemic (Table 6). Within the group of patients with a leukemic growth pattern, 51% later had a transformation into acute leukemia compared with only 23% for those with a nonleukemic growth pattern. In one study an attempt was made to establish a scoring system for myelodysplastic syndromes (Mufti et al. 1985). When patients with MDS were scored according to the hematological features bone marrow blasts $<5\%$, platelets $<100\times10^9$/liter, neutrophils $<2.5\times10^9$/liter,

Table 5. Frequency of chromosome aberrations and outcome in MDS patients. (Data from Hoelzer et al. 1984)

Total patients	Patients with		Patients developing ANLL with	
	Abnormal karyotype	Normal karyotype	Abnormal karyotype	Normal karyotype
529	249	280	43%	26%

Table 6. In vitro growth of hemopoietic stem cells and outcome in MDS patients. (Data from Hoelzer et al. 1984)

Number of patients	Patients with leukemic growth pattern	Patients developing ANLL with	
		Leukemic growth pattern	Nonleukemic growth pattern
441	194 (43%)	51%	23%

Leukemic growth pattern = reduced colony growth
increased micro-/macrocluster growth
increased cluster: colony ratio.

and Hb < 10.0 g/dl, a highly significant difference in survival between the arising groups was observed. These factors and, in addition, evaluation of the karyotype and the growth pattern in agar culture are already used in some studies to decide when and how a patient with MDS should be treated.

Treatment

Although a few patients with MDS have a long survival, the average survival time for all forms of MDS is only about 15 months. These results are no better than those which can be obtained in acute myeloid leukemia, emphasizing the need for improved therapeutic strategies for patients with MDS.

The decision when to treat a patient with MDS intensively is often very difficult. Several factors contribute to this uncertainty. Initially the diagnosis is usually not clear and is confirmed only by the course of the disease. Often the disease progresses very slowly and hemopoietic function is still sufficient. Furthermore, since normal hemopoietic stem cells are reduced the regeneration after intensive chemotherapy is delayed and posttherapeutic aplasias lead to severe complications. Also, owing to the higher age of most patients there is an increased risk of toxicity to nonhemopoietic organs.

The therapeutic possibilities for patients with myelodysplastic syndromes are listed in Table 7. Most important is still the supportive therapy, with substitution of erythrocytes and thrombocytes and treatment of infections. Androgens and glucocorticoids are often used but complete remissions can mostly not be obtained. However, improvements such as, e.g., correction of anemia in patients with RA, can be achieved. In a study where patients with preleukemia were treated with glucocorticoids (Bagby et al. 1980), only a small proportion of about 10% responded well, whereby in vitro colony growth could identify the steroid responsive and unresponsive patients. At the same time, the hazard of infectious complications connected with glucocorticoid therapy must be weighed carefully against the therapeutic benefit in these patients.

Chemotherapy

Intensive chemotherapy has up to now had disappointing results in patients with MDS. Often patients have prolonged posttherapeutic aplasia leading to fatal infections and in addition remissions are short. With improved cytostatic schedules for treatment of

Table 7. Therapy of myelodysplastic syndromes

1. Androgens	
2. Glucocorticoids	
3. Intensive chemotherapy	< 50 years
4. Bone marrow transplantation	< 50 years
5. Supportive therapy	< 50 years; > 50 years
6. Differentiation therapy	> 50 years
Low-dose Ara-C	> 50 years
Vitamin A and vitamin D analogues	> 50 years
7. Biological response modifiers	> 50 years
γ-interferon	> 50 years
GM-CSF	> 50 years

ANNL applied in MDS and with the general improvement in supportive therapy, results of treatment in MDS patients are slightly better (Tricot et al. 1986a). Thus intensive chemotherapy might become an approach in younger patients with excess of bone marrow blasts before transition to overt ANNL.

Bone Marrow Transplantation

A promising new approach seems to be bone marrow transplantation for younger patients with MDS. Since the first transplantation of a patient with MDS in 1979 (Bhadhuri et al. 1979), about 30 patients have been transplanted; of these, about two-thirds are still alive and remain in remission. Table 8 gives the results of the two largest series (Applebaum et al. 1984; Tricot et al. 1986a). The median age of these patients is 13 and 24 years; the oldest patient is, however, 54 years. Bone marrow transplantation seems at present to be the only chance of curing MDS and for the 10%-15% of patients below 50 years of age, transplantation should be carried out whenever possible.

Differentiation Induction

The concept of differentiation therapy is not, as in cytotoxic therapy, to destroy the leukemic cells but to induce maturation up to a stage where the cells are no longer capable of self-replication and thereby exhausting the proliferating malignant cells. It has been demonstrated in mouse leukemic cell lines (Sachs 1978) and in fresh human leukemic cells (Hoelzer et al. 1977) that the differentiation block can be overcome and that cells can be induced to differentiate into mature granulocytes with partially normal function. That phenotypically normal granulocytes in leukemic patients in remission can be descendants of a malignant clone has been shown convincingly at the molecular level (Fearon et al. 1986). Thus, differentiation induction as a form of therapy without the severe side effects of intensive chemotherapy is now a considered concept for elderly patients with acute myeloblastic leukemias and myelodysplastic syndromes.

Substances which can induce differentiation in mouse or human myeloid leukemic cells are listed in Table 9. There is a great variety of "inducers," including physiological regulator substances such as colony-stimulating factors (CSFs), analogues of vitamin A and vitamin D, biological response modifiers, cytostatic drugs in low dosage, polar compounds, or even tumor promoters. It is evident that the underlying mechanisms by which they induce differentiation must differ widely and there is more speculation than knowledge about their mode of action (Bloch 1984).

Low-dose cytosine arabinoside (Ara-C) is one of the substances which is currently used in the treatment of patients with MDS. However, up to now it has not been clear

Table 8. Bone marrow transplantation in MDS patients

Author/group	*N*	Age[a] (years)	Relapse	Outcome
Appelbaum et al. (1984) Seattle	10	13 (4-54)	2	6 alive in CR
Tricot et al. (1986) Leuven	7	24 (4-34)	1	4 alive in CR

[a] Median (range).

Table 9. Compounds that induce differentiation of myeloid leukemic blast cells

Physiological agents	CSF (pluripotent CSF, GM-CSF, M-CSF, G-CSF) Vitamin D Vitamin A analogues (retinoic acid) γ-interferon
Cytotoxic agents	Actinomycin D Adriamycin Methotrexate 5-Azacytidine Cytosine arabinoside (ara-C)
Polar agents	DMSO Butyric acid
Tumor promoters	12-0-Tetradecanoylphorbol-13-acetate (TPA)

Table 10. Low-dose ara-C in patients with ANLL or MDS

	N	CR	PR
MDS	109	28 (26%)	18 (17%)
ANLL	148	61 (41%)	15 (10%)
ANLL (MDS)	31	5 (16%)	2 (6%)
MDS > 65 years	47	15 (32%)	7 (15%)

Pooled data from the literature.

whether its action is cytostatic or differentiation inducing. From comparative in vivo and in vitro studies, it seems that both mechanisms are responsible for therapeutic success (Hoelzer et al. 1985). The remission rate with low-dose Ara-C in 109 patients with MDS (update of the literature, Table 10) is 26%; in acute nonlymphoblastic leukemia (ANLL) it is 41%. Interestingly in patients with overt acute leukemia evolving from an MDS, the remission rate is only 17%. From these results one must conclude that if low-dose Ara-C treatment is considered, it should be started before the transformation occurs. Here it seems noteworthy that in a randomized study it could clearly be demonstrated that low-dose Ara-C given by continuous infusions brought superior results in ANLL and MDS than did the mostly used subcutaneous bolus injections (Powell et al. 1986).

Of the vitamin analogues, 13-bis-retinoic acid (Swanson et al. 1986) has been used in the treatment of MDS. In the studies so far published, a complete remission rate of only 10% was achieved. In addition, one third to one-half of the patients showed a response. Treatment with vitamin D3 was not very successful in patients with MDS. The possibility that a combination of differentiation inducers can act synergistically and thereby improve therapeutic results is at present under study (Francis et al. 1985).

Another new approach in the treatment of patients with MDS is the use of biological response modifiers. There is some evidence that interferon might induce differentiation, most probably not directly but by activation of T cells. A further attempt is the use of cloned colony-stimulating factor (GM-CSF) which can enhance proliferation and differentiation of normal hemopoietic stem cells and can induce terminal differentiation of leukemic cells (Schlick and Ruscetti 1986); also here, pilot studies are under way.

References

Applebaum FR, Storb R, Ramberg RE, et al. (1984) Allogeneic marrow transplantation in the treatment of preleukemia. Ann Intern Med 100: 689-693

Bagby GC Jr, Gabourel JD, Linman JW (1980) Glucocorticoid therapy in the preleukemic syndrome (hemopoietic dysplasia). Identification of responsive patients using in vitro techniques. Ann Intern Med 92: 55-58

Bhadhuri S, Kubanek B, Heit W, et al. (1979) A case of preleukemia - reconstitution of normal marrow function after bone marrow transplantation (BMT) from identical twins. Blut 38: 145-149

Bennett JM, Catovsky D, Daniel MT, et al. (1982) Proposal for the classification of the myelodysplastic syndromes. Br J Haematol 51: 189-199

Bloch A (1984) Induced cell differentiation in cancer therapy. Can Treatm Rep 68: 199-205

Block M, Jacobson LO, Bethard WF (1953) Preleukemic acute human leukemia. JAMA 152: 1018-1028

Fearon ER, Burke PJ, Schiffer CA, et al. (1986) Differentiation of leukemic cells to polymorphonuclear leukocytes in patients with acute nonlymphatic leukemia. N Engl J Med 315: 15-24

Francis GE, Guimaraes JETE, Berney JJ, Wing MA (1985) Synergistic interaction between differentiation inducers and DNA synthesis inhibitors: a new approach to differentiation induction in myelodysplasia and acute myeloid leukemia. Leuk Res 9: 573-581

Hamilton-Paterson JL (1949) Preleukaemic anaemia. Acta Haematol (Basel) 2: 309-316

Heimpel H, Hoelzer D (1982) Grenzfälle der Behandlung akuter Leukämien. In: Scheurlen PG, Pees HW (eds) Aktuelle Therapie bösartiger Blutkrankheiten. Springer, Berlin Heidelberg New York, pp 58-68

Hoelzer D, Kurrle E, Schmücker H, Harriss EB (1977) Evidence for differentiation of human leukaemic blood cells in diffusion chamber culture. Blood 49: 729-744

Hoelzer G, Ganser A, Heimpel H (1984) "Atypical" leukemias: preleukemia, smoldering leukemia and hypoplastic leukemia. Recent Results Cancer Res 93: 69-101

Hoelzer D, Ganser A, Schneider W, Heimpel H (1985) Low-dose cytosine arabinoside in the treatment of acute nonlymphoblastic leukemia and myelodysplastic syndromes. Semin Oncol [Suppl 2] 12: 208-211

Mufti GJ, Stevens JR, Oscier DG, et al. (1985) Myelodysplastic syndromes: a scoring system with prognostic significance. Br J Haematol 59: 425-433

Powell B, Capizzi R, Muss H, et al. (1986) Low dose Ara-C (LoDAC) treatment of acute nonlymphocytic leukemia (ANNL) and myelodysplastic syndromes (MDS). Proc Am Soc Clin Oncol 5: 166

Sachs L (1978) Control of normal cell differentiation and the phenotypic reversion of malignancy in myeloid leukemia. Nature 274: 535

Schlick E, Ruscetti FW (1986) In vivo induction of terminal differentiation of malignant myelopoietic progenitor cells by CSF-inducing biological response modifiers. Blood 67: 980-987

Swanson G, Picozzi V, Morgan R, et al. (1986) Responses of hemopoietic precursors to 13-*cis* retinoic acid and 1,25 dihydroxyvitamin D_3 in the myelodysplastic syndromes. Blood 67: 1154-1161

Teerenhovi L, Lintula R (1986) Natural course of myelodysplastic syndromes - Helsinki experience. Scand J Haematol [Suppl 45] 36: 102-106

Todd WM, Pierre RV (1986) Pre-leukemia: a long-term prospective study of 326 patients. Scand J Haematol [Suppl 45] 36: 114-120

Tricot G, Bogaerts MA, Verwilghen RL (1986a) Treatment of patients with myelodysplastic syndromes: a review. Scand J Haematol [Suppl 1] 36: 121-127

Tricot G, Vlietinck R, Verwilghen RL (1986b) Prognostic factors in the myelodysplastic syndromes: a review. Scand J Haematol [Suppl 1] 36: 107-113

Yunis JJ, Rydell RE, Oken MM, et al. (1986) Refined chromosome analysis as an independent prognostic indicator in de novo myelodysplastic syndromes. Blood 67: 1721-1730

Incipient Malignant Lymphoma: Definition and Histopathology

J. Diebold and J. Audouin

Laboratoire d'Anatomie et de Cytologie Pathologiques, Faculté de Médecine
Broussais-Hôtel Dieu, 15, rue de l'Ecole de Médecine, 76270 Paris Cedex, France

A malignant lymphoma represents the uncontrolled proliferation of a family of lymphoid cells arising from the same initial cell (so-called monoclonal proliferation). The tumoral cells resemble those cells seen during the normal development of lymphoid tissue or during an immune response. This kind of proliferation can occur in any type of lymphoid tissue, in the bone marrow, and sometimes in other tissues.

Definition

Incipit is a Latin word which refers to the first words of a manuscript in paleography. Thus, an "incipient" malignant lymphoma can be defined as the beginning of a lymphoma, or the earliest manifestation of the disease. Other possible terms are *early* or *focal* lymphoma.

Proposed Morphologic and Clinical Criteria

The diagnosis of an early lymphoma is based on certain morphologic and clinical features. The morphologic criteria which can be proposed are the following:

1. Focal infiltration of a tissue
2. By sheets of homogeneous lymphoid cells
3. With limited modification or destruction of the normal tissue architecture

The clinical picture is that of a local lesion at the time of diagnosis. The absence of dissemination is often very difficult to demonstrate.

These criteria are valuable not only for non-Hodgkin's malignant lymphoma but also for Hodgkin's disease. The practical difficulty in the recognition of early or incipient lymphoma reflects the fact that these criteria are not universally accepted, and in some situations are probably inadequate. The difficulty in making the diagnosis also accounts for the rare number of true cases of early lymphoma in the literature.

Although the presence of a homogeneous cellular infiltrate in otherwise intact tissue is highly suspicious, this morphologic appearance may be deceptive. Cytologic examination is imperative and may permit identification of cells characteristic of one of the subtypes of malignant lymphoma (Lennert et al. 1978).

Recent Results in Cancer Research, Vol. 106

Other Criteria

Immunolabeling studies can be very useful in the detection of early lymphoma. This is essentially true for B-cell lymphomas. The demonstration of surface or cytoplasmic immunoglobulins with only one type of light chains is highly suggestive. However, such monotypic immunoglobulin secretion does not constitute proof of malignancy (Levy et al. 1983). It merely demonstrates cellular proliferation corresponding to the expansion of one cellular clone - and this is not unequivocally diagnostic of a malignant lymphoma (Bray and Alper 1983; Palutke et al. 1982).

For early T-cell lymphoma immunolabeling studies are not very useful. No specific markers are known that can be used to establish the monoclonality of T-cell proliferation. In Hodgkin's disease, immunolabeling technics are also somewhat disappointing. Some monoclonal antibodies label Reed Sternberg cells (for ex Ki 1, Leu M 1), but these reagents are not monospecific (Stein et al. 1985).

Perhaps in the future, molecular biological techniques such as in situ hybridization will prove helpful (Arnold et al. 1983).

Differential Diagnosis

The differential diagnosis of incipient or early lymphoma is not easy. The greatest difficulty arises in cases of reactive lymphoid hyperplasia. When lymphoid hyperplasia is organoid (e.g., presence of follicules with large germinal centers), the differential diagnosis is simple and includes only intrafollicular malignant lymphoma. In contrast, when lymphoid hyperplasia is diffuse diagnosis is very difficult and sometimes it is impossible to distinguish reactive changes from early small cell lymphoma.

So-called "pseudolymphoma" also poses a diagnostic problem. This name was proposed by Saltzstein (1969) to describe lymphoid hyperplasia with some atypical features mimicking malignant lymphoma but having a good prognosis. Immunolabeling studies have demonstrated that pseudolymphomatous lesions are composed of a variable proportion of peripheral helper or suppressor/cytotoxic T cells and polyclonal B cells (Knowles et al. 1982). The predominance of one light chain in the B-cell population may be a sign of emerging lymphoma (Bray and Alper 1983; Eimoto et al. 1985; Saraga et al. 1981). An increase of B-lymphocytes with a single class of surface immunoglobulins on frozen section may have the same significance (Palutke et al. 1982).

Such lesions can be recognized in various tissues: lymph nodes, the lung, the digestive tract and particularly the stomach, the salivary and lacrymal glands, the thyroid, and the orbit. The etiology is unknown, but in some cases viral infection or drug hypersensitivity reactions are suspected. Many pseudolymphomas are associated with autoimmune syndromes: rheumatoid arthritis, systemic lupus erythematosis, Sjögren's syndrome, Hashimoto's thyroiditis, and hemolytic anemia with autoantibodies. Some pseudolymphomas are considered to be prelymphomatous conditions (Lennert et al. 1979). The differential diagnosis is most problematic in distinguishing between pseudolymphomatous lesions with prelymphomatous potential and true incipient or early lymphoma. Prelymphomas were well reviewed by Lennert et al. at the meeting of the German Society of Pathology in 1979.

Examples of Early Non-Hodgkin's Lymphoma

Early lymphoma has been described in the stomach and accounts for up to 30% of mucosal and submucosal gastric lymphomas regardless of size (Ranchod et al. 1978; Lewin et al. 1978). The incidence of early lymphoma localized only to the mucosa was estimated at 20% in another series (Lim et al. 1977). Isaacson and Wright (1984) have described small foci of monotypic B cells invading normal submucosal lymphoid tissue. Some early lymphomas are associated with reactive lymphoid hyperplasia (Murayama et al. 1984; Scoazec et al. 1986; Brooks and Enterline 1983). Nine cases reported in the literature have documented the coexistence of a lymphoma with a gastric pseudolymphoma (Scoazec et al. 1986; Murayama et al. 1984; Brooks and Enterline 1983; Wolf and Spujt 1981; Faris and Saltzstein 1964). Direct proof of a relationship between the two lesions was not always provided. In other series, transitional features have been observed between follicular hyperplasia and pseudolymphoma on the one hand, and between pseudolymphoma and lymphoma on the other (Hyjek and Kelenyi 1982; van den Heule et al. 1979).

We have demonstrated small foci of cells containing monotypic immunoglobulin (mainly cytoplasmic mu kappa) in pseudolymphomatous, hyperplastic lymph nodes of patients with Sjögren's syndrome (Diebold et al. 1978). This was consistent with previous publications (Anderson and Talal 1972; Talal and Bunim 1964) and confirmed by others (Lennert et al. 1979). In some cases Waldenstrom's disease developed subsequently (Anderson and Talal 1972; Diebold et al. 1978). In lacrymal glands of patients with Sjögren's disease or in tumors of the orbit, we have also found malignant lymphomas of the lymphoplasmocytic type. These foci were present within a diffuse lymphoid infiltrate containing some follicles, the so-called pseudolymphomatous pattern (Dhermy et al. 1981 a, b). The same observation was made by Molenaar et al. (1983), who suggested that monoclonal lymphoplasmocytoid cells could first arise in germinal centers, then diffusely infiltrate tissue. The germinal centers would then become progressively effaced. Harris et al. also reported the discovery of monotypic lymphoid cell sheets in orbital diffuse lymphoid infiltrates, and these authors stress the importance of immunoperoxidase staining of frozen sections for the diagnosis of orbital malignant lymphoma.

In myoepithelial sialadenitis (MESA) often associated with Sjögren's syndrome or other types of autoimmune disease, Schmid et al. (1982) demonstrated the development of B-cell malignant lymphoma in many cases. The proliferative areas can be small and circumscribed; these regions contain B-lymphoid cells expressing a monotypic immunoglobulin in their cytoplasm. The lesion resembles a lymphoplasmocytic immunocytoma. Schmid et al. (1982) proposed the term "early lymphoma" for this type of atypical myoepithelial sialadenitis because some of these cases later evolved into malignant lymphomas either of immunocytoma or immunoblastic type.

The same morphologic and immunologic changes have been described in NZB mice with spontaneous autoimmune disease akin to Sjögren's syndrome (Talal 1974), and in mice with experimentally induced chronic graft-versus-host reactions (Grundmann and Hobi 1973). The mice showed initial reactive changes, then a prelymphomatous stage, which preceded the development of so-called reticulum cell sarcoma with intracytoplasmic monotypic immunoglobulin. These tumors probably correspond to lymphoplasmocytic lymphoma with transformation into immunoblastic lymphoma.

According to Klein (1980), initiation of a tumor is based upon a genomic change. Tumor progression depends upon genetic and epigenetic (or regulatory) changes. Thus, the initial process leads to the development of modified cells that are capable of dividing. They constitute a polyclonal population responsible for the so-called pseudolymphoma pattern, with prelymphomatous capacity. The epigenetic change which is responsible for the malignant transformation is not known. It could reflect a disturbance of suppressor T-cell function, or the expression of oncogenes, or the action of various environmental agents (radiation, viruses, drugs, etc.).

Classification According to Origin

In the histophathologic description of early lymphoma, two different situations should be distinguished (Fig. 1):

1. *The de novo development of a primary malignant lymphoma*. Some examples of early primary non-Hodgkin's malignant lymphoma include:
   1.1. The first histopathologic lesion in T-CLL is minimal, diffuse infiltration of the cords of the splenic red pulp by small lymphocytes with a large pale cytoplasm and intracytoplasmic azurophilic granules seen best on imprints. Surrounding tissue architecture is preserved. The infiltrating cells are Leu 7 positive, a phenotype expressed by natural killer cells.
   1.2. Intrafollicular malignant lymphoma represents the first stage of development of centroblastic, centrocytic lymphoma with a follicular pattern. The following criteria confirm the presence of the lymphoma: monomorphous aspect of the population despite the pleomorphism of the centrocytes, absence of mitosis and of macrophages with tingible bodies, disappearance of the pale and dark zone organization of the germinal centers, more or less advanced effacement of the mantle zone, and presence of a monotypic population expressing a membrane immunoglobulin with only one type of light chain.
   1.3. Minimal infiltration of the bone marrow by small clusters of plasma cells characterizes early myeloma (Fig. 2). The diagnostic criteria are the following: presence of small nests of plasma cells dispersed in between the myeloid cells, often near bone trabeculae and at a distance from the small vessels; presence of big plasma cells; presence of large nucleoli in some cells; and cells exhibiting the morphology of proplasma cells or sometimes of plasmoblasts. Here again immunolabeling studies on paraffin sections can aid in diagnosis by showing the monotypy of the intracytoplasmic immunoglobulin. In early myeloma, the cytologic criteria and the topography of the plasma cell clusters are very important for the distinction between true early myeloma and so-called benign monoclonal gammopathy.
   1.4. Early lymphoplasmocytoid lymphoma can also be recognized by the presence of monotonous sheets of lymphoplasmocytoid cells infiltration an organ or a tissue, e.g., lacrymal glands in a patient with Sjögren's syndrome. Here again, the monotypy of the intracytoplasmic immunoglobulin (e.g., mu, lambda) suggests the emergence of a lymphoplasmocytoid lymphoma from an original lymphoid infiltrate.
   1.5. Early high grade lymphoma may also be found. In one of our cases, a single tumor 2 cm in diameter was found in the fundus of the stomach. A diffuse infiltrate partly destroyed the mucosa and invaded the submucosa. Follicular hyperplasia of the lymphoid tissue was associated. The tumoral cells were large and exhibited the morphology of B immunoblasts. Some of them contained a small quantity of a monotypic immunoglobulin, mu kappa.

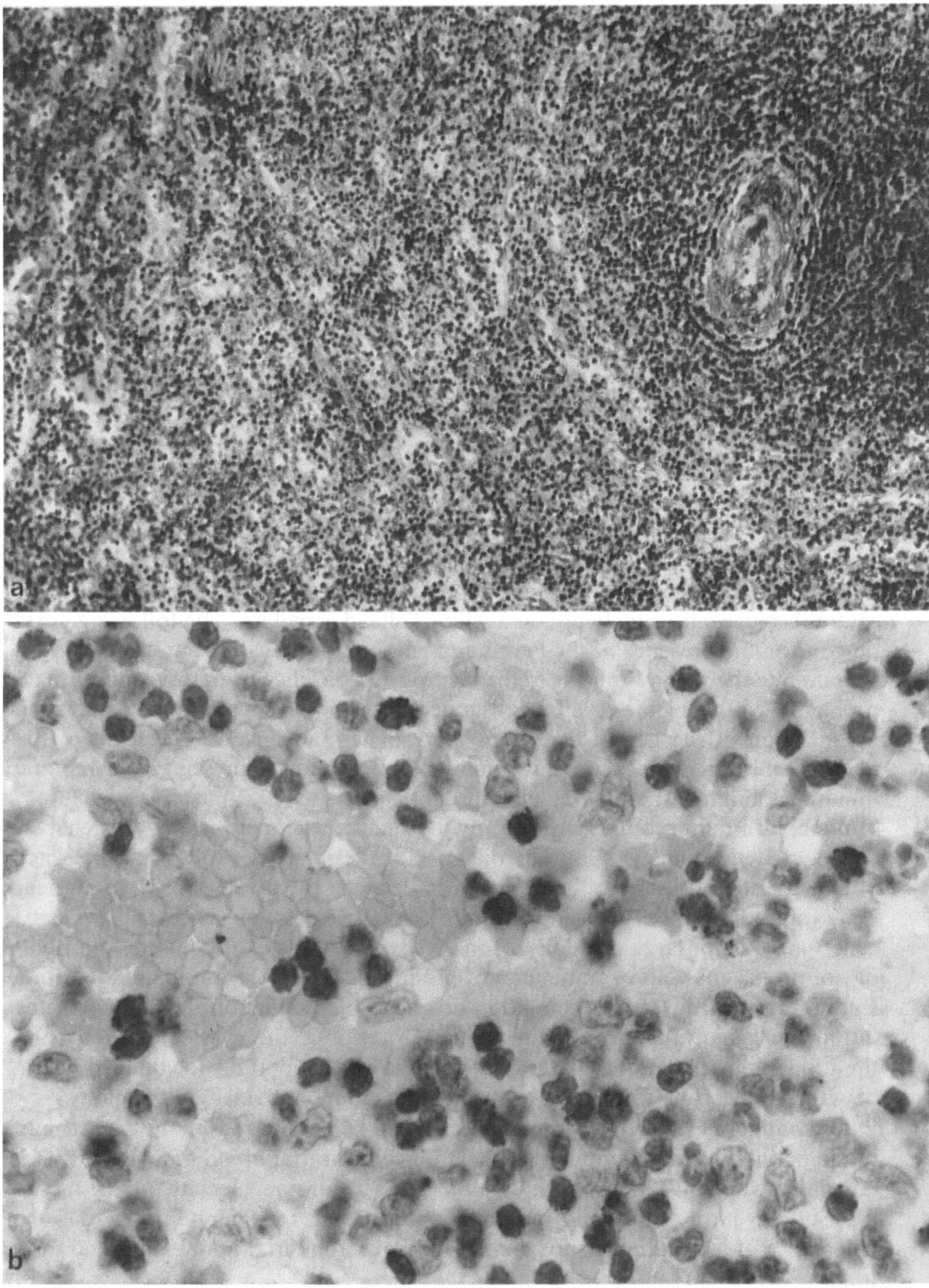

Fig. 1 a, b. Early involvement of the spleen by a T-cell chronic lymphatic leukemia with azurophilic granules. **a** The cords of the red pulp are infiltrated by small lymphoid cells. The architecture is well preserved. Notice the normal aspect of the malpighian corpuscle. Giemsa, × 195. **b** The lymphocytes in the cords have slightly irregular nuclei and a pale cytoplasm. The cytoplasm and the granules are heavily positive with the Leu 7 monoclonal antibody. This demonstrates the natural killer origin of the lymphoid cells. Immunoperoxidase on paraffin section: ABC technique, Leu 7, × 600

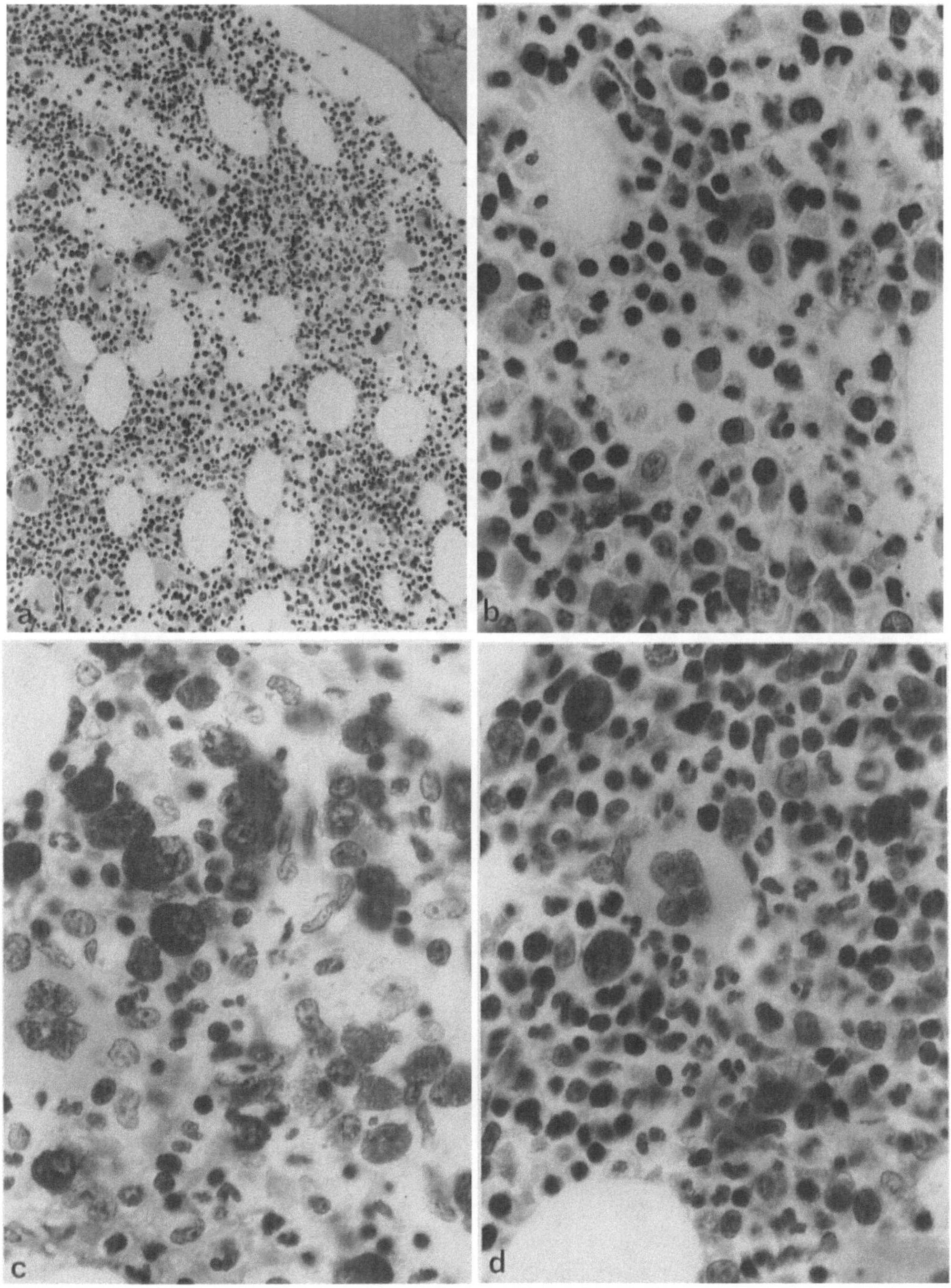

Fig. 2 a–d. Early bone marrow involvement by a myeloma. **a** The bone marrow exhibits a normal cellular density, without tumor and without a heavy diffuse infiltrate. Giemsa, × 160. **b** At a higher magnification, small nests of sometimes giant plasma cells and proplasmocytes are easily recognized. They are found dispersed between the normal myeloid cells at a distance from blood vessels, Giemsa, × 630. **c, d** Immunolabeling technique demonstrating the presence of intracytoplasmic immunoglobulin kappa **c** and gamma **d** chains. **c, d** immunoperoxidase on paraffin section ABC technique, polyclonal antibodies anti-Kappa, and anti-Gamma, × 630

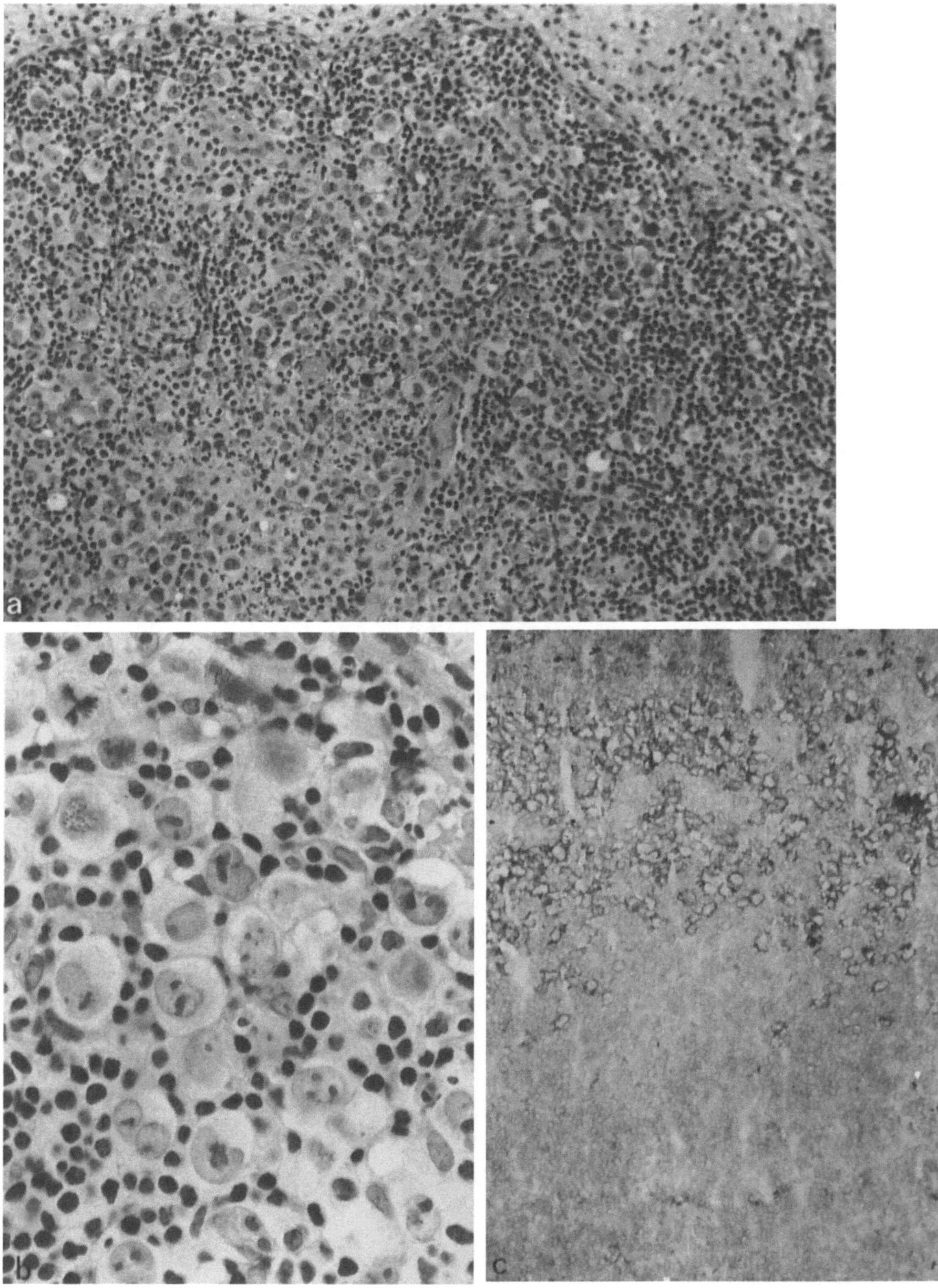

Fig. 3a–c. Early lymph node involvement by large anaplastic cells characteristic of malignant Ki 1 positive lymphoma. **a** Presence of small sheets of tumoral cells with focal destruction of the cortical area of a lymph node. H & E, × 220. **b** The tumoral cells have large, pale, sometimes irregular nuclei with multiple nucleoli and abundant pale cytoplasm. H & E, × 570. **c** The tumoral cells are heavily stained with the Ki 1 monoclonal antibody. Notice the presence of large areas free of tumor cells. Immunoperoxidase on frozen section ABC technique, Ki 1 monoclonal antibody, × 350

1.6. A new type of high-grade lymphoma was recently described by Lennert and his coworkers (Stein et al. 1985). We have seen a case with early involvement in small enlarged inguinal lymph nodes in a 40-year-old man (Fig. 3). Small nests of tumoral cells were found in the cortical areas and the lumina of some sinuses. The cells had a broad cytoplasm, irregular nuclei, and large nucleoli. Pseudometastatic patterns were sometimes present. The tumoral cells were negative with all the B, T, and histiomonocytic markers. They were labeled only with the Ki 1 monoclonal antibody.

2. *The localized development of a high-grade early lymphoma in a patient with a preexistent lymphoma of low-grade malignancy.* In most of these cases, this situation is recognized during treatment relapse. These lymphomas are made up of centroblasts or immunoblasts, a mixture of both, or of plasmoblasts. The primary lymphoma can be a B-CLL (so-called Richter's syndrome), a lymphoplasmocytic immunocytoma, a myeloma, a centroblastic centrocytic follicular lymphoma, or mycosis fungoides (Lennert et al. 1978).

Early Lesions of Hodgkin's Disease

In Hodgkin's disease, early involvement of lymph nodes can also be recognized. In the nodular sclerosing subtype, the first lesion in the so-called "cellular phase" is composed of lacunar Reed-Sternberg cells arranged in nests in the external part of the lymph node cortex (Lennert and Mohri 1974; Lukes 1971; Strum and Rappaport 1971). The interfollicular type of Hodgkin's disease described by Dorfmann can also be considered as the first manifestation of this type of malignancy (Lukes 1971). The development of a nodular Hodgkin's paragranuloma in a lymph node results in the progressive transformation of follicles. The germinal centers are enlarged and diffusely infiltrated by small lymphocytes. Small clusters of epithelioid cells appear in these transformed follicles. Tumorous cells look like small Reed-Sternberg cells (Poppema et al. 1979).

Conclusion

Small foci of tumoral lymphoid cells can be found in different types of tissues. They represent early or incipient lymphomas of different types depending upon their site of origin.

References

Anderson LG, Talal N (1972) The spectrum of benign to malignant lympho-proliferation in Sjögren's syndrome. Clin Exp Immunol 10: 199–211

Arnold A, Cossman J, Bakhshi A, Jaffee ES, Waldmann TA, Korsmeyer SJ (1983) Immunoglobulin-gene rearrangements as unique clonal markers in human lymphoid neoplasms. N Engl J Med 309: 1593–1599

Bray M, Alper MG (1983) Lambda light chain predominance as a sign of emerging lymphoma. Am J Clin Pathol 80: 526–528

Brooks JJ, Enterline HT (1983) Gastric pseudolymphoma. Its 3 subtypes and relation to lymphoma. Cancer 51: 476–486

Dhermy P, Diebold J, Tricot G, Offret G (1981a) Le lymphome malin lymphoplasmocytaire de l'orbite et de la conjonctive. J Fr Ophtalmol 4: 553-563

Dhermy P, Diebold J, Audouin J, Tricot G (1981b) Les pseudolymphomes des annexes oculaires. Leurs rapports avec le syndrome de Sjögren. J Fr Ophtalmol 4: 787-796

Diebold J, Zittoun R, Tulliez M, Reynes M, Tricot G, Bernadou A, Audouin J (1978) Pseudolymphoma and lymphoproliferative syndromes in Gougerot-Sjögren syndrome. Sem Hop Paris 54: 1033-1040

Eimoto E, Futami K, Naito H, Takeshita M, Kikuchi M (1985) Gastric pseudolymphoma with monotypic cytoplasmic immunoglobulin. Cancer 55: 788-793

Faris TD, Saltzstein SL (1964) Gastric lymphoid hyperplasia: a lesion confused with lymphosarcoma. Cancer 17: 207-212

Grundmann E, Hobi HP (1973) Lymphoretikuläre Sarkome bei immunologisch geschädigten Mäusen. Z Krebsforsch 79: 298-303

Harris NL, Harmon DC, Pilch BZ, Goodman ML, Bhan AK (1984) Immunohistologic diagnosis of orbital lymphoid infiltrates. Am J Surg Pathol 8 (2): 83-92

Hyjek E, Kelenyi G (1982) Pseudolymphomas of the stomach: a lesion characterized by progressively transformed germinal centers. Histopathology 6: 61-68

Isaacson P, Wright DH (1984) Extranodal malignant lymphoma arising from mucosa-associated lymphoid tissue. Cancer 53 11: 2515-2524

Klein G (1980) Immune and non-immune control of neoplastic development: contrasting effects of host and tumor evolution. Cancer 45: 2486-2499

Knowles DM, Halper JP, Jakobiec FA (1982) The immunologic characterization of 40 extranodal lymphoid infiltrates: usefulness in distinguishing between pseudolymphoma and malignant lymphoma. Cancer 49: 2321-2335

Lennert K, Mohri N (1974) Histologische Klassifizierung und Vorkommen des Morbus Hodgkin. Internist (Berlin) 15: 57-65

Lennert K, Mohri N, Stein H, Kaiserling E, Muller-Hermelink HK (1978) Malignant lymphoma other than Hodgkin's disease. Springer, Berlin Heidelberg New York (Handbuch der speziellen pathologischen Anatomie und Histologie, vol I/3B)

Lennert K, Knecht H, Berkert M (1979) Vorstadien maligner Lymphome. Prelymphom Verh Dtsch Ges Pathol 63: 170-196

Levy N, Nelson J, Meyer P, Lukes RJ, Parker JW (1983) Reactive lymphoid hyperplasia with single class (monoclonal) surface immunoglobulin. Am J Clin Pathol 80: 300-308

Lewin KJ, Ranchod M, Dorfman RF (1978) Lymphomas of the gastrointestinal tract. A study of 117 cases presenting with gastrointestinal disease. Cancer 42: 693-707

Lim FE, Hartman AS, Tan EGC, Cady B, Meissner WA (1977) Factors in the prognosis of gastric lymphoma. Cancer 39: 1715-1720

Lukes RJ (1971) Criteria for involvement of lymph node, bone marrow, spleen and liver in Hodgkin's disease. Cancer Res 31: 1755-1767

Molenaar WM, Schwarze EW, Lennert K (1983) An immunologic study of germinal centers in 4 ophthalmic immunocytomas. Virchows Arch [Pathol Anat] 399: 141-148

Murayama H, Kikuchi M, Eimoto T, Doki T, Doki K (1984) Early lymphoma coexisting with reactive lymphoid hyperplasia of the stomach. Acta Pathol Jpn 34: 679-686

Palutke M, Schnitzer B, Mirchandani I, Tabaczka PM, Franklin R, Eisenberg L, Kahp S, Carrillo G (1982) Increased numbers of lymphocytes with single class surface immunoglobulins in reactive hyperplasia of lymphoid tissue. Am J Clin Pathol 78: 316-323

Poppema S, Kaiserling E, Lennert K (1979) Hodgkin's disease with lymphocyte predominance nodular type (nodular paragranuloma) and progressively transformed germinal centers. A cytohistological study. Histopathology 3: 295-308

Ranchod M, Lewin RJ, Dorfman RF (1978) Lymphoid hyperplasia of the gastrointestinal tract. A study of 26 cases and review of the literature. Am J Surg Pathol 2: 283-400

Saltzstein SL (1969) Extranodal malignant lymphomas and pseudolymphomas. Pathol Annu 4: 159-185

Saraga P, Hurliman J, Ozzello L (1981) Lymphomas and pseudolymphomas in the alimentary tract: an immunohistochemical and clinicopathologic correlation. Hum Pathol 12: 713-723

Schmid V, Helbron D, Lennert K (1982) Development of malignant lymphoma in myoepithelial sialadenitis (Sjögren's syndrome). Virchows Arch [Pathol Anat] 395: 11-43

Scoazec JY, Brousse N, Potet F, Jeulain JF (1986) Focal malignant lymphoma in gastric pseudolymphoma. Histologic and immunohistochemical study of a case. Cancer 57: 1330–1336
Stein H, Mason DY, Gerdes J, O'Connor N, Wainscoat J, Pallesen G, Gatter K, et al. (1985) The expression of the Hodgkin's disease associated antigen Ki-1 in reactive and neoplastic lymphoid tissue. Evidence that Reed Sternberg cells and histiocytic malignancies are derived from activated lymphoid cells. Blood 66: 848–858
Strum SB, Rappaport H (1971) Interrelationship of the histologic types of Hodgkin's disease. Arch Pathol 91: 127–134
Talal N (1974) Autoimmunity and lymphoid malignancy in New Zealand black mice. R Clin Immunol 2: 101–120
Talal N, Bunim JJ (1964) The development of malignant lymphoma in the course of Sjögren's syndrome. Am J Med 43: 50–65
Van den Heule B, van Kerkem C, Heimann R (1979) Benign and malignant lymphoid lesions of the stomach: a histological reappraisal in the light of the Kiel classification for non-Hodgkin's lymphomas. Histopathology 3: 309–320
Wolf JA, Spujt HJ (1981) Focal lymphoid hyperplasia of the stomach preceding gastric lymphoma: case report and review of the literature. Cancer 48: 2518–2523

Subject Index

MIX
Papier aus verantwortungsvollen Quellen
Paper from responsible sources
FSC® C105338

If you have any concerns about our products,
you can contact us on
ProductSafety@springernature.com

In case Publisher is established outside the EU,
the EU authorized representative is:
Springer Nature Customer Service Center GmbH
Europaplatz 3, 69115 Heidelberg, Germany

Printed by Libri Plureos GmbH
in Hamburg, Germany